Introduction to Metal-Ceramic Technology
Second Edition

Introduction to METAL-CERAMIC TECHNOLOGY

Second Edition

W. Patrick Naylor, DDS, MPH, MS

Associate Dean for Advanced Education
Professor of Restorative Dentistry
School of Dentistry
Loma Linda University
Loma Linda, California

With contributions by
Arlo H. King, CDT
Lumberton, New Jersey

Quintessence Publishing Co, Inc

Chicago, Berlin, Tokyo, London, Paris, Milan, Barcelona,
Istanbul, Moscow, New Delhi, Prague, São Paulo, and Warsaw

To my wife, Penelope, for her continued support, patience, hours of reviewing, and understanding during the revision of this work.

Library of Congress Cataloging-in-Publication Data

Naylor, W. Patrick.
  Introduction to metal-ceramic technology / W. Patrick Naylor ; with contributions by Arlo H. King. -- 2nd ed.
       p. ; cm.
  Includes bibliographical references and index.
  ISBN 978-0-86715-460-3 (hardcover)
  1. Dental ceramic metals. I. King, Arlo H. II. Title.
  [DNLM: 1. Metal Ceramic Alloys. 2. Dental Porcelain. 3. Technology, Dental--methods. WU 180 N333i 2009]
  RK653.5.N39 2009
  617.6'95--dc22
                          2008049256

© 2009 Quintessence Publishing Co, Inc

Quintessence Publishing Co, Inc
4350 Chandler Drive
Hanover Park, IL 60133
www.quintpub.com

Editors: Bryn Goates and Lisa C. Bywaters
Cover, internal design, and production: Patrick Penney

Printed in China

Table of Contents

In Memoriam

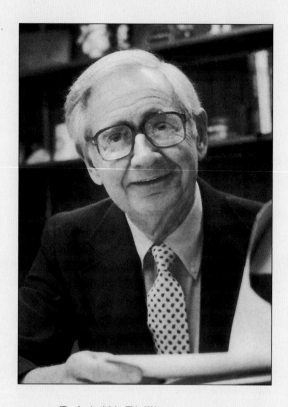

Ralph W. Phillips, MS, DSc
Research Professor Emeritus of Dental Materials
Indiana University School of Dentistry
Indianapolis, Indiana
January 12, 1918–May 17, 1991

This book is dedicated to the memory of my mentor, teacher, and friend, Dr Ralph W. Phillips, who passed away unexpectedly in May, 1991, before he was able to see this book in final form. Ralph Phillips was an expert of international renown whose contributions to dental materials science and to dentistry in general are immeasurable. His death was a tragic loss for those of us who turned to him for guidance and insight.

This dedication is a small tribute to a man who left an indelible mark on the dental profession.

Preface

For this second edition, every chapter was revised and updated to include relevant topics not included in the first edition and to expand the chapter content in a meaningful way. Mr Arlo King (Dentsply Prosthetics) contributed immensely to this edition with the industry perspective.

Readers will note that much of the technical data on dental porcelains and metal-ceramic alloys published in the first edition was retained and enhanced with detailed information on more contemporary products. This level of detail will aid readers of older published scientific literature where it was less common for authors to provide actual chemical makeup and percentage composition on the products that were evaluated. The importance of being aware of the elements in materials was highlighted in reports in 2008 of lead contamination of dental restorations outsourced to offshore laboratories in China.[1] It is vital that clinicians and dental laboratories purchase recognized products of known origin from reputable manufacturers.

Among the other major changes is the inclusion of relevant references at the close of each chapter with synopses of selected journal articles and textbooks. Also, key statements in each chapter appear in text boxes to emphasize salient points throughout the book. The nature and extent of the revisions appearing in this second edition are as follows:

- Chapter 1. The history of the metal-ceramic restoration is expanded to offer a richer and clearer perspective on how this technology evolved.
- Chapter 2. The chemistry of dental porcelain and the contributions of several leading pioneers in the development of metal-ceramic technology are expanded substantially. Subjects such as fluorescence, metamerism, and opalescence are explained. Classification of dental porcelains has been updated to reflect contemporary usage and clarify designations not found in many leading dental materials textbooks. The compositions of the components in several modern-day dental porcelain systems are presented in tables.
- Chapter 3. Contemporary classification is suggested along with a modification to the 1984 American Dental Association classification system. The composition of various alloys is included along with expanded lists of important physical properties. Some older articles in the literature refer to alloys by name but fail to identify their classification or major elements; these tables will help readers gain a broader appreciation of the alloys being discussed or evaluated. The section on biocompatibility is expanded with emphasis on the intraoral and extraoral indications of an allergic response to constituent elements such as nickel and beryllium. The occupational risks posed to dental laboratory technicians are also explored.
- Chapter 4. Expanded to provide more details, reference specific statements, and broaden the explanation of the rationale for the steps in substructure design. The ovate pontic is mentioned as an alternative to the modified ridge lap design.
- Chapter 5. Spruing, investing, and casting have not changed since the first edition, but the content is better referenced and the terminology better defined.
- Chapter 6. The theories that explain the nature of the porcelain-metal interface remain the same today, but more statements have been referenced to reflect the evidence-based rationale for the subjects covered in this chapter.
- Chapter 7. More references and improved formatting of the technical steps associated with presoldering and postsoldering.
- Chapter 8. Content is better correlated to contemporary dental porcelain systems. Firing schedules of a few representative products appear in appendix A. The use of visual indicators for assessing the accuracy and appropriateness of temperature settings is explained.
- Chapter 9. Reproducing the variation in natural teeth is explained through an emphasis on outline form, surface texture, and level of glaze. New photographs illustrate how differences in appearance can be identified and captured in porcelain.
- Glossary. Expanded to reflect chapter revisions
- Appendices. Revised and updated in support of the changes made in the text.

1. Furlong A. Lead in dental lab work? ADA urges scrutiny. Am Dent Assoc News 2008;39 (5):1, 22.

Acknowledgments

Many of the historical articles reviewed for this second edition were graciously loaned to me from the personal library of Dr Charles J. Goodacre, Dean of the Loma Linda University School of Dentistry and Professor of Restorative Dentistry. I offer my sincere thanks to Dr Goodacre for his willingness to share this information for the benefit of the dental community at large.

Special thanks are extended to the following individuals: Ms Anita Bobich, Program Director of the dental laboratory technology program at Pasadena City College (Pasadena, CA), who provided welcomed comments and recommendations to improve each chapter, as well as Dr Veeraraghavan Sundar (Dentsply Prosthetics) and Mr Tridib "TD" Dasgupta (Ivoclar Vivadent) for their technical reviews.

I would also like to recognize the following companies for providing products for photographing: Dentsply Prosthetics, Ivoclar Vivadent, Vident, and Whip Mix. Corporate contacts who kindly provided assistance were Ms Jill Piechota (Ivoclar Vivadent), Mr Patrick Boche (Creation International), and Ms Tony Testa (Dentsply Prosthetics).

In addition, I wish to recognize Ms Jennifer Osborne for her administrative role and thank Ms Rebecca Mintz for her help in gathering the research materials used for the updating. A particular note of gratitude is extended to Mr Ryan Becker for the added photographs and transformation of the artwork into a more realistic and contemporary appearance.

Last, I would be remiss if I did not acknowledge the leadership and staff of Quintessence Publishing for allowing me to update this book and for providing editorial and graphic support throughout the publication process.

Preface to the First Edition

The metal-ceramic restoration is one of the most widely used restorative combinations in dentistry today. Unfortunately, there are few publications available that provide introductory level, skill-oriented technical information on the processes involved in fabricating this very popular prosthesis. *Introduction to Metal-Ceramic Technology* was written specifically for dental technology students, dental students, and graduate classes.

Following a brief historical review of the evolution of porcelain in dentistry, chapter 1 introduces the reader to the technical language of metal-ceramic technology. Each of the subsequent eight chapters adds new information to this foundation and literally builds on the preceding material. By the end of the text (chapter 9), the reader will have learned the basic techniques of porcelain application.

A concerted effort has been made to include sufficient information of a theoretical nature to permit the reader to understand why certain procedures, techniques, or equipment are used. The skill of physically constructing an esthetic metal-ceramic restoration is an *art*: however, understanding the rationale for the processes involved requires a knowledge of the true *science* of dental technology.

It is hoped that this text has successfully merged art with science in such a way that the reader is able to meet the challenges of this exciting aspect of dental technology with confidence.

CHAPTER 1

History and Overview

Historical Perspective

One of the more interesting facets in the annals of dental technology is how the centuries-old artistry of making porcelain evolved into processes that continue to revolutionize modern-day dentistry. The creation of porcelain works of art and fine china were stepping stones in a journey that literally took thousands of years before a few pioneers saw potential dental applications for these simple ceramic materials. In fact, it was not until the 19th century that applications for porcelain in dentistry evolved into what eventually would lead to metal-ceramic technology. From the late 1800s until today the pace of change has been extraordinary, thanks in large part to the continued introduction of new products and techniques. You need only examine the origin of dental porcelain to gain an appreciation of just how far ceramic technology has come.

At the same time, it is important to recognize the contributions of different nations, cultures, and individuals responsible for the advancements now enjoyed by patients, dental laboratory technicians, and clinicians the world over.

From earthenware to stoneware to porcelain

In his historical account of the development and evolution of dental ceramics, Jones described the role of Chinese artisans in transforming crude fired clay objects into delicate and functional pieces of transparent porcelain.[1] The earliest traces of the origins of ceramics were porous fragments of mud and clay fired at low temperature. These rudimentary products, described as *earthenware*, were estimated to date back to approximately 23,000 BC.[1] Firing in primitive kilns at temperatures up to 900°C allowed the clay particles

to fuse only at points of contact, which yielded a rather porous final result.[2]

Thousands of years later in 100 BC, the Chinese discovered how to produce more refined pieces fired at higher temperatures. The resultant stoneware was not only stronger than its earthenware predecessor but also impervious to water due to improvements in manufacturing.[1,2] Early earthenware was porous and hence more suited for holding nonliquids. In contrast, stoneware was fired routinely at temperatures that allowed glass formation to seal the ceramic surface.[2]

Anyone who has ever attempted to chronicle the history of ceramic materials knows that the Chinese also are credited with the subsequent development of porcelain as early as AD 1000.[1] So refined was this "China stone" or "China ware" that strong, functional, transparent containers were produced with walls only a few millimeters thick. To this day the terms *china* and *porcelain* are often used interchangeably when referring to high-quality ceramic items.

Key European contributors

Despite repeated attempts, European artisans were unsuccessful in their own efforts to unravel the secrets of Chinese ceramic technology. In fact, the best that researchers could do was to produce materials akin to Chinese stoneware. While this was an improvement over porous and crude earthenware, these early European ceramic products reportedly failed to approach the quality, strength, and translucency of fine oriental porcelains.

In what Jones described as "an early example of industrial espionage," Francois Xavier d'Entrecolles, a Jesuit priest, ingratiated himself with Chinese potters around 1717 to learn the porcelain manufacturing process.[1] Father d'Entrecolles lived in what was considered China's porcelain center, the city of King-te-tching, where he was able not only to obtain Chinese porcelain products but also to acquire essential descriptions of the manufacturing methods.[2] With the help of the French scientist René-Antoine Ferchault de Réaumur, the composition of Chinese porcelain was found to consist of approximately 50% clay (kaolin or hydrated aluminum silicate), 25% to 30% feldspar (sodium and potassium–aluminum silicates), and 20% to 25% quartz (silica).[2] Within a few years, Europeans also began making fine translucent porcelains.[3] Despite d'Entrecolles' achievement, ceramics were not immediately recognized as a material of potential value to dentistry in the early 18th century. But in less than 60 years, that would change.

There is evidence to indicate that in the late 18th century, an edentulous French apothecary by the name of Alexis Duchâteau was troubled by stained and odiferous ivory dentures, a condition probably not uncommon among the general population of that time.[1] Armed with his skills as an apothecary, Duchâteau attempted to make a set of porcelain dentures for himself. Much to his dismay, those initial efforts were less than successful.[4] It was not until he teamed up with the Parisian dentist Nicolas Dubois de Chémant that the two were finally able to construct complete dentures from a material they referred to as "mineral paste" in approximately 1774.[3,4] Satisfied with the improved fit of his new dentures, Duchâteau returned to his apothecary shop. But Dubois de Chémant became intrigued by his experimentation and went on to reformulate the original mineral paste. He focused his efforts on enhancing the color, increasing the dimensional stability, and improving the attachment of the "mineral teeth" to the denture base.

Dubois de Chémant eventually patented his porcelain formulation and in 1788 published a pamphlet on his work. Yet it was not until 1797 that his more definitive text, *A Dissertation on Artificial Teeth*, appeared in print. For many years that followed, Dubois de Chémant's "mineral paste dentures" were also referred to as "incorruptible teeth" or more simply as "incorruptibles."[4,5] Dubois de Chémant's porcelain formulation enabled denture wearers to have "clean and hygienic dentures."[5] However, not everyone hailed Dubois de Chémant's decision to patent the porcelain paste. Some of his contemporaries regarded his actions as nothing more than the theft of Duchâteau's original invention.[1] In fact, the work of Duchâteau and Dubois de Chémant may have been preceded by another French dentist, Pierre Fauchard, who is generally considered the father of modern dentistry.[1]

Evidently, Fauchard and others reported using what they referred to as "baked enamel" prior to 1760 and perhaps as early as the 1720s.[1] Fauchard's writings described the use of porcelain for the construction of dentures in 1723, but 5 years passed before he actually published his philosophy on dentistry

in 1728 in a book entitled *Le Chirurgien dentiste, ou, Traité des dents (The Surgeon Dentist, or, Treatise on the Teeth)*.[4] Then in 1746, some 18 years later, Fauchard released an expanded second edition of his book. The two-volume work was 863 pages in length and contained more subject matter and improved illustrations. According to Ring, Fauchard's writings influenced dentistry well into the next century.[4]

The next notable advancement came around 1806 from Italian dentist Giusseppangelo Fonzi who reportedly devised a method to mass-produce individual porcelain denture teeth; however, he did not publicize this achievement until 1808.[1] Evidently, Fonzi devised a technique for placing platinum pins in the back of the porcelain teeth, so they could then be soldered to a metal denture base.[1,3] Fonzi's individualized porcelain teeth were referred to as "terro-metallic incorruptibles"[3] or "terro-metallic teeth."[1]

It is believed that sometime around 1837 English goldsmith Claudius Ash began manufacturing fine porcelain teeth.[4] Ash later created an artificial tooth that could be placed over a post in either a complete denture or a fixed partial denture. The "tube tooth," as it came to be known, went on to enjoy wide popularity in its day.

Arrival of porcelain in America

Accounts describing the path of porcelain technology through Europe and across the Atlantic to the United States differ slightly among dental historians.[1,4,6,7] Nonetheless, it is generally agreed that, like their European counterparts, the American artisans' first use of porcelain in dentistry was in the fabrication of complete dentures. French dentist Antoine Plantou is credited with introducing individual porcelain teeth to America around 1817.[1] Yet it was Philadelphia jeweler Samuel W. Stockton who saw the widespread potential of this application. Around 1830, he became the first American to mass-produce porcelain denture teeth in the United States.[1]

Creation of translucent porcelain with enhanced color

The porcelain used to fabricate dentures was described as an opaque white material with the appearance of commercial ceramic products used in industry.[8] Then in 1838, American dentist and Philadelphia native Dr Elias Wildman revamped the formula, bringing both translucency and tooth colors to dental porcelain.[3,8] The next major milestone in the enhancement of translucency and color development did not occur until 1949 with the introduction of vacuum firing by the Dentists Supply Company (now Dentsply).[3,9]

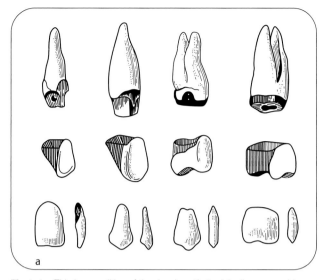

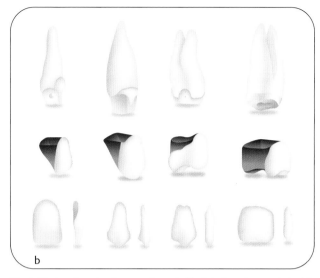

Fig 1-1a This is a rendition of the drawings that originally appeared in one of Land's 1886 articles.[12] Note the use of facings on platinum foil much like contemporary cast metal-ceramic substructures.

Fig 1-1b Land's restorations as shown in Fig 1-1a have been colorized in an attempt to portray what the ceramic veneers may have looked like.

Evolution of modern applications

The road from porcelain dentures and denture teeth to the contemporary technology of metal-ceramics was also a long and winding journey, often littered with disappointments and outright failures. Historical accounts have singled out and credited several key individuals with achieving additional milestones in ceramic technology. This evolutionary process reflected the combined talents of many inquiring minds and very determined researchers. While it is impossible to identify and recognize all those responsible for the development of metal-ceramic restorations, it is important to appreciate how this technology evolved. Therefore, the writings of several early pioneers will be recognized by referencing their articles published in leading scientific journals of the time.

Contributions of Dr Charles H. Land

In the nearly five decades that followed Wildman's improved formulation, dental porcelain remained primarily a material for use in complete denture prosthodontics.[8] That eventually changed, and dental porcelain entered the world of restorative dentistry thanks in large part to the creative mind of one man—Dr Charles H. Land.

The idea of fusing porcelain to a thin platinum foil is credited to Land, a Detroit dentist, who patented the concept sometime between 1886 and 1888.[1,4,10,11] Around this same period, Land published reports describing his technique for fitting what he referred to as "enamel fronts" to prepared teeth.[12] These prefabricated porcelain "fronts," or facings, were ground to fit a 30-gauge platinum foil matrix adapted to prepared teeth. Land also described using a low-fusing porcelain he developed to make restorations for a maxillary anterior tooth for which a porcelain facing was attached to the "prepared base" of a platinum-and-iridium alloy (Fig 1-1a).[12,13] The facings were then fused to the foil matrix with body porcelain in a "Land's Gas Furnace."[12] The resulting restoration of platinum foil and porcelain facing was described by Land as an "enameled metallic coating" or "metallic enamel coating." Shortly after the turn of the 20th century, Land published another article in which he again referred to different types of restorations: "enameled metallic caps" and "enameled caps or jacket crowns."[10] Capon acknowledged that Land's technique of burnishing platinum foil to prepared teeth and using the adapted foil as a substrate onto which dental porcelain was fused in a gas furnace was entirely different from any techniques recognized up to that time.[14] It is also necessary to point out that although the designations "enameled metallic caps" and "enameled caps" appear similar, the restorations themselves were quite different.

Enameled metallic caps

Unlike porcelain facings that were ground to fit a foil matrix of pure platinum, enameled metallic caps had a metal substructure fabricated from an alloy of platinum and iridium. Land veneered these platinum-iridium substructures with the low-fusing porcelain he had developed.[10] The porcelain was built up, fired, and shaped to final contour (see Fig 1-1a).

3

Re-creations of the drawings that Land published in 1886, with color added, resemble restorations that might be seen today (Fig 1-1b).

It is important to note that when Land retained the word *metallic* in the name, as in *enameled metallic cap,* he apparently was describing a primitive metal-ceramic restoration. However, Land reportedly had a great deal of difficulty with his low-fusing porcelain. The high levels of borax and pulverized glass apparently rendered the material susceptible to deterioration in the oral cavity.[1]

Jacket crowns (enameled caps)

The enameled caps Land described actually referred to all-porcelain jacket crowns that relied on a platinum-foil matrix used solely as a supporting foundation during the fabrication process. In other words, the porcelain was applied to the matrix, shaped, and fired. Once the porcelain portion of the restoration had been built to final form, the metal matrix was removed, leaving what Land described as a "complete coat of artificial enamel."[10] This final restoration was merely a "hollow veneer or shell" of dental porcelain, but it reportedly replicated a natural tooth. The designation *enameled cap* appeared to be Land's way of describing an all-porcelain restoration that replaced the natural enamel (coronal) structure of a tooth.

Land portrayed this treatment approach to the dental profession and fellow clinicians as a way to offer patients a "much better artistic effect" coupled with "the preservation of a large amount of tooth structure."[12,15] This same technique served as the basis for the platinum foil–porcelain, pin-retained inlays that Land advocated in lieu of large metallic intracoronal restorations.[10,11,13]

In addition to improved esthetics, Land had a remarkable appreciation for the differences in thermal conductivity between metal restorations and "metallic coatings," and he understood the important clinical implications of these differences.[13] Vital teeth with large, all-metal restorations were found to undergo greater thermocycling (alternating hot and cold changes) than did his metallic-coating restorations. Land reported that such temperature fluctuations could be potentially harmful to healthy pulpal tissues. In addition, he noted that nonvital teeth with large metal restorations were prone to root "checking and fracture."[13] Land's observations even extended to an appreciation of the periodontal health of teeth when he stated that "inflammation of the membrane"— likely a reference to the periodontal ligament—can occur and may lead to tooth loss.[13] Land published a subsequent report as part of his continuing effort to bring "this new mode of practice to the notice of the dental profession."[16]

By promoting the use of enamel coatings for complete crowns and partial veneer restorations, Land became a stri-

dent advocate of conservative dentistry. His writings could be interpreted as a plea to the dental profession to preserve as much healthy tooth structure as possible, appreciate pulpal health, and design and construct porcelain restorations for complete or partial coverage. As far back as 1887, Land is quoted as stating, "in nearly all the modern systems of crown-work there seems to be too much good tooth material cut away, and I think a careful investigation will demonstrate this new process to be far superior, making it possible to save the greater portion of the crown, it not being necessary to cut beneath the gum."[16] In this same paper, Land not only promoted his new porcelain process, but he also offered his patented discovery to advance the dental profession.

A few years later in an 1889 presentation before the First District Dental Society of the State of New York, Land, reporting that he had been "restoring teeth with porcelain" for 5 years, shared his findings with the group.[15] He again advocated not removing the entire clinical crown but retaining coronal tooth structure and constructing restorations made by fusing porcelain to metal. Land felt this treatment was especially valuable when restoring teeth in children. These early writings reflect an astute awareness of esthetics, dental materials science (the potential damaging effects of thermal changes on vital and nonvital teeth), the importance of conservative tooth preparation, and the need to maintain periodontal health. Land published other articles in which he reported that the enameled caps he placed in his patients had survived 8, 10, and 12 years.[10]

> Famed aviator Charles A. Lindbergh Jr was the grandson of Dr Charles H. Land.[18]

According to a 1927 article by Capon entitled "Enameling Plugs and Restoring the Contour of Defective Teeth by the Application of Enameled Caps," Dr B. W. Wood is reported to have "presented an article" in 1862 that described a technique for enameling a metallic cap.[14] Capon acknowledged that Wood did not provide any details of his technique, and he did not mention where Wood made his presentation or if it was ever published.[14] However, Capon felt Wood's work should be recognized as "the basis of our porcelain jacket of today."[14]

The "father of porcelain dental art"

Nearly two decades after Land described his enameled metallic caps, Spalding reported that there were two prevailing techniques of that time to replace human enamel: *(1)* bake porcelain on a platinum foil matrix (0.001-inch thick), remove the foil, and cement the porcelain restoration to the tooth; and *(2)* grind a denture tooth to create a facing that is then baked on a platinum foil matrix.[17] Spalding clarified that the first technique was used on premolar and molar teeth, whereas the second technique was popular for restoring incisors and canines. Clearly, Land's plea to the dental profession to use enameled metallic coatings was heard and had gained popularity.

Then in 1905, Zeigler published a tribute in which he recognized Land as the "father of porcelain dental art."[18] He noted that "Dr Land has not only outgrown, but outrivaled any other claims as to the origination of porcelain art."

While Land's discoveries and technical procedures led to the development of the modern-day porcelain jacket crown, he stood largely alone in his day as the one individual who guided the dental profession toward wider applications for porcelain, preservation of tooth structure, improved esthetics, and the need to protect and preserve periodontal tissue.

Recognizing limitations

Land's discoveries and technical procedures foreshadowed the modern-day porcelain jacket crown. Nevertheless, his demonstration of the need for a restoration with a metallic foundation and a veneer of dental porcelain—and the actual creation of such a restoration—are less acknowledged. As early as 1886 Land described a "platinum overcoat" to cover prepared anterior and posterior teeth that received porcelain facings (see Fig 1-1).[12] Land mechanically fitted a piece of thin, 30-gauge platinum to a prepared tooth to create what he described as a "hollow shell."[12]

It was apparent that Land appreciated the limitations of a platinum foil matrix because he recognized that porcelain would not bond to a high-noble metal. In 1903 he wrote, "we must realize that a vitreous mass, like all our porcelain bodies, does not strongly adhere to non-oxidizable metals and will readily peel off."[10] Despite this inherent weakness, however, Land continued to fabricate this type of crown in his private practice, as featured in his published illustrations. His drawings combine a metal foundation of platinum foil with porcelain facings and even include a porcelain occlusal surface for posterior teeth (see Fig 1-1).[10,11,12,13] Land referred to cases in which he treated both anterior and posterior teeth with restorations using these different crown designs.

Clearly, Land's achievements and contributions laid the groundwork for the eventual development of methods to bond porcelain to metal and the creation of the metal-ceramic restoration. The illustrations of rudimentary metal and porcelain crowns placed by Land in the late 1800s are strikingly similar to substructures fabricated today (see Fig 1-1b). In fact, Land's metal and porcelain crowns should be considered precursors to the modern-day metal-ceramic restoration—a fact not generally recognized.

> "Dr Land has not only outgrown, but outrivaled any other claims as to the origination of porcelain art."

Evolution of the metal-ceramic restoration

After numerous refinements of the early formulations of low-fusing porcelain and years of trials and tribulations, the technology for the metal-ceramic restoration eventually emerged. It was not until the 1950s that reports appeared in the literature revealing the successful pairing of porcelain-fused-to-gold for fixed restorations.[19,20] Foremost among the 20th-century writing in the area of metal-ceramic technology was Dr S. Charles Brecker's article entitled "Porcelain Baked to Gold—A New Medium in Prosthodontics."[19] Published in the *Journal of Prosthetic Dentistry,* this article probably has been more widely read than Land's reports in respected 19th-century journals such as the *Independent Practitioner* and *Dental Cosmos.* Therefore, contemporary students of dental laboratory technology are unlikely to have seen Land's illustrations or to be familiar with his writings of more than a century ago.

Contributions of Dr S. Charles Brecker

Brecker's article remains one of the most widely referenced publications on the emergence of a "new medium in prosthodontics," that being the "porcelain baked to a gold" alloy or "porcelain-fused-to-gold" restoration.[19] Brecker contended that a gold alloy restoration provided a superior foundation for porcelain than either an iridium-platinum alloy or a palladium alloy.

The fabrication technique described in Brecker's article differed from Land's methodology in that Brecker actually cast a gold crown, or "thimble," to a platinum matrix (0.001-inch thick) burnished to a die, whereas Land mechanically adapted the foil to the prepared tooth. With the Brecker technique, the platinum foil–gold substructure was then returned to the prepared tooth for adjustment to ensure a proper fit that is able to "slip on and off with strong finger pressure." Once it was returned to the laboratory, the casting was cleaned with water and dried in a furnace to rid the surface of any contaminants. Next, a "refractory wetting agent (red cadmium compound)," or what might best be described as a *bonding agent*, was mixed with water, applied, and fired in a furnace to 982°C. Opaque porcelain, added in two thin coats, reportedly was able to bond to the treated substructure and mask the color of the underlying metal. Body porcelain was applied, carved, and fired. This process was repeated until the desired final restoration contours were achieved.

In 1956 this "porcelain-fused-to-gold restoration" was deemed new and destined to replace the "acrylic-faced gold crown" so popular at the time.[19] Brecker also suggested its use when a patient's occlusion would not permit the placement of a porcelain jacket crown. Sensitive to the need for esthetics, Brecker illustrated a case where a porcelain-fused-to-gold restoration, with a facial porcelain veneer, was fabricated without displaying a facial metal collar. The platinum foil was adapted over the facial margin of the die, making it possible to "butt the porcelain against the bared shoulder like a porcelain jacket crown."[19] Brecker acknowledged that platinum with "about 10 per cent iridium added for stiffness" was an alloy combination used in dentistry for some time.[19] That statement is consistent with Land's mention of the use of a "telescope cap of platinum and iridium" in 1903.[10,11] But the early platinum-iridium and palladium alloys used by Becker were difficult to cast, and the resultant substructures reportedly left much to be desired in terms of fit.[1]

Metal-ceramic restoration in contemporary dentistry

More than a century ago Land wrote about his use of metal as a foundation for porcelain, and more than 50 years have passed since Brecker published his frequently quoted article on the "porcelain-fused-to-gold restoration."[12,13,19] From 1956 to 1962, improvements were made in ceramic materials and the technical procedures required to produce a porcelain-fused-to-gold crown.[1] Largely, the development of gold alloys and compatible porcelains resulted in the harmonious creation of an esthetic veneering material (dental porcelain) on a rigid metallic foundation composed of a noble alloy that was ductile yet strong and tough. By 1962, M. Weinstein, S. Katz, and A. B. Weinstein patented an improved dental porcelain for gold-based alloys, followed by a second patent by M. Weinstein and A. B. Weinstein in that same year.[21,22] Soon, many newer products emerged, and the porcelain-fused-to-metal (PFM) restoration, or what is now referred to as the *metal-ceramic restoration*, exploded in popularity.

It may have required centuries to introduce porcelain to dentistry, but it took mere decades to transform a rudimentary metal-ceramic restoration into a sophisticated mainstay of modern dental therapy the world over. Today the dental marketplace is inundated with a variety of dental porcelains and an array of ceramic casting alloys with a wide range of compositions and costs. Appreciating subtle differences in handling characteristics between the various porcelains and alloy types is no longer a simple task. In fact, dental alloy formulations vary so widely that classifying them has become complex. Likewise, it also is apparent that success in contemporary dental technology requires both a refinement of artistic skills and an understanding of materials science.

The first edition of *Introduction to Metal Ceramic Technology* cited the results of a 1986 survey that indicated the metal-ceramic restoration was the most popular restorative combination of all materials available in fixed prosthodontics for the construction of a complete crown.[23] One potential reason given for this popularity was that the technology behind this metal-porcelain system had advanced greatly in the brief interval since its introduction. In a subsequent article published nearly 17 years later, the same author released the results of a survey he conducted on the types of restorations made by a large commercial laboratory over a 6-month period.[24] Some 65% of the 363,000 crowns fabricated during this brief period were metal-ceramic restorations. Only 23% were all-ceramic restorations. More recently, all-ceramic products have come into their own to challenge the metal-ceramic restoration in very demanding clinical situations. This trend will undoubtedly continue as new and improved all-ceramic products enter the marketplace.

In all, the metal-ceramic restoration remains a vital component of dental technology and is likely to continue as an integral part of dental laboratory services in the future.[25] Moreover, metal-ceramic restorations have a track record of success spanning decades. With the increasing use and success of dental implants, fewer fixed partial dentures will be needed in the future. This trend will likely translate into an increased need to fabricate multiple single-unit restorations. Mastering the skills required in metal-ceramic technology can continue to serve as a springboard for individuals interested in learning more sophisticated laboratory procedures in fixed prosthodontics, especially in the face of the wider use of all-ceramic systems and the increased placement of dental implants.

Art and Science of Dental Technology

Dental technology, like clinical dentistry, has evolved from the image of a trade or craft to a profession with its own unique demands and challenges. Those who excel in this field do so because of an ability to understand the theoretic aspects of dental technology and to acquire the visual acuity and manual dexterity needed to put these theories into practice. These individuals not only master the technical procedures but also develop an understanding of the materials and techniques they use routinely. Highly skilled dental ceramists are able to transform simple ceramic powders into lifelike restorations that mirror natural teeth in every physical sense. Such talent is acquired over years of dedicated training, practice, experimentation, and life-long learning.

For a better understanding of how art and science are intertwined in dental technology, consider the important issue of esthetics. In complete denture prosthodontics, the

Table 1-1 Factors affecting esthetics in prosthodontics

Type of treatment	Level of control	Comments
Complete denture prosthodontics		
Tooth form (mold)	Maximum	Wide selection
Tooth color (shade)	Maximum	Wide selection; can mix shades
Gingival form	Maximum	Can create natural contours; can modify at try-in
Gingival characterization	Maximum	Can characterize (stain) denture base acrylic resin internally or externally
Dental materials	Maximum	Many types of denture base acrylic resins available; can choose veined or nonveined acrylic resin; several base shades from which to choose
Removable partial denture prosthodontics		
Patient expectations	Reduced	A priority
Prosthesis design	Reduced	Balanced with esthetic requirements
Dental materials	Reduced	Important to select most appropriate materials
Fixed prosthodontics		
Patient requirements	Limited	Treatment options driven by patient needs
Controllable factors	Limited	Clinical requirements dictate selection of shade, outline form, surface texture, size, occlusal plane, and tooth position
Dental materials	Limited	Select materials best suited for each case

dentist and technician generally have maximum control over the techniques required to produce lifelike restorations (Table 1-1). For example, they have great latitude in shade and mold selection and in positioning teeth when restoring an entire dentition. In such cases, even the denture base acrylic resin can be contoured to appear more natural and characterized to create a custom blend of patterns that more naturally reflect the colors of the patient's gingival tissues (Figs 1-2 and 1-3).

The same techniques required to produce lifelike complete dentures can also be applied when restoring only a portion of the natural dentition via a removable partial denture (RPD) (Fig 1-4). In these instances, however, it is more difficult to select tooth shade and mold because the artificial teeth you are creating, or adding, must blend with the surrounding natural dentition. The patient's remaining natural teeth and gingival tissues dictate tooth length, width, and shade as well as the shade of the denture base material; therefore, there is reduced control in the prosthesis fabrication process owing to increased patient demands and a need to balance proper prosthesis design with the patient's esthetic requirements (see Table 1-1). As a result, compromises are more common, be they in the design of the denture or in the selection of materials for the prosthesis.

For instance, fabricating one or two anterior crowns adjacent to unrestored natural teeth is an example of one of the most exacting professional challenges in prosthodontics (Fig 1-5). By any measure, both clinician and technician have limited control of the variables involved in this case (see Table 1-1). Patient requirements for such factors as esthetics, cost, and time dominate, while the number of factors under the control of either the dentist or technician are reduced in comparison to the complete and partially edentulous patient. The very choice of materials used to make crowns imposes increased limitations from a purely technical standpoint. Therefore, selection of the most appropriate dental materials for each case is critical.

As will be discussed in subsequent chapters, all-ceramic crowns are not suitable for every patient or every clinical situation. In spite of its limitations, the metal-ceramic restoration has been enormously successful. What is remarkable is that most technicians fabricate metal-ceramic restorations without the benefit of seeing the patient for whom they are intended. As such, dental technicians—who, by virtue of their training and experience, have mastered the technical skills needed to manipulate dental porcelain—are frequently identified as *ceramists* or *dental ceramists*. Designations such as these are bestowed with a mixture of reverence and envy

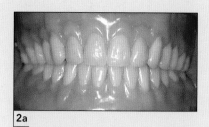 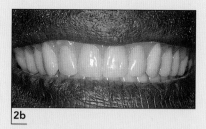 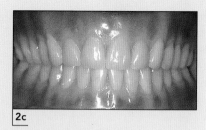

Fig 1-2a Complete maxillary and mandibular wax trial dentures with denture teeth of an appropriate mold (size and shape) and shade.

Fig 1-2b Note how the high value of the wax strongly suggests the need for custom characterization of the denture base resin.

Fig 1-2c The appearance of the definitive maxillary and mandibular complete dentures, following custom characterization of the denture base resin, illustrates the possibility of maximum control over materials and techniques.

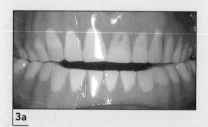 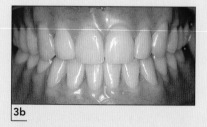 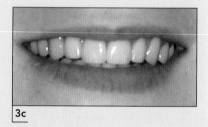

Fig 1-3a These maxillary and mandibular complete dentures have short, severely worn acrylic resin denture teeth and a poor occlusal relationship.

Fig 1-3b The dentures were remade in the correct occlusal relationship with new teeth and properly contoured denture bases.

Fig 1-3c The postoperative appearance of the patient with definitive prostheses looks more natural.

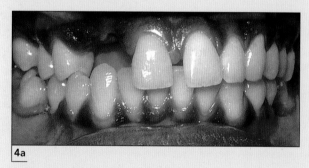 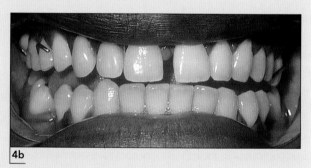

Fig 1-4a Preoperative appearance of a patient missing the maxillary right canine and lateral incisor.

Fig 1-4b Postoperative appearance of the patient with a characterized maxillary transitional partial denture replacing the right canine and lateral incisor.

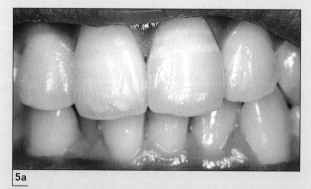 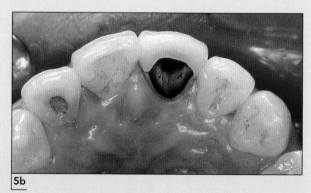

Fig 1-5a Facial view of a metal-ceramic crown with a porcelain labial margin. (Ceramics by Mr Larry Costin.)

Fig 1-5b Lingual view of metal-ceramic crown in Fig 1-5a designed to restore the lingual surface in metal yet retain interproximal porcelain.

because they set these individuals apart from their coworkers. What makes a skilled ceramist unique is an ability to transform dental porcelain powders into vital-looking restorations that replicate natural teeth.

The common thread in the previously mentioned clinical cases is an ability to re-create the position, form, texture, and color of the surrounding oral tissues. Such work reflects the artistic skills of the dental technician and dentist (ie, the *art* of dental technology). However, artistic talent alone is no guarantee of success, and it is best used when accompanied by a working knowledge of dental materials (ie, the *science* of dental technology). Blending the *art* and the *science* of metal-ceramic technology can result in successfully planned and fabricated metal-ceramic crowns and fixed partial dentures.

Metal-Ceramic Terminology

You may find that some of the descriptions and instructions in the following chapters require an expanded vocabulary of technical terms unique to the materials used or the procedures described. A working knowledge of this terminology will help you avoid confusion and potential misunderstandings. An even more extensive glossary of technical terms can be found in the back of the book. In some instances, pertinent terms have been defined at the beginning of several chapters. Where appropriate, the *Glossary of Prosthodontic Terms*[26] has been used as a reference to ensure that the terminology in this text is consistent with that used in the specialty of prosthodontics.

Instances may arise when you detect differences in the interpretation of certain terms in this text as compared with other publications, including the *Glossary of Prosthodontic Terms*. In these cases, an attempt will be made to identify such distinctions. The selected interpretation will be explained and used as consistently as possible throughout the text. It is for you to weigh the merits of both explanations, make a personal interpretation, and select the definition that you think best describes the term in question.

For example, opinions differ on how to properly describe the restorative combination of metal and porcelain. Several popular designations include *porcelain-fused-to-metal* (PFM) *restoration*, *ceramo-metal restoration*, *porcelain-bonded-to-metal* (PBM) *crown*, *porcelain veneer crown* (PVC), and finally, the term used in this text, *metal-ceramic restoration*. All these terms are acceptable in that they describe the same restoration and can be used interchangeably. However, the designation *metal-ceramic* has been selected to describe either a single crown or a fixed partial denture just as the term *all-ceramic* is preferred to identify ceramic crowns and fixed

partial dentures with nonmetallic substructures. Some preliminary terminology follows.

- **Metal-ceramic restoration** A fixed restoration that employs a metal substructure veneered by a ceramic material.
- **Porcelain-fused-to-metal (PFM)** Popular alternative designation for the metal-ceramic restoration.
- **Bonding** Mechanisms by which dental porcelain fuses or adheres to a metal substructure (see chapter 7); also known as *porcelain bonding*.
- **Coping** Metal substructure of single-unit crowns designed for bonding to dental porcelain; copings are made for individual units or attached to pontics to create a fixed partial denture.
- **Framework** A fixed partial denture with a one-piece substructure composed of either several copings attached to a pontic or multiple single units connected as one.
- **Oxidation** Process by which a cast metal substructure is heat treated in a porcelain furnace to elevated temperatures (980°C to 1,050°C), typically in a reduced atmosphere (vacuum), to produce an oxide layer for porcelain bonding and to cleanse the porcelain-bearing surfaces of contaminants (see chapter 7); also known as *oxidizing*. Because this process also can eliminate entrapped gaseous contaminants, it was formerly called *degassing*. (Author's note: Alloys are available that do not have to be oxidized in a reduced atmosphere. In fact, manufacturers of a few base metal alloys claim that oxidation of castings is optional, although such a recommendation is not typical. Therefore, it is vital to adhere to an alloy manufacturer's instructions for all phases of processing.)
- **Substructure** Foundation of a single-unit crown or fixed partial denture for metal-ceramic and all-ceramic restorations.

Components of the Metal-Ceramic Restoration

In its simplest form, a metal-ceramic crown or fixed partial denture has two major components: *(1)* a metal substructure and *(2)* a porcelain veneer. The surface oxide layer that lies between the metal substructure and the porcelain veneer could be considered a separate component, but it is more an integral part of the metal. Even the dental porcelain veneer has several discreet layers, yet it functions as one mass. Consequently, the metal-ceramic restoration is best considered a composite entity with a metal substructure (coping or framework), a layer of opaque porcelain, dentin and enamel veneers, and a surface glaze (Fig 1-6).

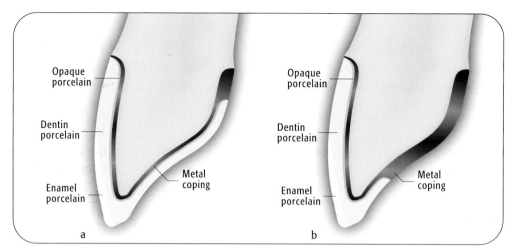

Fig 1-6 *(a)* The components of a complete porcelain veneer restoration include the metal coping, the oxide layer, the opaque layer, the dentin veneer, the enamel veneer, and the external glaze. *(b)* A partial porcelain veneer crown contains all the components of a complete porcelain veneer restoration but relies on more metal to restore the occluding surfaces (lingual/occlusal).

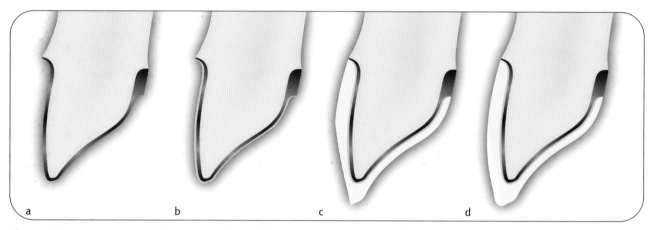

Fig 1-7 *(a)* A coping has been metal finished and oxidized. *(b)* The opaqued metal substructure. *(c)* The dentin porcelain has been cut back for the application of enamel powders. *(d)* The final buildup with enamel porcelain, which is applied and contoured. Note: The location to terminate the enamel cutback coronally on the facial surface depends on the appearance of the tooth to be restored.

Metal substructure

Conventional low-fusing dental porcelain alone lacks the strength required of an all-ceramic restoration, so a metal substructure is added to support the porcelain veneer. The thickness of the metal coping for a single crown or a fixed partial denture can vary from 0.2 to 0.5 mm, depending on the type of casting alloy used and the amount of tooth structure removed by the dentist (Fig 1-7a).

Oxide layer

Metal-ceramic alloys are oxidized after the porcelain-bearing area of the restoration has been properly finished and cleaned. The metallic oxides that form on the alloy's surface during this heat-treatment procedure play a key role in bonding the dental porcelain to the underlying metal substructure. Because noble elements do not oxidize, an alloy's base metal constituents are principally responsible for forming the oxide layer. Differences in alloy composition require that oxidation techniques be alloy specific.

Ideally this oxide layer should be no more than a discrete monomolecular film on the alloy surface for any metal-ceramic alloy, irrespective of compositional differences (see Fig 1-7a). The chemical nature of that film generally varies among different alloy systems as is discussed in chapter 3. Furthermore, the role these oxides play in bonding dental porcelain to metal is explained in chapter 7.

Opaque porcelain layer

Because dentin and enamel porcelains must possess some degree of translucency to mimic natural tooth structure, they lack the ability to mask the dark color of the underlying metal substructure. The opaque porcelains were formulated to serve three major functions: *(1)* to establish the porcelain-metal bond, *(2)* to mask the color of the metal substructure, and *(3)* to initiate development of the selected porcelain shade.

The precise dimension of a fired opaque layer varies among different brands of dental porcelain and in combination with the color of the oxidized metal substructure to which it is applied.[27–29] A uniform thickness of 0.2 to 0.3 mm generally is regarded as ideal[29,30] (Fig 1-7b). Furthermore, all brands of opaque porcelains are vacuum fired onto the metal substructure in a dental porcelain furnace (see chapter 8).

Dentin porcelain veneer

While the development of the porcelain shade (color) begins with the opaque layer, the major color contribution is derived from the pigmented metal oxides in the dentin body porcelain (see Figs 1-6 and 1-7c). This initial layer of dental porcelain imparts the dentin shade associated with, but not confined to, the gingival two-thirds of a tooth. During the fabrication process, the layer of dentin porcelain is overbuilt slightly, cut back, and overlaid with enamel porcelain in those sections of the restoration where greater translucency is desired. For more accurate shade duplication, estimates of the combined thickness of fired dentin and enamel porcelains range from a minimum of 0.5 to 1.0 mm[30,31] to a maximum of 1.5 to 2.0 mm depending on the location of the restoration being measured.[31,32]

Porcelain that is built (stacked) and fired above this 2-mm maximum height is considered unsupported by metal and more prone to fracture.[32] Within thick, unsupported porcelain sections, harmful stresses can form that increase the risk of crack propagation and subsequent fracture of the veneer. For uniformity of shade and maximum strength, it is highly desirable to have an even thickness of porcelain covering the metal substructure.

> Estimates of the combined thickness of fired dentin and enamel porcelains range from a minimum of 0.5 to 1.0 mm to a maximum thickness of 1.5 to 2.0 mm.

Enamel porcelain veneer

The enamel porcelain veneer has intentionally not been labeled the *incisal layer* to avoid implying that these porcelains must be restricted to the incisal third of a buildup. It is appropriate to place enamel porcelain wherever natural enamel translucency is required—even if that placement is outside the incisal third of an anterior crown or the occlusal third of a posterior metal-ceramic restoration.

In general, enamel porcelains are used largely in the incisal and interproximal areas, but they need not be limited to these areas in every porcelain buildup (see Fig 1-7c). The desired final esthetic outcome of the restoration determines the placement and amount of the cutback for enamel porcelain. To re-create the appearance of natural translucency and the vitality of natural tooth structure, the dentin buildup should support the incisal edges as well as individual cusp tips. The enamel layer is applied and vacuum fired with the dentin buildup. It is unwise to fire the dentin and enamel layers separately because the blending of shades will not be as subtle and realistic as when these two materials are fired together (Fig 1-7d).

External glaze

The luster of a natural tooth is reproduced by the development of a sheen over the external surface of the fired porcelain (see Fig 1-5). The final processing step in the fabrication of a metal-ceramic restoration is to heat the completed work to a temperature (recommended by the porcelain manufacturer) sufficient to produce what is often referred to as an *autoglaze*, *self-glaze*, or *natural glaze*. An alternative glazing method, and one that is perhaps used more often, is to apply and fire artificial glazing porcelain (overglaze) to re-create this natural sheen and seal the exterior ceramic surface in the process.

The most common practice for both techniques is to air-fire the restoration and hold it at a high temperature until the desired degree of luster and maturation are attained. Details of the step-by-step procedure of glazing a metal-ceramic restoration are included in chapter 9.

In some instances, a simple steplike mechanical polishing on a lathe using a rag wheel with a fine diamond paste or other polishing agent (eg, Brasso [Reckitt Benckiser] mixed with flour of pumice) can help transform a glassy surface into a more natural-appearing finish.

Summary

A brief history of ceramics, a discussion of dental technology, the definition of key terminology, and an introduction to the components of the metal-ceramic restoration have been discussed. It is now appropriate to take a closer look at dental porcelains. Chapter 2 provides an overview of the chemistry of metal-ceramic porcelains as we know them today. The various types of porcelain powders are identified and described in terms of both composition and use.

References

1. Jones DW. Development of dental ceramics. An historical perspective. Dent Clin North Am 1985;29(4):621–644.

2. van Noort R. Introduction to Dental Materials, ed 3. London: Mosby, 2008.

3. Kelly JR, Nishimura I, Campbell SD. Ceramics in dentistry: Historical roots and current perspectives. J Prosthet Dent 1996;75(1): 18–32.

4. Ring ME. Dentistry: An Illustrated History. New York: Abrams, 1985.
   This well-illustrated text is the definitive reference on the evolution of dentistry.

5. Herschfeld JJ. Charles H. Land and the science of porcelain in dentistry. Bull Hist Dent 1986;34(1):48–54.

6. Hagman HC. History of ceramics, Part I. Dent Lab Rev 1980; 55(12):34, 36.

7. Hagman HC. History of ceramics, Part II. Dent Lab Rev 1980; 55(13):34–36.

8. Clark EB. Requirements of the jacket crown. J Am Dent Assoc 1939;26:355–363.
   Clark describes Wildman's improvement of dental porcelain, the "Land crown," and the four requirements for a successful all-porcelain jacket crown.

9. Southan DE. The development and characteristics of dental porcelain. Aust Dent J 1970;15(2):103–107.

10. Land CH. Porcelain dental art. Dental Cosmos 1903;45(6):437–444.
    Land discusses his papers on "enamel coatings" and the broader applications for porcelain.

11. Land CH. Porcelain dental art: No. II. Dental Cosmos 1903;45(6): 615–620.
    Land describes the technique for fabricating an all-porcelain crown using a platinum foil matrix and calls it a "new art." He blames overextended gingival crown margins and bacteria for gingival irritation and the absence of healthy tissue.

12. Land CH. A new system of restoring badly decayed teeth by means of an enameled metallic coating. Independent Pract 1886;7: 407–409.
    Land introduces the "enameled metallic coating" restoration as a more esthetic treatment modality that preserves more tooth structure than do alternative techniques of the time.

13. Land CH. Metallic enamel coatings and fillings. Independent Pract 1886;7:413–414.
    Land outlines the fabrication of platinum foil–backed crowns and "fillings" with platinum pins for mechanical retention. Advantages of "enamel coatings" include reducing thermal insults to pulp, lowering the risk of root checking or fracture, and preventing injury to surrounding periodontal tissues.

14. Capon WA. Porcelain—Its properties. J Am Dent Assoc 1927; 14(8):1459–1463.
    Capon credits Wood with the first description of an enameled metallic cap—"the basis of our porcelain jacket of today."

15. Land CH. Clinic report. First District Dental Society, State of New York. Dental Cosmos 1889;31:191–192.
    Land reports restoring teeth with porcelain as early as 1884 and emphasizes the importance of preserving coronal tooth structure and avoiding gingival impingement.

16. Land CH. Metallic enamel sections. A new system for filling teeth. Independent Pract 1887;8:87–90.
    Land advocates preservation of coronal tooth structure and elimination of subgingival preparations.

17. Spalding EB. Report to the First District Dental Society, State of New York. Dental Cosmos 1904;46:467.
    Spalding reports methods for natural enamel replacement in both anterior and posterior teeth.

18. Zeigler H. The father of porcelain dental art. Dominion Dent J 1905; 17:30–31.
    Zeigler pays tribute to Charles H. Land.

19. Brecker SC. Porcelain baked to gold—A new medium in prosthodontics. J Prosthet Dent 1956;6(6):801–810.
    Brecker describes the "porcelain baked to gold restoration" using a gold alloy and a bonding agent.

20. Johnston JF, Dykema RW, Cunningham DM. The use and construction of gold crowns with a fused porcelain veneer—A progress report. J Prosthet Dent 1956;6(6):811–818.

21. Weinstein M, Katz S, Weinstein AB [inventors]. Fused porcelain-to-metal teeth. US patent 3,052,982. Aug 1962.

22. Weinstein M, Weinstein AB [inventors]. Porcelain-covered metal-reinforced teeth. US patent 3,052,983. Sept 1962.

23. Christensen GJ. The use of porcelain-fused-to-metal restorations in current dental practice: A survey. J Prosthet Dent 1986;56(1):1–3.
    This 1983 survey found that the porcelain-fused-to-metal restoration was most widely used for crowns with a nickel-based alloy.

24. Christensen GJ. The confusing array of tooth-colored crowns. J Am Dent Assoc 2003;134:1253–1255.
    This laboratory survey found that 65% of the restorations made in a 6-month period were porcelain-fused-to-metal crowns, which was slightly lower than data from 3 years earlier.

25. McLean JW. Evolution of dental ceramics in the twentieth century. J Prosthet Dent 2001;85(1):61–66.

26. Glossary of prosthodontic terms. J Prosthet Dent 2005;94(1):10–92.

27. Avila R, Barghi N, Aranda R. PFM color changes caused by varied opaque firings [abstract 1249]. J Dent Res 1985;64(special issue): 313.
    The authors found that opaque porcelains can be fired up to 60°C above and 40°C below recommended firing temperature without adversely affecting the color of the veneering body porcelain.

28. Naylor WP. Non-Gold Base Dental Casting Alloys. Vol II: Porcelain-fused-to-metal alloys [ADA173766]. Brooks AFB, TX: School of Aerospace Medicine, 1986.
    This second volume provides an overview of dental porcelain; nongold based metal-ceramic alloys; and techniques for spruing, investing, and casting.

29. Terada Y, Sakai T, Hirayasu R. The masking ability of an opaque porcelain: A spectrophotometric study. Int J Prosthodont 1989;2(3): 259–264.

30. Barghi N, Lorenzana RE. Optimum thickness of opaque and body porcelain. J Prosthet Dent 1982;48:429–431.
    The authors concluded that opaque blockout of the metal substructure does not always result in the desired shade and that excessive opaque porcelain has little effect on color. They also found that excessive body porcelain can influence the final shade.

31. Shillingburg HT, Jacobi R, Brackett SE. Fundamentals of Tooth Preparation. Chicago: Quintessence, 1987.

32. Yamamoto M. Metal-Ceramics: Principles and Methods of Makoto Yamamoto. Chicago: Quintessence, 1985.
    This text, one of the most detailed works on ceramic and metal-ceramic technology ever written, includes extensive technical information.

CHAPTER 2

Chemistry of Dental Porcelain

The quality and range of available ceramic products have far surpassed those initial efforts that resulted in crudely constructed porcelain dentures, nonreinforced all-porcelain crowns, and primitive metal-ceramic restorations. Today, dentists and dental laboratory technicians have the luxury of fabricating prostheses from a wide range of esthetic materials of differing compositions suited to a variety of applications.

With this wide array of products comes the added complexity of understanding distinctions among diverse chemistries. It can be equally as challenging to appreciate the role of the metal-ceramic restoration alongside alternative technologies. Although all-ceramic restorations are increasingly popular, successful outcomes can still be achieved with well-made, metal-ceramic prostheses (Fig 2-1). This chapter reinforces the value of the continued use of the metal-ceramic restoration.

Terminology

Given the complexity of this subject, it is important to introduce some key terminology used in conversation, scientific writing, and product descriptions related to ceramics and, in particular, dental porcelains. The terms used to describe the materials applied to substructures (metallic or nonmetallic) and to formed (pressed) restorations may include *ceramics*, *glass*, *glass-ceramic*, *dental ceramic*, *porcelain*, and *dental*—or *feldspathic*—*porcelain*.

Ceramics

The designation *ceramics* can accurately identify anything from earthenware to glazed porcelain (or *china*) to dental restorations. According to one definition, *ceramics* describes the "art or technology of making objects of clay and similar materials treated by firing."[1] In dentistry, the term refers to inorganic crystalline materials that are fired at high temperature (sintered). Unfortunately, *ceramics* characteristically takes on a broad meaning—too nonspecific to represent a particular dental product or even a particular category of nonmetallic materials. It applies equally both to products that veneer a metal substructure and to those that comprise an entire restoration (substructure and veneer).

From a materials science perspective, ceramics are "compounds that contain metallic and nonmetallic elements."[2,3] In general, ceramics are brittle, hard, inert, insulating (electric and thermal), and refractory, and each characteristic is responsible for specific features, as demonstrated in the following examples[2]:

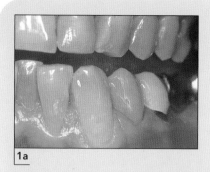 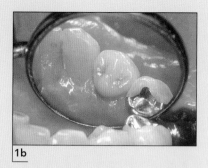 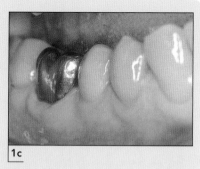

Fig 2-1a The classic problems associated with poorly made metal-ceramic crowns are exhibited on this mandibular left second premolar: unsatisfactory color, high value, and metal display following gingival recession. The all-ceramic crown (IPS Empress, Ivoclar Vivadent) on the adjacent first premolar blends well with the surrounding unrestored natural teeth.

Fig 2-1b Occlusal view of the all-ceramic crown and the metal-ceramic restoration in Fig 2-1a.

Fig 2-1c In contrast, the metal-ceramic crown on the mandibular right second premolar mirrors the appearance of the unrestored first premolar, which demonstrates that metal-ceramic restorations can be both esthetic and functional.

- **Brittle** Describes materials that are weak structurally and require protection or strengthening to function in the oral environment.
- **Hard** Describes materials that resist wear and mechanical forces but potentially can do more harm than good to other restorative materials and to human tooth structure.
- **Inert** Describes materials that are considered biocompatible because they do not break down (undergo dissolution) in the oral cavity; such products do not release elements that dissolve in the saliva, migrate into adjacent gingival tissues, nor enter organs in the human body.
- **Insulating** Describes materials that do not transmit electric current or temperature change and that help to protect sensitive pulpal and gingival tissues.
- **Refractory** Describes materials that withstand high temperatures, within certain limits, without undergoing structural (dimensional) change.

Glass

A *glass* is an amorphous (also referred to as *noncrystalline*) inorganic material in which atoms and molecules are not arranged in a regular lattice structure as they are in crystalline solids. Most glasses used in dentistry are in the silicate family and are based on silica (silicon dioxide, SiO_2) (Sundar V, personal communication, 2007), which is found in nature as *quartz*.

Glass ceramic

As the name implies, a *glass ceramic* is a material that retains a noncrystalline *glass phase* along with a partially crystallized (or devitrified) *ceramic phase* (Sundar V, personal communication, 2007). Crystal nucleation and growth in the glass matrix also is controlled.[3] The incorporation of crystalline ceramics within the glass matrix renders a material stronger and tougher than the glass phase alone.

Dental ceramics

Just as *ceramics* is an all-encompassing term that applies to many different materials, the designation *dental ceramics* is also sufficiently ambiguous to apply to all types of ceramic dental products. Everything from denture teeth to all-ceramic restoratives to metal-ceramic porcelains can be labeled as *dental ceramics*. The term should be defined in communications (eg, dental laboratory work authorizations) to indicate a specific product or at least a class of materials. Anusavice defined the term as an inorganic compound of metallic and nonmetallic elements "formulated to produce the whole or part of a ceramic-based prosthesis."[3]

Porcelain

Typically, *porcelain* refers to those ceramic materials initially derived from a combination of kaolin, quartz, and feldspar sintered at high temperatures[4] (Fig 2-2).

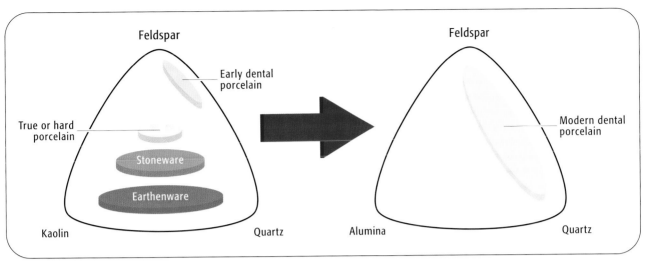

Fig 2-2 Schematic comparing the composition of earthenware, stoneware, porcelain, and early dental porcelain *(left)* that led to the development of modern dental porcelain *(right)*, in which kaolin was eliminated and alumina was added.

Table 2-1	Components of early dental porcelains[6] and contemporary high-fusing porcelains	
Ingredient	Early dental porcelains (wt%)	High-fusing porcelains (wt%)
Feldspar	78.0	75.0 to 85.0
Quartz	–	12.0 to 22.0
Alumina	–	≤ 10.0
Kaolin*	15.3	≤ 3.0
Potash silicate	4.7	–
Dehydrated borax	2.0	–

*Kaolin is rarely included in contemporary metal-ceramic porcelains.

Dental porcelains

From a materials science perspective, dental porcelains are made up of an amorphous glass matrix and at least one crystalline phase such as leucite[3] (K_2O-Al_2O_3-$4SiO_2$). In the early to mid-1800s, dental porcelain was not widely popular due, in part, to the unsatisfactory esthetics attributed to small quantities of kaolin (Table 2-1).[5,6] Evidently, ceramic restorations of the day were noticeably opaque and white.[7] Their appearance changed markedly around 1838 when Dr Elias Wildman devised a formulation that more closely approximated tooth color and translucency by increasing the amount of feldspar and eliminating the kaolin.[5,7] Hence, metal-ceramic porcelains were also referred to as *feldspathic porcelains*[8] or *feldspathic glasses*.[9] Yamamoto

described metal-ceramic porcelains as *crystallized glass*,[10] acknowledging the glass matrix and complex crystalline phase present in modern-day dental porcelains.

Contemporary dental porcelains retain a composite struc-ture of glasses, ceramics, or glass-ceramics. Crystalline ceramic and glass-ceramic components are added to strengthen and toughen the glass phase and to ensure that the veneering materials are compatible with their substruc-ture. Metallic oxides are needed to opacify glasses and to add color.

Historically, dental porcelains have been classified based on their fusion temperature (ie, melting range) as *high*, *medium*, and *low fusing*. These three categories of porcelain have vastly different applications in dentistry, and other clas-sification methods are needed.

Differences in Low-Fusing Dental Porcelains

Surprisingly, refinements to the original chemistry took well over a hundred years to evolve into modern-day dental applications. During this time, low-fusing porcelain served as the foundation for two different developments: (1) the metal-ceramic restoration and (2) the all-porcelain restoration.

Metal-ceramic restorations

The evolution of the metal-ceramic restoration reached a milestone around 1838 when Wildman reformulated porcelain to reduce opacity and increase translucency and color.[11,12] The next breakthrough occurred over a century later, in 1949, when the Dentists Supply Company (now Dentsply) introduced vacuum firing. Sintering in a vacuum—that is, in a reduced atmosphere—significantly improved porcelain translucency and color development.[7,12] The problem of restoration breakage was largely resolved by the addition of a small quantity of alumina (aluminum oxide, Al_2O_3) for strength. Next, Brecker reported a method for actually *bonding* low-fusing feldspathic porcelain to a metal substructure using a gold-based alloy.[13] After this development, the range of metal-ceramic alloys increased rapidly with the introduction of the patented Weinstein porcelain.[14] The Weinstein formulation demonstrated that the controlled addition of leucite crystals could raise the typically low coefficient of thermal expansion (CTE) of feldspathic porcelain to a level high enough to maintain a stable bond, or attachment, between the ceramic veneer and the underlying metal.[14,15]

As mentioned in chapter 1, Land created what he described as an *enameled crown* by placing dental porcelain on a platinum foil substrate. Land himself acknowledged that no mechanical or chemical attachment formed between the porcelain and metal.[16,17] In contrast, Brecker developed a method that permitted a chemical bond to form between the two substances.[13] Another distinction between the techniques used by Land and Brecker is that Land adapted metal foil to the prepared teeth whereas Brecker cast metal substructures indirectly using the lost-wax technique

> Around 1965, McLean and Hughes developed the aluminous porcelain that is used in making porcelain jacket crowns.

All-porcelain restorations

The second major application of low-fusing porcelain led to the refinement of the all-porcelain restoration. To understand the significance of this development requires a review of the contributions of Land and the subsequent achievements of Dr John McLean.[15–20]

Land's all-porcelain jacket crowns

The all-porcelain crowns that Land created in the late 1800s were made entirely of low-fusing feldspathic porcelain.[11,21] Land apparently made these early crowns simply by air-firing the low-fusing feldspathic porcelain used to make complete dentures and individual denture teeth. Although his restorations were heated on a platinum foil substructure, the foil was removed because there was no expectation of a chemical bond between metal and veneer.[22] These restorations lacked the strength and toughness of contemporary porcelains, and structural failures were common.[5] Consequently, the porcelain inlays and feldspathic all-ceramic crowns that Land advocated did not gain widespread popularity. The lack of acceptance was probably related to the clinical failure of restorations due to their inherent weakness.[5]

McLean's aluminous porcelain jacket crowns

More than 60 years following Land's groundbreaking efforts, McLean introduced aluminous porcelain to dentistry.[19,20] McLean created a special aluminous "core" porcelain containing between 40% and 50% (by weight) of added alumina.[3,8,18,23]

McLean found that incorporating a large volume of alumina created a strong core material that retained the inherently low CTE of low-fusing dental porcelain.[19,20] The decision to add alumina also meant that the aluminous core substructure could be fired and veneered with thermally compatible low-fusing body porcelains. It is important to point out that the corresponding dentin aluminous porcelains are simply low-fusing feldspathic porcelains that contain only 5% to 10% alumina, whereas the enamel powders are predominantly alumina free.[8] McLean's improvements enabled the aluminous porcelain jacket crown to emerge as a viable restoration for anterior teeth for many years.[19,20]

What differentiates dentin and enamel aluminous porcelains from their metal-ceramic counterparts is their low linear CTE that is well matched to aluminous core porcelain. From a purely physical standpoint, the CTE for an aluminous porcelain ranges from 6.5 to $8.5 \times 10^{-6}/°C$, which is slightly more than one half the CTE of most metal-ceramic alloys (13.5 to $15.5 \times 10^{-6}/°C$).[8,24,25] It is this compatibility of CTEs that permits dentin and enamel aluminous porcelains to veneer all-ceramic substrates. In fact, some of the new non-

Table 2-2	Classification of dental porcelains by fusion temperature

Type	Temperature range		
	Anusavice[3]	Craig[4]	O'Brien[27]
High-fusing	1,288°C to 1,371°C (2,350°F to 2,500°F)	1,315°C to 1,370°C (2,400°F to 2,500°F)	1,288°C to 1,371°C (2,350°F to 2,500°F)
Medium-fusing	1,093°C to 1,260°C (2,000°F to 2,300°F)	1,090°C to 1,260°C (1,994°F to 2,300°F)	1,093°C to 1,260°C (2,000°F to 2,300°F)
Low-fusing	871°C to 1,066°C (1,600°F to 1,950°F)	870°C to 1,065°C (1,598°F to 1,949°F)	660°C to 1,066°C (1,220°F to 1,950°F)
Ultra low-fusing	< 850°C (< 1,562°F)		

cast ceramic systems are either strengthened feldspathic porcelains or improved aluminous porcelains. As will be described in greater detail in chapter 3, the large difference in CTEs between aluminous porcelains and ceramic alloys makes them incompatible.

Contemporary metal-ceramic porcelains

The application of dental porcelains in metal-ceramic technology evolved from a series of breakthroughs: the elimination of kaolin, the addition of alumina, the introduction of vacuum firing, and the incorporation of a leucite-containing component.[5,7,14,15,24,26] These changes vastly improved the esthetics, increased the strength, and raised the CTE of metal-ceramic porcelains (to ensure metal–dental porcelain compatibility), thereby enabling them to be used for numerous dental applications.

Improved esthetics

Wildman's reformulation and the introduction of vacuum firing vastly improved the esthetic qualities of dental porcelain.[5] Further advancements in esthetics included the use of vacuum firing to enhance the translucence of the fired ceramic and the incorporation of metallic oxides for color development.[5] Metallic oxides not only provide a level of opacity sufficient to mask an underlying metal substructure but also enable restorations to possess sufficient color to match or blend with adjacent natural teeth.

Improved strength

Vacuum firing during sintering strengthens ceramic.[26] The addition of calcined alumina at the expense of an equivalent amount of quartz, credited to McLean and Hughes, also improves porcelain through a process known as *dispersion strengthening*.[7,19]

Increased linear CTE

Leucite crystals in the glass matrix have a high CTE (20 to 25×10^{-6}/°C).[3] The source of leucite in Weinstein's famed 1962 porcelain patent was "Component No. 1"—a mixture of six different oxides.[24] Thermal compatibility between the ceramic veneer and metal substructure is vital to the maintenance of a stable bond.

To better appreciate feldspathic porcelains in general, it is helpful to understand how dental porcelains may be classified.

Classification of Dental Ceramics

Recognizing the subtle distinctions among porcelain products enhances appreciation for metal-ceramic technology in dentistry. There are several ways to classify dental porcelains.[3] In this text, the focus is on four methods: *(1)* fusion temperature, *(2)* fabrication method, *(3)* crystalline phase (ie, chemistry), and *(4)* clinical application.[4]

Fusion temperature

Fusion temperature refers to the temperature range over which ceramic particles fuse together because the melting process does not occur at a discreet temperature. In fact, the mixed ingredients gradually undergo pyroplastic flow (also known as *slumping*) over a span of several hundred degrees. The temperature at which porcelains begin to transform from a solid to a glass—a supercooled liquid—is referred to as the *glass transition temperature* or *glass temperature* (T_g).[27] At this temperature, there is also a significant increase in the ceramic's CTE.

It was not long ago that only three major categories of dental porcelain were identified using fusion temperature (Table 2-2):

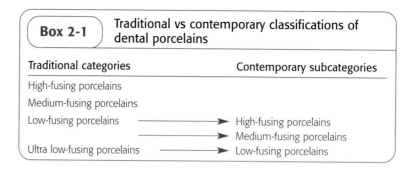

(1) high fusing, (2) medium fusing, and (3) low fusing.[4,27] In fact, using the fusion temperature range to classify different porcelains is a practice that dates to the 1940s,[4] when the number of dental ceramic products was far more limited than it is today. These three types of porcelain have their own unique properties, but the high-fusing and medium-fusing porcelains are similar in both composition and microstructure. In terms of actual use, denture teeth are made from the high-fusing materials, whereas the medium-fusing porcelains most often are used to produce prefabricated pontics (historically known as *trupontics*). Metal-ceramic porcelains and aluminous porcelains emerged from the traditional low-fusing porcelains.

It was not until Brecker's work in the 1950s on bonding porcelain to gold-based alloys and the emergence of the Weinstein formulation in 1962 that low-fusing porcelains containing leucite became thermally compatible with metal-ceramic alloys.[13–15] These porcelains can accommodate the relatively higher expansion (and contraction) of metal-ceramic alloys and, consequently, differ more in terms of composition and physical properties than do the high-fusing and medium-fusing porcelains.

More recently a new group—ultra low-fusing porcelains—was added to this classification.[3]

Ultra low-fusing porcelains

The ultra low-fusing porcelains were designed to veneer a metal substructure at even lower firing temperatures. With the Finesse ceramic system (Dentsply), for example, the opaque porcelain is sintered at a high temperature of 800°C (1,472°F), and a second dentin firing occurs at 750°C (1,382°F). Correction porcelain is then heated at the even lower temperature of 710°C (1,310°F).

> The majority of metal-ceramic porcelains fall within the traditional low-fusing category, though the number of ultra low-fusing products has seen a notable increase.

> What has emerged is a more contemporary "classification-within-a-classification" that is used by industry but which may not be found in dental materials textbooks. In this new classification, there are three subcategories within the traditional low-fusing porcelain category.

In addition, quartz-based rather than feldspar-based porcelains are available. One such product, HeraCeram (Heraeus Kulzer), is sintered below 850°C (1,562°F) and has been described as a *synthetic* material.[28]

In reading the product literature accompanying some metal-ceramic porcelains, it is apparent that dental manufacturers have adopted a more contemporary approach to classifying ceramics traditionally defined as low-fusing or ultra low-fusing porcelains.

Contemporary classification of low-fusing porcelains

According to many dental materials textbooks, low-fusing porcelains have a fusion temperature range from 870°C to 1,066°C (1,598°F to 1,950°F), with temperatures below 850°C (1,562°F) used to define ultra low-fusing porcelains[3] (see Table 2-2). Other books simply reduce the low-fusing porcelains' temperature range to 660°C (1,220°F), so ultra low-fusing products fall within this category.[27]

What has emerged is a contemporary "classification-within-a-classification" that is used by industry but which may not be found in dental materials textbooks. In this new classification, there are three subcategories *within* the traditional low-fusing porcelain category (Box 2-1). These subcategories are also labeled *high-fusing*, *medium-fusing*, and *low-fusing* porcelains, and differentiation is based on the temperature range. Thus, the *high-fusing* subcategory of the low-fusing porcelains includes ceramics that are fired above a temperature of approximately 900°C (eg, Ceramco 3, Dentsply). Low-fusing porcelains sintered from 850°C to 900°C (eg, IPS d.SIGN [Ivoclar Vivadent], Vita VM 13 [Vident]) fall into the *medium-fusing* subcategory, and the newer ultra low-fusing porcelains fired below 850°C (Finesse) are

Table 2-3 Contemporary classification of low-fusing porcelains

Low-fusing subcategories*	Products	Firing temperature
High-fusing > 900°C (1,652°F)	Ceramco 3 (Dentsply)	960°C
	Duceram Kiss (Dentsply)	920°C
	IPS InLine (Ivoclar Vivadent)	910°C
Medium-fusing 850°C to 900°C (1,562°F to 1,652°F)	Imagine Reflex (Wieland Dental & Technik)	900°C
	Vita VM 13 (Vident)	880°C
	HeraCeram (Heraeus Kulzer)	870°C
	IPS d.SIGN (Ivoclar Vivadent)	870°C
Low-fusing < 850°C (1,562°F)	Duceragold Kiss (Dentsply)	780°C
	Finesse (Dentsply)	760°C

*Temperatures used to establish subcategories of low-fusing porcelains are approximate. Variations in descriptions may occur because there are no established, industry-wide standards to categorize dental porcelains.

placed in the *low-fusing* subcategory.[3] The subcategories for several contemporary low-fusing porcelains are given in Table 2-3.

Statements about high-fusing metal-ceramic porcelains in product literature likely refer to what dental textbooks classify as traditional low-fusing porcelains (sintered between 870°C and 1,066°C). This high-fusing subcategory of low-fusing porcelains should not be confused with the high-fusing ceramics used to make porcelain denture teeth (see Table 2-2 and Box 2-1).

A mastery of the skills needed to create a metal-ceramic restoration will greatly aid those who wish to expand their training to all-ceramic systems. Look at the various steps in the production of an IPS Empress or IPS Empress 2 (Ivoclar Vivadent) restoration. From wax-up to final glaze, the process parallels that required to produce a metal-ceramic restoration with the exception that the substructure is heat-pressed ceramic rather than cast metal. The skills mastered in metal-ceramics can be transferred to this newer technology with only minimal additional training.

Fabrication method

Thanks largely to the development of contemporary high-strength all-ceramic materials, a classification system emerged to categorize products by their fabrication method. Today, ceramic restorations are made not only by sintering but also by heat pressing, machining, and slip casting. For some restorations, a substructure is created with one of these fabrication methods while the body of the restoration is constructed using the conventional metal-ceramic technique of sintering.

With traditional ceramic techniques, porcelain powders—including opaque, dentin, enamel, and effect porcelains—are mixed with water or modeling liquid and incrementally layered onto a metal substructure. The buildup is dried slowly and vacuum fired. Thus, sintering is a fabrication category for most metal-ceramic porcelains.

> Mastery of the skills needed to fabricate a metal-ceramic restoration will greatly aid those who wish to expand their training to all-ceramic systems.

Crystalline phase

The physical differences in the microstructure of dental porcelains also can serve as a means of differentiation. Low-fusing metal-ceramic porcelains have two principal phases: *(1)* an amorphous feldspathic glass matrix that surrounds *(2)* dispersed *crystalline* particles.[4,10] The glass matrix can be thought of as the glue that binds the mass together. The various crystalline components give porcelain its strength, opacity, color, and increased CTE, which ensures thermal compatibility with metal-ceramic alloys.

The greater the volume of the glass matrix, the greater the translucency of the fired porcelain—although there is a trade-off. With a larger glass matrix and increased translucency comes a weaker ceramic structure and a reduced crystalline phase. Although dentin, enamel, and translucent porcelains have a similar chemical composition, they exhibit

<table>
<tr><td colspan="2">Table 2-4   Classification of dental porcelains by clinical application</td></tr>
<tr><td>Clinical application</td><td>Type of ceramic</td></tr>
<tr><td>Porcelain denture teeth</td><td>High-fusing feldspathic porcelains (manufactured)
Medium-fusing feldspathic porcelains (manufactured)</td></tr>
<tr><td>All-ceramic systems</td><td>Based on alumina, feldspar, fluorapatite, leucite, lithium disilicate, lithium phosphate, mica, spinel, or zirconia (heat-pressed, machined [CAM], sintered, and slip-cast)</td></tr>
<tr><td>Metal-ceramic porcelains</td><td>Low-fusing feldspathic porcelains (sintered)
Ultra low-fusing feldspathic porcelains (sintered)</td></tr>
</table>

CAM = computer-assisted manufacture

vast differences in the ratio of matrix volume to crystals volume. For example, dentin porcelain contains more of the crystalline phase and less of the glass matrix than does fired enamel porcelain.

Most of the newer, all-ceramic systems have a chemistry different from the feldspar-based high-fusing, medium-fusing, low-fusing, and ultra low-fusing porcelains. Their crystalline phases may contain large volumes of alumina, feldspar, fluorapatite, leucite, lithium disilicate, lithium phosphate, mica, spinel, and zirconia (zirconium dioxide).

Clinical application

As mentioned previously, dental ceramics also can be classified based on three major applications (Table 2-4):

1. Porcelain denture teeth are manufactured from traditional high-fusing feldspathic porcelain, whereas prefabricated pontics are produced from medium-fusing feldspathic porcelain.
2. All-ceramic systems use materials containing the crystalline phases mentioned above (from alumina to zirconia). All-ceramic substructures or, in some instances, entire all-ceramic restorations can be heat pressed, machined (computer-assisted manufacture [CAM]), sintered, or slip cast.
3. Metal-ceramic porcelains consist of traditional low-fusing and ultra low-fusing feldspathic porcelains (see subcategories in Box 2-1).

Chemical Components of Dental Porcelain

The principal chemical components in contemporary dental porcelains include crystalline minerals such as feldspar, quartz, and alumina in a glass matrix[3,4] (see Fig 2-2). The exact proportions of each component vary with the type of porcelain (high, medium, and low fusing) and the brand, but general compositional ranges are known (Tables 2-5 to 2-7).

Feldspar

As mentioned previously, feldspar is the ingredient primarily responsible for forming the glass matrix,[4] and it lends itself well to the fritting and coloring processes. Naturally occurring feldspar does not exist in a pure form but as a mixture of two substances: (1) potassium aluminum silicate (K_2O-Al_2O_3-$6SiO_2$), also called *potash feldspar* or *orthoclase*; and (2) sodium aluminum silicate (Na_2O-Al_2O_3-$6SiO_2$), also called *sodium feldspar* or *albite*.[29] The ratio of potash feldspar to sodium feldspar differs in a given batch of material. This difference is important to porcelain manufacturers because the two types of feldspar impart quite different handling characteristics to porcelain.

Potash feldspar

Potash feldspar is found in most present-day formulations because of the translucent quality it adds to fired restorations. When melted between 1,250°C and 1,500°C (2,280°F to 2,730°F), potash fuses with quartz to become a glass.[29] The potash form of feldspar not only increases the viscosity, or thickness, of the molten glass but also aids in controlling the porcelain's pyroplastic flow during sintering. In other words, it reduces fluidity and helps to maintain the form of the porcelain buildup while it is being heated to maturity in the furnace.

Sodium feldspar

Sodium feldspar lowers the fusion temperature of porcelain, causing it to be more susceptible to pyroplastic flow. Sodium feldspar does not contribute to translucency, and it

| Table 2-5 | Composition (wt%) of opaque porcelains* |

	Contemporary products				Historical products		
Compound	Ceramco 3	Finesse	IPS d.SIGN paste	Vita VM 13	Vita VMK 68 (Vident)	Will-Ceram (Williams)	Duceram (Dentsply)
SiO_2	52.0–57.0	45.2	30.0–40.0	40.0–44.0	48.0–59.0	50.0	50.9
ZrO_2	–	24.0	15.0–40.0	3.0–5.0	–	–	–
Al_2O_3	10.0–14.0	6.1	8.0–12.0	11.0–14.0	16.3–20.0	17.0	12.6
K_2O	7.0–11.0	10.2	5.0–10.0	7.0–10.0	8.4–10.3	11.1	11.1
Na_2O	3.0–5.0	7.2	2.0–6.0	4.0–6.0	5.7–7.0	5.2	3.3
SnO_2	15.0–20.0	–	–	0–1.0	4.3–5.25	18.0	18.5
TiO_2	–	–	0.1–0.3	4.0–7.0	2.7–3.3	0.3	–
B_2O_2	–	1.4	0.5–1.5	–	1.2–2.5	–	1.6
Li_2O	0–2.0	1.6	–	–	–	–	1.0
CaO	0–1.0	1.4	0–2.0	1.0–2.0	1.2–1.45	–	–
F_2	–	–	–	–	0–0.5	–	0.5
Sb_2O_3	–	–	–	–	–	–	0.5
BaO	–	1.4	0–1.0	0–1.0	–	–	–
CeO_2	–	0.7	0.4–0.7	13.0–16.0			
P_2O_5	–		0–0.5	< 1.0			
Glycol	–	–	25.0				
Pigments	0–10.0	0–15.0	0–25.0				

*Weight percentages as reported by the manufacturers.

is considered a less attractive substitute for potash feldspar.[30] Because the linear CTE of leucite (25×10^{-6}/°C according to McLaren[31] and greater than 20×10^{-6}/°C according to Craig[4]) is much higher than that of feldspar (7.7×10^{-6}/°C according to McLaren and Anusarice[3,31]), low-fusing dental porcelains can be formulated that are compatible with the higher-expanding metal-ceramic alloys.[3,4,31]

Glass modifiers such as the potassium, sodium, and calcium oxides act as fluxes to increase a porcelain's CTE.[8] The addition of these alkali also enables dental porcelains to approach the higher CTE level of metal-ceramic alloys. The fluxes increase the porcelain's CTE by breaking up oxygen cross-linking. Unfortunately, if too much oxygen cross-linking is disrupted, the glass may recrystallize (or devitrify). Recrystallization (also referred to as *devitrification*) is likely to occur with high-expansion dental porcelains and can weaken the restoration, produce a cloudy appearance, and make the porcelain more difficult to glaze.[8] With contemporary porcelains, recrystallization seldom occurs if the manufacturer's recommended firing schedule is followed.

Quartz

Quartz (SiO_2), also known as silica, has a high fusion temperature and serves as the framework around which the other ingredients can flow. By stabilizing the porcelain build-up at high temperatures, quartz helps prevent the porcelain from undergoing pyroplastic flow on the metal substructure during sintering and strengthens the fired porcelain.[30]

Alumina

The third component of dental porcelain, alumina (Al_2O_3), is the hardest and strongest oxide. Naturally occurring alumina has water molecules attached to it. Using a calicination process similar to that used to refine gypsum products, "hydrated" alumina is transformed to pure alumina.[19] During the initial stages of calcination, the chemically bound water in the alumina trihydrate is removed to yield "calcined" alumina. A second calcination at 1,250°C converts the alumina to its alpha form, which is then ground to a fine powder for use in dentistry.[8]

| Table 2-6 | Composition (wt%) of body porcelains* | | | | | | |

	Contemporary products				Historical products		
Compound	Ceramco 3	Finesse	IPS d.SIGN	Vita VM 13	Vita VMK 68	Will-Ceram	Duceram
SiO_2	62.0–66.0	58.4–59.0	50.0–65.0	59.0–63.0	54.7–67.0	60.9	65.3
Al_2O_3	12.0–14.0	7.0–8.0	8.0–20.0	13.0–16.0	17.4–22.0	14.4	14.6
K_2O	9.0–11.0	12.4–13.5	7.0–13.0	9.0–11.0	8.7–10.6	14.0	10.8
Na_2O	4.0–6.0	9.3–10.5	4.0–12.0	5.0–7.0	6.6–8.1	4.0	6.4
SnO_2	–	–	–	< 0.5	4.30–5.25	–	–
CaO	1.0–3.0	2.0	0.1–6.0	1.0–3.0	1.7–2.1	–	1.0
TiO_2	–	–	0–4.0	< 0.5	0.25–0.29	0.3	–
F_2	–	–	1.0–3.0	–	0–0.5	–	0.5
Sb_2O_3	–	–	–	–	–	–	0.5
Li_2O	0–1.0	1.6–2.0	0–3.0	–	–	–	0.3
BaO	0–2.0	1.8–2.0	0–3.0	2.0–4.0	–	–	0.3
MgO	–	–	–	< 1.0	–	–	0.3
ZrO_2	–	< 1.0	0.3–5.0	< 0.5	–	0.1	–
P_2O_5	–	0–5.0	–	< 1.0			
ZnO	–	0–5.0	–	–			
B_2O_3	–	1.5–2.0	0–3.0	1.0–3.0			
CeO_2	0–2.0	1.0–1.1	0–3.0	< 0.5			
Tb_2O_3	0–2.0	1.0	–	–			
SrO	–	0–3.0	–	–			
Pigments	0–0.6	< 1.0–5.0	0–3.0				

*Weight percentages as reported by the manufacturers.

Refined alumina is only slightly soluble in low-fusing porcelain, but it is an important addition because it increases the overall strength and viscosity of the melt.[8] It also has a low linear CTE (9×10^{-6}/°C) compared to metal-ceramic alloys (13.5 to 15.5×10^{-6}/°C).[2,29] As mentioned previously, manufacturers add glass modifiers (eg, oxides of potassium, sodium, and calcium) to raise the CTE.

Kaolin

Mention is made of kaolin (Al_2O_3-$2SiO_2$-$2H_2O$ or *hydrated aluminum silicate*) solely for historical benefit. It has long since disappeared from the composition of metal-ceramic porcelain, yet it continues to be mentioned in dental materials textbooks. Kaolin initially was added to act as a binder and to increase the moldability of the unfired porcelain.[30] It gave the mixed porcelain greater mass and enabled the porcelain to be carved. Because kaolin is also opaque, it was added in very small quantities, if at all (see Fig 2-2).

Fritting and frits

To create the powders for bottled dental porcelain, the crystalline minerals (eg, feldspar, quartz, alumina) are mixed with glass modifiers (ie, oxides of potassium, sodium, and calcium) and other ingredients, then sintered to very high temperatures. A vitreous (glasslike) phase is produced and preserved by quickly quenching the mass in cold water. The molten glass shatters on contact with the cold water to form unique noncrystalline solids called *frits*; this process is referred to as *fritting*.

Frits can be refined to the specific particle size established by individual manufacturers for their brand of porcelain. Metallic oxides, acting as opacifiers and pigments, are mixed with the powders before bottling to provide a multitude of optical qualities.[8] A complete porcelain kit might contain bottles of opaque, dentin, and enamel porcelain powders, along with numerous color concentrates such as opaque and dentin color modifiers, external colorants (or stains), and a colorless glaze.

Table 2-7 Composition (wt%) of stains*

Compound	Contemporary products				Historical products		
	Ceramco 3	Finesse	IPS d.SIGN	Vita VM 13[†]	Vita VMK 68	Will-Ceram[‡]	Duceram
SiO_2	72.0–77.0	56.0–59.0	50.0–65.0	56.0–58.0	60.0–67.8	65.0–70.0	62.0
B_2O_3	–	1.0–3.0	–	9.0–10.0	11.4–14.0	10.0–15.0	–
Na_2O	13.0–16.0	9.0–12.0	4.0–12.0	4.5–6.0	5.6–6.8	7.0–9.0	12.0
Al_2O_3	0–2.0	5.0–8.0	8.0–15.0	6.0–7.0	5.0–6.7	5.0–7.0	–
CaO	3.0–6.0	1.0–3.0	0.0–5.0	4.0–5.0	4.5–5.5	–	–
K_2O	–	12.0–15.0	7.0–13.0	3.0–4.0	3.2–4.0	3.0–4.0	10.0
BaO	–	1.0–3.0	–	1.5–2.0	1.4–1.8	–	12.0
ZnO	–	–	1.0–5.0	–	0.5–0.7	–	–
Sn_2O	–	–	–	4.0–5.0	–	–	2.0
F_2	–	–	–	–	–	–	2.0
P_2O_5	–	–	–	< 0.5	–	–	–
B_2O	–	–	–	–	–	1.0–2.0	–
C_2O	–	–	–	–	–	0.5–1.5	–
ZrO_2	–	–	0.5–5.0	0.5–1.0	–	–	–
Li_2O	–	1.0–3.0	0–4.0	–	–	–	–
TiO_2	–	–	0–4.0	0.5–1.0			
Tb_2O_3	–	0–2.0					
CeO_2	–	0–2.0	0–3.0				
SrO	–	–	0–3.0				
F	–	–	0–2.5				
Glycol			30.0–40.0				
Pigments	3.0–30.0	3.0–32.0	~10.0–25.0				

*Weight percentages as reported by the manufacturers.
[†]Vita Akzent stains can be used with all the Vita veneering ceramic products.
[‡]Mole percentages as reported by the manufacturer.

The manufacturing process can be altered to effect changes in the properties of the porcelain: its viscosity, melting range, chemical durability, thermal expansion, and even its resistance to recrystallization. These alterations may partly explain variations in the handling characteristics among brands of porcelains.

Phases of dental porcelains

Feldspar melts around 1,150°C, transforming the mass into a molten glass phase and a leucite phase.[4] On cooling, the leucite crystals form and are interspersed throughout the glass matrix. As much as 75% to 85% of the total volume is comprised of the glass matrix. The volume of leucite may range from 10% to 20%[4] to 15% to 25%,[32] but some report it to be as high as 30% to 40%.[5]

Leucite

Recall that leucite is a potassium aluminum silicate, with the same chemical components as potash feldspar, formed by a process in which heated feldspar is transformed into an amorphous glass phase accompanied by the precipitation of refractory leucite crystals.[11,15,33] This process in which a material melts to create a liquid and a different crystalline material is referred to as *incongruent melting*.[3]

Although leucite crystallization occurs within the glass matrix when the porcelain is fired between 700°C and 1,200°C,[34] additional leucite ceramic may be added artificially to the frit during manufacturing. Therefore, contemporary veneering materials can contain up to 35%, by weight, of this ceramic (Sundar V, personal communication, 2007). The crystalline phase of leucite raises the linear CTE of metal-ceramic porcelain and plays a minor role in strengthening and toughening dental porcelain.

Factors such as the amount of potash, the firing temperature, and the length of time the porcelain is held at high temperature also affect the extent of crystal formation.[34,35] Repeated firings and slow cooling can either increase or decrease the leucite content in the glassy matrix depending on the brand of porcelain.[12] In fact, leucite crystals are known to form with each firing, thereby raising the porcelain's CTE through a process referred to as *secondary crystallization*.[36]

Conversely, overheating or firing at too high a temperature can cause leucite crystals to dissolve into the glass matrix.[10] Such a change reduces the volume of the crystalline phase, lowers the linear CTE of the dental porcelain veneer, and weakens the ceramic. Faithful adherence to the manufacturers' recommended firing instructions is important to the creation and maintenance of a stable metal-ceramic bond. In addition, porcelain furnaces should be calibrated and checked on a regular schedule. Should porcelain cracking or bond failures occur, attention should first be directed to how the porcelain is being processed in the dental laboratory before inquiring as to whether there is a manufacturing problem with the ceramic or the casting alloy

Given the importance of thermal expansion compatibility and contemporary manufacturing methods, leucite could be considered another key ingredient of dental porcelain. Without it, the CTEs between the ceramic veneer and the metal substructure would be incompatible or, at the very least, unfavorable stresses would occur at the porcelain-metal interface.

Low-Fusing Porcelains for Metal-Ceramic Restorations

The large number of US, Japanese, and European manufacturers and distributors of low-fusing dental porcelains makes for a very competitive market. Commercial products differ in terms of chemical composition, particle size distribution, handling characteristics, shrinkage, esthetics, and cost. The precise formulations of porcelains vary as well (see Tables 2-5 to 2-8).

Because of the competitive nature of the dental porcelain market in the United States, many porcelain systems are available in all or several of the most popular shade systems. Figure 2-3 includes a variety of porcelain shade guides, including specialized guides for Ceramco 3 and for the Vita 3D-Master system (Vident) that allow users to create intermediate shades with a 1:1 mixture of adjacent porcelain shades. Because shade tabs have a neck region that is darker than the indicated body shade, removing the neck

and repolishing the adjusted area may help with the selection of body shades (Fig 2-4).

Other porcelain products available for use include opacious dentins and high-fusing shoulder porcelains. *Opacious dentins* (also marketed as *opaceous*, *deep*, or *base dentins*) are more pigmented than conventional dentin porcelains. High-fusing shoulder powder and porcelain margin powder are sintered at temperatures higher than regular body porcelains and were developed for the creation of porcelain margins.

Opaque porcelains

By and large, opaque porcelains serve three primary functions: *(1)* they wet the metal surface and establish a metal-porcelain bond; *(2)* they mask the color of the metal substructure; and *(3)* they initiate development of the selected shade.

Metal-porcelain bond

The metal-porcelain attachment is established when the opaque layer is fired, which causes chemical bonds to form with oxides on the metal surface. Further discussion of the mechanism of metal-porcelain attachment is covered in chapter 6.

Masking metal

The opacity provided by opaque porcelains is due to insoluble oxides such as tin dioxide (SnO_2), titanium dioxide (TiO_2), zirconium dioxide (ZrO_2), cerium dioxide (CeO_2), or zircon (ZrO_2-SiO_2) (see Table 2-5). Other oxides that might be included in an opaque porcelain include rubidium oxide (Rb_2O), barium oxide (BaO), and/or zinc oxide (ZnO).[8,29,37] Such oxides have high refractive indices, so they scatter light. Between 8% and 15% of an opaque powder is composed of metallic oxides, and some particles may be less than 5 μm in size.[8]

The masking power of opaque porcelain is influenced by small differences in particle-size distribution[38] and by the amount and color of the oxidized metal casting[25] (Fig 2-5). Some casting alloys produce a discrete layer of light-colored surface oxides, which allows a thin opaque layer to effectively mask the metal surface. A casting alloy of a different composition might generate a thick, dark oxide layer[25] and require a thicker opaque covering. This phenomenon is explained in more detail in chapter 7.

The thickness of the opaque layer needed to cover the metal and the surface oxides differs among brands of porcelain and even varies for different shades within the same

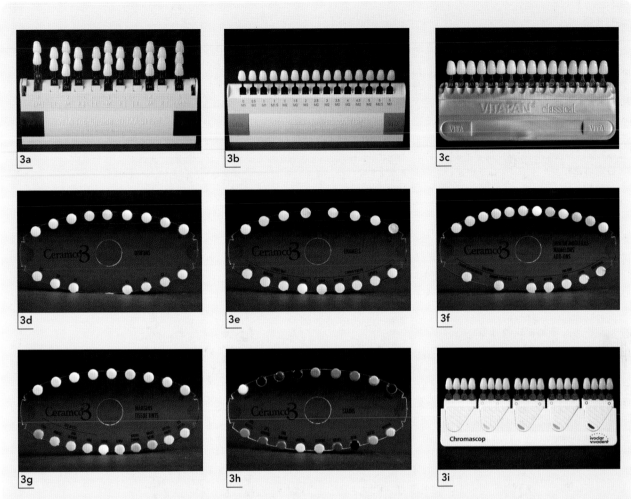

Fig 2-3 Shade guides used in metal-ceramic technology. *(a)* Vita 3D-Master. *(b)* Vita Bleachguide 3D-Master (Vident) for lightened teeth. *(c)* Vitapan Classical (Vident). *(d)* Ceramco 3 for dentin porcelains; *(e)* enamel porcelains; *(f)* dentin modifiers, mamelons, and add-on porcelains; *(g)* porcelain margins and gingival tissues; and *(h)* stains. *(i)* Chromascop (Ivoclar Vivadent).

Fig 2-4a Shade tabs usually have a characterized neck *(left)* that can be removed so the viewer focuses on the basic body shade *(right)*.

Fig 2-4b With the darker neck removed from each shade tab, it is easier to compare the body shade on a shade tab to the color of the tooth to be restored.

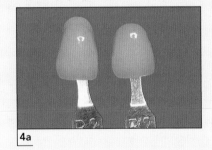

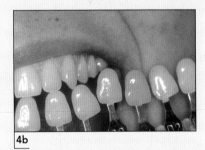

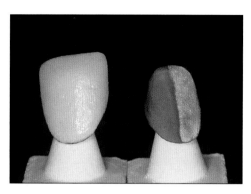

Fig 2-5a An oxidized base metal alloy casting used to evaluate the masking ability of one layer of opaque porcelain on the right half of the coping.

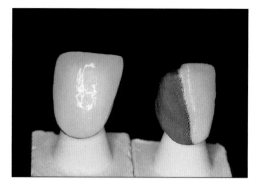

Fig 2-5b The same restoration in Fig 2-5a after firing a second opaque layer with the dentin and enamel porcelains on the test half of the coping. The opaque porcelain was able to mask the dark oxide layer.

porcelain system.[38,39] Studies suggest a minimum thickness of 0.2 mm[39] and a maximum thickness of 0.5 mm[27] due to the wide variability among opaque porcelains and the requirements of different shades. In practice, many opaque porcelains adequately block the color of the metal and initiate shade development when only 0.2 to 0.3 mm thick.[39] However, proper technique is required during the application process to obtain a uniform thickness of the opaque layer within this recommended range. When mixing the opaque powder with its special liquid, it is advisable to use a glass rod rather than a metal instrument. The coarse opaque powder can abrade the metal and possibly contaminate the mix.

Shade development

Opaque porcelains create the foundation for a body shade, and they can be altered by color modifiers and other additives to simulate natural fluorescence. Porcelain systems may include opaque porcelains with concentrated colorants identified as *opaque modifiers.* These color modifiers contain a higher percentage of metallic oxides for more saturated color. Typically, opaque modifiers are mixed with standard opaque porcelains to achieve internal shade modifications.

Body porcelains

Body porcelain is the preferred designation to collectively describe four principal types of porcelain powders used to create a restoration: dentin porcelains, enamel porcelains, translucent porcelains, and body modifiers[29] (see Table 2-6).

These powders are mixed with either distilled water or a special liquid (provided with the porcelain kit) that helps prevent the buildup from drying out rapidly.

Dentin porcelains

As explained in chapter 8, the bulk of the crown buildup for most metal-ceramic restorations is in the dentin material. Therefore, dentin porcelain is the major determinant of the shade of any porcelain restoration. In many porcelain kits, there is a separate dentin porcelain for every shade, although several shades may share the same enamel porcelain, and all shades use the same translucent powders.

The term *dentin porcelain* is generally preferred for this group of materials, although occasionally they are described as *body*, *gingival*, or *cervical* powders. Use of the terms *gingival porcelain* and *cervical porcelain* is discouraged because several porcelain systems contain separate gingival or cervical powders with a chemical composition that differs from the makeup of the principal dentin shade powders. These include the opacious dentins, or deep dentins, mentioned previously. Typically, these cervical porcelains are less translucent, more saturated with color, and intended primarily for placement in the gingival third or in interproximal areas. However, dentin porcelains are routinely incorporated into areas of a restoration other than the gingival third of a crown. In fact, many restorations require that dentin porcelains extend to the incisal third or occlusal surface to support incisal edges or individual cusps.

Because body porcelains have the same chemical and physical properties, they may be intermixed freely if custom shades are desired. They differ in final appearance due to differences in the metallic oxides each contains.

Enamel porcelains

Contemporary porcelain systems are complex, and manufacturers offer a wide assortment of enamel porcelains. Enamel porcelains are usually in the violet to gray range and impart a combination of true translucency and the illusion of translucency by virtue of their grayish or sometimes bluish hue. For example, Vident offers Vita Effect Enamel porcelains to create a range of translucent effects (eg, pink translucent, yellowish translucent, reddish translucent, red translucent, orange translucent) for the cervical, middle, and incisal portions of a restoration. Although occasionally referred to as *incisal porcelains*, enamel porcelains are not restricted to any single area of the tooth and can be extended into the gingival third of a porcelain buildup. When fired, enamel porcelains are more translucent than are dentin porcelains.[8]

Translucent porcelains

In addition to optional enamel effect porcelains, translucent materials are provided in practically all porcelain systems, although some technique manuals neglect to describe their use in a basic buildup. As appreciation has increased for the depth and natural translucency provided by a veneer of translucent porcelain, more manufacturers have begun to include these products in their kits.

Translucent porcelains are not transparent; they do not allow the transmission of *all* light. They can be applied over nearly the entire buildup surface to give depth and a natural enamel-like translucency without substantially altering the body shade.

Body modifiers

A group of related materials, referred to as *body modifiers*, are color concentrated and were designed to aid in internal color modification. Modifiers can be used full strength for vivid characterization, or they can be diluted by mixing with dentin and enamel powders for more subtle shade alterations. Remember, all body porcelains—whether they be dentin porcelains, enamel porcelains, translucent porcelains, or body modifiers—may be mixed freely for custom shading because they have the same basic chemical and physical properties.

It is important to remember the following characteristic of each body porcelain: dentin porcelains are color *predominant;* enamel and translucent porcelains are color *reduced;* and body modifiers are color *intense.*[25] All these powders are basically the same material, but they differ in their optical qualities because of the amounts and types of metallic oxide pigments they contain. A partial listing of representative color effects and their corresponding metallic oxides include the following examples[25]:

- *Yellow*—the predominant color in most teeth is derived from either indium or praseodymium (lemon), both of which are stable pigments
- *Vanadium*—zirconium or tin oxide diluted with chromium is also used but is less stable
- *Green*—developed from chromium oxide but avoided in dental porcelain because it has the characteristic color of glass
- *Pink*—derived from either chromium tin or chrome alumina and used to eliminate the greenish hue in the glass, thereby creating a warm tone to the porcelain; stable only to a temperature of 1,350°C (2,462°F) and, therefore, useful in low-fusing porcelains
- *White*—created through the use of opacifiers such as cerium dioxide, titanium dioxide, and zirconium dioxide, which is the most popular
- *Black*—produced by iron oxide
- *Gray*—derived from platinum gray or by diluting iron oxide
- *Blue*—obtained from cobalt salts and used for enamel shading

Stains and glazes

Unlike the opaque and body porcelains, stain powders contain less silica or alumina and more sodium and potassium oxides in combination with special colorant oxides[29] (see Table 2-7). The high concentrations of metallic oxides increase their fluidity at temperatures above 1,600°F.

Stains are created by mixing the metallic oxides with low-fusing glasses—not to dilute the color intensity but to ensure that their fusion point is *below* the maturation temperature of the dentin and enamel porcelains.[8] Stains also permit surface characterization and color modification for custom shade matching or harmonizing (see Figs 2-1c and 2-6).

Glazes are generally *colorless* low-fusing porcelains that possess considerable fluidity at high temperature. They fill small surface porosities and irregularities and, when fired, help to re-create the external sheen or glossy appearance of a natural tooth (see Fig 2-6c).

To the highly skilled ceramist, color development begins with the opaque layer, is enhanced by the body porcelains, and is then highlighted by a natural glaze or overglaze. Surface stains and glazes do not provide the finite optical qualities of a matured dental porcelain's natural glaze; they are surface characterizations and, as such, refract light differently than internal color modifiers veneered by dentin or enamel porcelain. As an example, incisal translucency looks far more natural when achieved with enamel or translucent

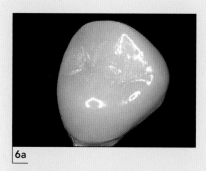
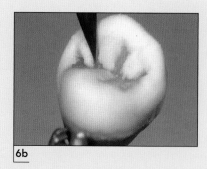
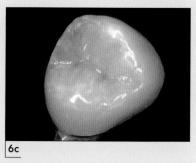

Fig 2-6a The occlusal morphology of this porcelain restoration lacks definition and appears ill defined.

Fig 2-6b The occlusal morphology is redefined in the subsequent buildup and then fired. Note how a pointed brush can be used to create the desired form.

Fig 2-6c An occlusal view of the same restoration after characterization with surface stains covered by an applied glaze.

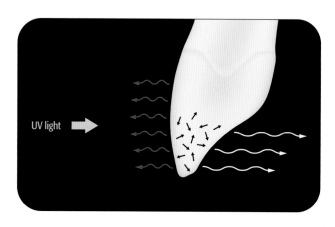

Fig 2-7 Fluorescence occurs in a dark environment when the shorter wavelengths of UV light are reflected toward the viewer as blue or bluish white light.

porcelain than with a layer of fired blue surface stain. Despite these limitations, stains are often invaluable because they enable immediate color corrections to compensate for minor shade discrepancies (see Fig 2-1c).

Optical qualities

Fluorescence

The term *fluorescence* refers to the process by which an object absorbs light at one wavelength and reflects it at another wavelength.[27] For example, teeth absorb light in the 300 to 400 nm ultraviolet (UV) range and reflect that light back toward its source at a higher wavelength, 400 to 450 nm. In the visible light spectrum, the color blue lies in the 450 to 500 nm range.[10] Thus, fluorescence is the phenomenon that occurs in UV light, whereby a viewer with no limitations to color perception sees the reflected UV light as blue or bluish white (Fig 2-7). Put another way, fluorescence

occurs when UV light is absorbed[8] and reflected back to the viewer as blue or bluish-white light.[36] Dentin exhibits more fluorescence than does enamel.[36]

Not all porcelains fluoresce, and not all fluorescent porcelains are equivalent. In fact, in a dark or dimly lit setting illuminated with fluorescent lighting, some metal-ceramic restorations may appear dark compared to adjacent natural teeth. For this reason, modest quantities of rare earth oxides, such as cerium oxide, europium, terbium, and ytterbium, are added to porcelain to mimic the natural fluorescence of human enamel.[4,8,40] This composition adjustment also reduces the potential for metamerism to occur.[33]

Metamerism

The change in appearance of an object under varying light sources is known as *metamerism*.[5] When two objects match in color under one light but differ in color under another light, they may be referred to as a *metameric pair*.[27] For example, when examined in daylight, a metal-ceramic

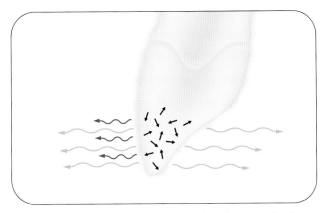

Fig 2-8 Opalescence is observed in daylight when shorter wavelengths are reflected to the viewer as blue or bluish white light. Longer wavelengths appear as an orange or orange-yellow color as some wavelengths pass through the enamel and others are reflected back to the observer.

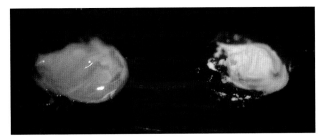

Fig 2-9 Red and blue color tags are readily available to customize each dentin and enamel mix. Note how the addition of a red color tag *(left)* intensifies the dentin porcelain mix. When making customized porcelain build-ups, color tags allow the technician to readily identify where specific body, modifier, and effect porcelains are placed relative to one another. Without color differentiation, it is difficult to track the placement of multiple shades of porcelain and internal color development until *after* a restoration has been fired.

crown may match or blend well with the adjacent natural teeth. Should the light source change from daylight to fluorescent lighting or even to UV lighting, the artificial crown may reflect light differently and no longer match the color of the surrounding natural teeth.

Opalescence

While a dark environment and UV light are needed for fluorescence to be detected, the opposite is true for opalescence. In fact, for opalescence to be observed, there must be sufficient daylight for light waves to be refracted in two ways. Lower energy light is reflected back toward the viewer as blue or blue-white wavelengths. At the same time, higher energy light waves pass through translucent material and appear to the observer as orange-yellow[33] or orange-amber[36] (Fig 2-8).

These opal effects have to do with the light-scattering abilities of translucent porcelain, so opalescent formulations are typically found in the enamel and translucent powders of major porcelain brands.[12] Opal porcelains are available to reproduce the natural opalescence of teeth. In a test of several brands, the flexural strength and modulus of opal porcelains and opal body porcelains were compared to their regular body porcelain counterparts.[41] No statistically significant differences were found between layered opal body porcelains and regular body porcelains for the two brands evaluated.[41] In contrast, the dentin in human teeth typically demonstrates greater fluorescence than the enamel. However, both enamel

> Enamel and translucent areas of teeth are more likely to demonstrate greater opalescence than dentin tooth structure.[36]

and the translucent areas of teeth are more likely to demonstrate greater opalescence than will dentin tooth structure.[36]

Readers who would like more in-depth information about opal porcelains should read Yamamoto's 1989 article on this subject.[42]

Color coding dental porcelain powders

Several porcelain systems rely on organic dyes to color code the porcelain powders.[25] By convention, dentin powders are pink and enamel powders are blue. The organic colorants burn off on heating, so the porcelain literally turns white in color before the firing cycle is finished. These dyes do not affect the shade of the fired restoration in any way.

Some brands of dental porcelain are not color coded for identification, and all the shades of dentin and enamel porcelain appear white. When distilled water is added, the dentin and enamel mixes look virtually the same. With these systems, the manufacturer may include *color tags*, which are red and blue liquid colorants for custom coloring of each individual mix (Fig 2-9). Colored organic food dyes also can be used to create a wide range of color effects when special shade modifications are involved. These liquids are color intense, and only small amounts are needed to create the desired effects.

Some technicians prefer to use multiple color tags to highlight modifiers and areas of custom shading and characterization during the buildup process. Through custom

---

color tagging, mixtures of shade A2 and A3.5 porcelains on the same glass mixing slab can be transformed into two distinct intensities of pink (see Fig 2-9). Without such differentiation, the two porcelain mixtures would have the same color, and identification of the different shades would be based on their position on the mixing slab or on marking the shade or modifier numbers directly on the mixing slab.

Once the porcelain mix is color coded, the technician establishes the proper consistency by adding additional distilled water or a special modeling liquid. Special liquids are useful because they do not dry out as rapidly as distilled water. This is particularly helpful during the buildup of multiple single units or for fixed partial dentures. Tap water should never be used with dental porcelain because it contains impurities that could contaminate the dental porcelain and potentially discolor the fired restoration.[25]

Starter or trial kits

Many dental manufacturers offer what are called *starter* or *trial* porcelain kits to introduce a new product and make it easier to try an alternate brand of porcelain. A typical kit contains instructions and bottles of the basic components of the larger, more complete system: opaque porcelain, opaque liquid, and the corresponding dentin and enamel porcelains.

Most major manufacturers are happy to furnish ceramists with any number of shades that they might want to purchase in order to acquaint them with the handling characteristics and esthetics of a new ceramic system.

Requirements of a porcelain for bonding to metal

At least two features make low-fusing porcelains suitable for bonding to metal: *(1)* they have a high CTE (13.5 to 15.5 ×

$10^{-6}/°C$), and *(2)* they melt below the melting range of the alloy. High-fusing, medium-fusing, and aluminous porcelains are not thermally compatible with metal-ceramic casting alloys. Therefore, these porcelains would not remain attached to the metal substructure. To achieve the required thermal compatibility, the porcelain veneers should have a CTE slightly *lower* than that of the metal-ceramic alloy to which they are attached (see chapter 7).

The temperature range over which the porcelain fuses should be well below the melting range of the alloy that serves as the substructure. Otherwise, high temperature can distort the metal and alter the fit of a restoration.

Nondiscoloring dental porcelains

A number of companies market metal-ceramic porcelains that are reportedly "nongreening"; that is, they can be fired on silver-containing alloys without risk of discoloring the ceramic veneer (Box 2-2). It is difficult to substantiate claims of resistance to discoloration without subjecting a nongreening porcelain to multiple firings on a high-silver–content alloy. Therefore, it may be advisable to conduct an in-house laboratory assessment of this claim prior to fabricating actual clinical cases.[43] Consider buying a porcelain trial kit to verify the resistance to "greening" before making any major purchase of a new porcelain system or a new silver-containing alloy. Refer to the discussion on palladium-silver alloys in chapter 3 for more information on porcelain discoloration.

Please note that following an in-house evaluation, the porcelain furnace must be purged of any residual silver contamination prior to resuming work with metal-ceramic porcelain.

Porcelain firing schedules

The number of dental porcelains suitable for fusing to metal-ceramic alloys introduced into the US market continues to grow at an extraordinary rate, and there is no indication that this trend will abate. While the basic process of sintering opaque porcelains, body porcelains, and stains is the same among most brands, the actual firing techniques (temperatures and times) vary markedly. Consequently, firing schedules for a few metal-ceramic porcelains can be consulted in appendix A. These schedules were prepared with the assistance of the porcelain manufacturers or distributors. In addition, the calibration and performance of porcelain furnaces vary widely, so the temperature settings may have to be adjusted to accommodate variance in individual units.

Converting temperatures from Fahrenheit to Celsius

The temperatures for porcelain firing schedules in appendix A are presented in both degrees Fahrenheit and degrees Celsius to accommodate US and foreign products. To make additional conversions, refer to the temperature conversion chart in appendix B or use the following formulas:

$$°C = \tfrac{5}{9}(°F - 32)$$
$$°F = \tfrac{9}{5}(°C + 32)$$
or
$$°F = 1.8(°C) + 32$$

Converting the rate of rise in firing schedules

The formulas listed above are used only for converting a given temperature in degrees Fahrenheit or Celsius to its corresponding value in degrees Celsius or Fahrenheit, respectively. However, when the rate of rise in a porcelain firing schedule is converted from one scale to another, the calculations are somewhat different. For example, when a restoration is fired from 1,200°F to 1,800°F in 6 minutes, the *rate of rise* is determined by dividing the temperature increase (600°F) by the time (6 minutes) to obtain the rate: 100°F per minute. Conversely, in degrees Celsius the temperature change would be from 649°C to 982°C. This represents a 333°C increase in temperature over the 6 minutes, or a 55.5°C per minute rate of rise. Therefore, a 100°F rate of rise is equivalent to a 55°C rate of rise. By convention, most manufacturers list the conversion as 100°F (55°C) and do not round the 55.5°C to 56°C.

The quickest way to convert the rate of rise from degrees Celsius to degrees Fahrenheit is to multiply the degrees Celsius by 1.8 and *not* add the 32. Remember, this applies *only* to calculating the rate of rise.

Summary

At this point, you should know how to classify dental porcelains and be able to describe their chemical composition. You should also know something about the components and functions of the different types of low-fusing porcelains. Finally, you should be aware that the various brands of dental porcelains differ in their handling characteristics, their ability to mask the oxide layer, and their recommended firing schedule, yet they are all derived from the same basic ingredients.

References

1. Dictionary.com Unabridged, v 1.1. Available at: http://dictionary.reference.com/browse/ceramic. Accessed 22 June 2007.
2. Van Vlack LH. Elements of Materials Science and Engineering, ed 5. Reading, MA: Addison Wesley, 1985.
3. Anusavice KJ. Phillips' Science of Dental Materials, ed 11. Philadelphia: Saunders, 2003. *Part of chapter 21 (pages 655 to 680) covers the history of dental ceramics and issues related to metal-ceramic technology.*
4. Craig RG. Restorative Dental Materials, ed 12. St Louis: Mosby, 2006.
5. van Noort R. Introduction to Dental Materials, ed 3. London: Mosby, 2008. *An overview of dental ceramics (chapter 3.4) and metal-ceramic technology (chapter 3.5).*
6. Jones DW. Development of dental ceramics. An historical perspective. Dent Clin North Am 1985;29:621–644.
7. Southan DE. The development and characteristics of dental porcelain. Aust Dent J 1970;15:103–107.
8. McLean JW. The Science and Art of Dental Ceramics. Vol I: The nature of dental ceramics and their clinical use. Chicago: Quintessence, 1979. *This classic text is comprehensive and detailed; technical sections are best read after gaining a general understanding of dental ceramics.*
9. McLean JW. The Science and Art of Dental Ceramics. Vol II: Bridge design and laboratory procedures in dental ceramics. Chicago: Quintessence, 1980. *The in-depth explanations of how to perform many laboratory procedures are invaluable.*
10. Yamamoto M. Metal-Ceramics: Principles and Methods of Makoto Yamamoto. Chicago: Quintessence, 1985. *One of the most detailed works on ceramics and metal-ceramic technology, this book describes the mechanics and rationale for various techniques.*
11. Clark EB. Requirements of the jacket crown. J Am Dent Assoc 1939;26:355–363. *Refer to chapter 1 for summary.*
12. Kelly JR, Nishimura I, Campbell SD. Ceramics in dentistry: Historical roots and current perspectives. J Prosthet Dent 1996;75:18–32.
13. Brecker SC. Porcelain bakes to gold—A new medium in prosthodontics. J Prosthet Dent 1956;6:801–810. *Refer to chapter 1 for summary.*
14. Weinstein M, Katz S, Weinstein AB [inventors]. Fused porcelain-to-metal teeth. US patent 3,052,982. Aug 1962.
15. Weinstein M, Weinstein AB [inventors]. Porcelain-covered metal-reinforced teeth. US Patent 3,052,983. Sept 1962.
16. Land CH. A new system of restoring badly decayed teeth by means of an enameled metallic coating. Independent Pract 1886;7:407–409. *Refer to chapter 1 for summary.*
17. Land CH. Metallic enamel coatings and fillings. Independent Pract 1886;7:413–414. *Refer to chapter 1 for summary.*

18. Land CH. Clinic report. First District Dental Society, State of New York. Dental Cosmos 1889;31:191–192.
Refer to chapter 1 for summary.

19. McLean JW, Hughes TH. The reinforcement of dental porcelain with ceramic oxides. Brit Dent J 1965;119(6):251–267.
Classic article on ceramic oxide (alumina) as a strengthener and the development of aluminous porcelain for the porcelain jacket crown.

20. McLean JW. A higher strength porcelain for crown and bridge work. Brit Dent J 1965;119(6):268–272.
Description of aluminous porcelain core substructure design and porcelain jacket crown construction.

21. Land CH. Porcelain dental art. Dental Cosmos 1903;45(6):437–444.
Refer to chapter 1 for summary.

22. Land CH. Porcelain dental art: No. II. Dental Cosmos 1903;45(6): 615–620.
Refer to chapter 1 for summary.

23. McLean JW. The alumina reinforced porcelain jacket crown. J Am Dent Assoc 1967;75:621–628.
The porcelain jacket crown is indicated for anterior and posterior restorations using aluminous core porcelain with 40% to 50% aluminum oxide.

24. Mackert JR Jr, Butts MB, Fairhurst CW. The effect of the leucite transformation on dental porcelain expansion. Dent Mater 1986; 2:32–36.
Close agreement found between the predicted and measured thermal expansion of the leucite-containing "Component No. 1" of the Weinstein patent.

25. Naylor WP. Non-Gold Base Dental Casting Alloys. Vol II: Porcelain-fused-to-metal alloys [ADA173766]. Brooks AFB, TX: School of Aerospace Medicine, 1986.
Refer to chapter 1 for summary.

26. Vines RF, Semmelman JO. Densification of dental porcelain. J Dent Res 1957;36(6):950–956.
Techniques described to reduce porosity and increase dental porcelain density: vacuum firing, diffusible atmosphere firing, and pressure methods.

27. O'Brien WJ. Dental Materials and Their Selection, ed 4. Chicago: Quintessence, 2008.

28. Chu SJ. Use of a synthetic low-fusing quartz glass-ceramic material for the fabrication of metal-ceramic restorations. Pract Proced Aesthet Dent 2001;13(5):375–381.
Physical and optical properties are described for low-fusing synthetic porcelains: superior surface smoothness, reduced shrinkage, stable CTE, low wear resistance, and opalescence.

29. Lacy AM. The chemical nature of dental porcelain. Dent Clin North Am 1977;21:661–667.
A concise and easy-to-read overview of dental porcelains of the time.

30. Muia PJ. The Four Dimensional Tooth Color System. Chicago: Quintessence, 1982.
Includes a discussion on fluorescence and the basic components of dental porcelain.

31. McLaren EA. Utilization of advanced metal-ceramic technology: Clinical and laboratory procedures for a lower-fusing porcelain. Pract Perodontics Aesthet Dent 1998;10:835–842, 884.

Discusses the fabrication of metal-ceramic restorations, high CTE of leucite compared with feldspar, benefit of high–gold content metal-ceramic alloy substructures, and ultra-low fusing porcelains.

32. Denry IL. Recent advances in ceramics for dentistry. Crit Rev Oral Biol Med 1996;7:134–143.

33. Leinfelder KF. Porcelain esthetics for the 21st century. J Am Dent Assoc 2000;131:47S–51S.
Includes discussions of all-ceramic systems, low-fusing porcelains, leucite, fluorescence and opalescence, metal-ceramic restorations, and luting agents.

34. McLean JW. Evolution of dental ceramics in the twentieth century. J Prosthet Dent 2001;85:61–66.

35. Chu S, Ahmad I. A historical perspective of synthetic ceramic and traditional feldspathic porcelain. Pract Proced Aesthet Dent 2005;17:593–598, 600.
The evolution of dental porcelain is followed by a comparison of feldspathic and synthetic ceramics with mention of fluorescence and the role of leucite.

36. Zena R. Evolution of dental ceramics. Compend Contin Educ Dent 2001;22(suppl 12):12–14, quiz 19.
HeraCeram reportedly does not undergo secondary crystallization with repeated firings that can increase its CTE and lead to cracking or bond failures.

37. Binns DB. The chemical and physical properties of dental porcelain. In: McLean JW (ed). Dental Ceramics: Proceedings of the First International Symposium on Ceramics. Chicago: Quintessence, 1983:41–82.
Provides a comparison of feldspathic and synthetic ceramics with mention of fluorescence and the role of leucite.

38. Woolsey GD, Johnson WM, O'Brien WJ. Masking power of dental opaque porcelains. J Dent Res 1984;63:936–939.
Particle size might have a greater effect on the masking ability of opaque porcelain rather than the amount of tin oxide or titantium oxide.

39. Barghi N, Lorenzana RE. Optimum thickness of opaque and body porcelain. J Prosthet Dent 1982;48:429–431.
The necessary thicknesses of opaque (0.3 mm) and body porcelains (0.5 to 1.0 mm) varies among six different shades from two different brands.

40. Raptis NV, Michalakis KX, Hirayama H. Optical behavior of current ceramic systems. Int J Periodontics Restorative Dent 2006;26:31–41.
Five prosthodontists conclude that maxillary anterior all-ceramic crowns have better light transmission than the metal-ceramic restorations.

41. Hart DA, Powers JM. Flexural strength and modulus of opalescent porcelains [abstract 271]. J Dent Res 1994;73:135.
Opalescent/body porcelain is compared with opal porcelains.

42. Yamamoto M. A newly developed "Opal" ceramic and its clinical use, with special attention to its relative refractive index. Quintessence Dent Technol 1989;9–33.
Yamamoto discusses opalescence, light transmission in ceramics and natural teeth, and the opal porcelains he developped.

43. Naylor WP. A practical laboratory test for detecting porcelain discoloration in silver-containing metal ceramic alloys. Quintessence Dent Technol 1990/1991;13:83–90.

CHAPTER 3

Casting Alloys for Bonding to Dental Porcelain

Literally hundreds of dental casting alloys are available for fabricating metal-ceramic crowns and fixed partial dentures. All of these alloys reportedly bond to dental porcelain, yet they can differ widely in physical and mechanical properties, cost, and appearance.

Individuals who work with various types of casting alloys should have a broad understanding of their chemical compositions, general properties, and handling characteristics, as well as their reported advantages and disadvantages. This information is helpful in appreciating the capabilities and limitations of a particular alloy and how it might differ from similar products on the market.

This chapter begins with definitions of important terms and proceeds to an overview of the different ways to categorize alloys, including the American Dental Association (ADA) classification system. Descriptions of numerous recognized types of metal-ceramic alloys are presented as are the functions of constituent metals. Lastly, the subject of the biocompatibility of casting alloys is discussed, especially as it relates to base metal alloys containing nickel and beryllium.

> All noble metals are precious,
> but not all precious metals are noble.

Chemistry of Metal-Ceramic Alloys

Traditional Type III and IV gold-based crown-and-bridge alloys cannot be used for the substructure of a metal-ceramic restoration for the following reasons:

1. They are not thermally compatible with low-fusing porcelains because their coefficients of thermal expansion (CTEs) differ too much to permit the bonding of porcelain to metal.

2. They have a lower melting range than dental porcelains. Consequently, these alloys would begin to melt before the dental porcelain reached its proper maturation temperature.

3. They are not chemically compatible with porcelain; they do not form the oxides that are needed for bonding to dental porcelain.

To understand the chemistry of metal-ceramic alloys, it is important to define a few key terms.

Related terminology

The following terms are used frequently in reference to metal-ceramic alloys, so it is important to know their definitions to ensure that they are used appropriately.

- **Noble** This term is applied to metals that are corrosion- and oxidation-resistant because of an inherent chemical inertness.[1] The seven noble metals used in dentistry are gold and the six members of the platinum group: platinum, palladium, iridium, osmium, rhodium, and ruthenium. Some authors include silver among the noble metals except when it is used in dentistry—silver has a tendency to oxidize in the oral cavity.[2,3,4] Apparently, there are variations of nobility, leaving the term *noble* somewhat difficult to define.
- **Non-noble** If noble metals do not oxidize, then non-noble metals would be expected to form oxides. *Non-noble metal* is considered an acceptable alternative to the preferred term *base metal*.
- **Precious** This term is applied to metals that, by virtue of their scarcity, possess a relatively high intrinsic commercial value based on supply and demand. Several examples likely to be found in dental casting alloys include gold, silver, the six members of the platinum group (listed previously), beryllium, gallium, and indium, to name only a few. Although all noble metals are precious, not all precious metals are noble.
- **Semiprecious** (*obsolete*) Though it is one of the most frequently used terms, *semiprecious* is a misleading characterization. The prefix *semi-* implies that half of the alloy is precious and the other half is not precious. Also, there is no accepted definition related to alloy composition, making the description valueless. Therefore, the use of this term is discouraged.[3,4]
- **Nonprecious** This designation refers to metals that are not scarce and do not possess a high intrinsic value. Clinicians and dental laboratory technicians often use *nonprecious alloy* to describe metals that oxidize readily and have no commerical value. The technically preferred term is *base metal*.[4]
- **Base metal** This is the preferred designation for metals and alloys that undergo oxidation and have little or no intrinsic value. Examples of base metal–ceramic alloys used in dentistry are those that contain nickel, chromium, cobalt, and aluminum. They are also known as *non-noble alloys*.

What is a metal-ceramic alloy?

At least six principal features distinguish an alloy for bonding with porcelain from both crown-and-bridge and removable partial denture alloys. A metal-ceramic alloy:

1. Must be able to produce surface oxides for chemical bonding with dental porcelains (Fig 3-1). The major elements in base metal alloys, for example, are non-noble, which means they possess a natural tendency to oxidize when subjected to the elevated temperatures of a porcelain furnace. Noble alloys behave in the opposite manner. In fact, because noble elements (eg, gold and the platinum group) do not oxidize, trace amounts of base metals must be added for oxidation to take place (see chapter 6 on porcelain bonding).
2. Should be formulated so that its CTE is *slightly* greater than that of the porcelain veneer. On cooling, the ceramic veneer is placed under compression to maintain the metal-porcelain attachment. Even though oxides form and the metal chemically bonds to the porcelain, the ceramic veneer may fracture if the metal and porcelain are thermally incompatible (Fig 3-2). Thermal compatibility must be maintained during the heating and cooling processes and requires strict adherence to the porcelain manufacturers' firing instructions using a calibrated porcelain furnace.

> Several methods for classifying alloys exist, but the classification system revised by the ADA in 1984 remains a universally accepted standard.

3. Must have a melting range that is considerably higher than the fusing range of the dental porcelain that veneers it. This temperature separation is necessary so the porcelain buildup can be sintered to a temperature high enough to ensure a proper level of maturity and subsequently glazed without the risk of distorting or melting the metal substructure or altering the porcelain-metal compatibility.
4. Must not undergo distortion as a result of repeated firing at the maximum temperatures of the porcelain. The ability to withstand repeated exposure to high temperatures without dimensional change is often referred to as *high temperature strength* or *sag resistance*.[2]
5. Must fulfill the first four requirements and satisfy the technician's need for ease of handling. Processing should not be too technically demanding. Any alloy that is difficult to melt, cast, finish, and polish could lose favor despite its excellent bond strength, dimensional stability, and thermal properties.
6. Should be biocompatible. The safety of the technician, the clinician, and the patient must not be put at risk as a result of using a casting alloy containing elements linked to unfavorable human responses, particularly if satisfactory alternative alloys are available. Biocompatibility is discussed in more detail later in this chapter.

Fig 3-1 A casting must be metal finished *(left)*, air-particle abraded *(middle)*, and oxidized *(right)* to form the surface oxides for chemical bonding to dental porcelain.

Fig 3-2a When an alloy and a dental porcelain are not compatible, cracks can appear in the restoration *(left)* or a portion of the ceramic may debond *(right)*.

Fig 3-2b In another example of incompatibility, the porcelain can sometimes literally pop off the metal substructure during fabrication.

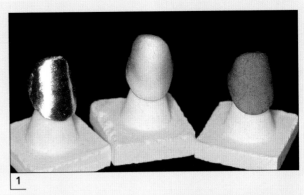

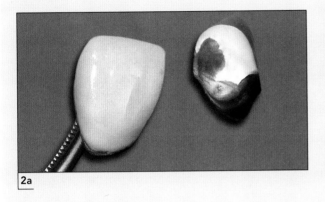

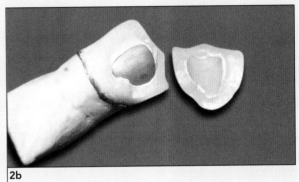

Classification of Dental Casting Alloys

Several methods for classifying alloys exist, but the classification system revised by the ADA in 1984 remains a universally accepted standard.[3] In fact, several descriptions of alloys can be found in both the dental literature and the marketing information supplied by manufacturers. It is a challenge to keep track of all the "new and improved" alloys that enter the marketplace. Moreover, grouping similar materials for comparative purposes is made difficult if an alloy's composition is not fully disclosed by a manufacturer.

The aim of each classification method itself may vary. One system may be based on function, while another may be based on factors such as color, composition, cost, and use. Examples of frequently encountered classification systems are described in the following sections.

Classification based on function

One of the oldest and simplest methods used to categorize casting alloys was devised by the National Bureau of Standards in 1932.[2,5] The gold-based crown-and-bridge metals of that time were organized according to function into only four

categories and were described as a Type I, II, III, or IV alloy. The alloys in each classification, or type, were arranged according to their gold and platinum group composition as well as by their associated Vickers hardness number (VHN).[2] Evidently, many of these early formulations suffered one major limitation: they tarnished in the oral cavity. Once it was learned that castings with a gold content below 65% to 75% tarnished, the classification system for crown-and-bridge alloys was modified in 1948 to include specific composition guidelines within the four types. However, it was not until 1960 that a fifth category was established for metal-ceramic alloys.

With the development and introduction of silver-, palladium-, nickel-, cobalt-, and iron-based alloys, comparisons using hardness were no longer valid. Alloys that have similar VHNs but which are based on different metals do not necessarily possess comparable strength characteristics nor function similarly. Metal-ceramic alloys, in particular, do not lend themselves to categorization as Type I, II, III, or IV because they vary in function, composition, and hardness.

Classification based on color or composition

A second method of classification describes alloys according to their color and principal element or elements.[2] The

Table 3-1	1984 ADA classification for dental alloys[3]

Classification	Content (%) requirement*
High-noble	Noble metal ≥ 60 and gold ≥ 40
Noble	Noble metal ≥ 25[†]
Predominantly base	Noble metal < 25

*Noble metals include gold, platinum, palladium.
[†]There is no upper limit to accommodate high noble–metal content alloys with less than 40% gold.

number of subcategories in this system varies in different sources from four to eleven.

- *Yellow golds*—yellow in color, with greater than 60% gold content
- *White golds*—white in color, with greater than 50% gold content
- *Low golds*—usually yellow in color, with less than 60% gold content (usually 42% to 55%)
- *High-palladium*—white in color, predominantly palladium; may contain small quantities of gold (2%) and limited amounts of either copper or cobalt
- *Silver-palladium*—white in color, predominantly silver (55% to 71%) with substantial amounts of palladium (25% to 27%) to provide added nobility and to help control tarnish; may contain small amounts of copper or gold
- *Palladium-silver*—white in color, predominantly palladium with a substantial quantity of silver (up to 40%)

One obvious limitation of this classification method is the inability to differentiate between the metal-ceramic alloys and the traditional Type I, II, III, and IV crown-and-bridge metals. For example, some published reports have inadvertently criticized the palladium-silver alloys based on research using crown-and-bridge silver-palladium alloys.[4,6,7] This distinction is significant because the palladium-silver alloys are formulated to bond to dental porcelain, whereas the silver-palladium alloys are alternatives to Type III and IV gold alloys.

ADA classification system

In 1984, the ADA Council on Dental Materials, Instruments and Equipment published a revised classification system for cast alloys based on noble metal content (Table 3-1).[3] This system does not distinguish metal-ceramic from crown-and-bridge alloys and was devised solely for identification in dental procedure codes, where the intrinsic value of the metals in castings provided to patients would influence the amount of reimbursement from insurance carriers.

Obviously, such a classification was not intended to indicate usage or suggest performance levels. Therefore, the ADA system does not group, order, or otherwise arrange the multitude of alloys that have flooded the dental market. Nor does it attempt to identify subcategories in each of the major divisions based on appearance, chemical makeup, physical properties, or other distinguishing features. Alloys are placed into one of only three categories; thus a major limitation of the ADA classification, from a technical perspective, is that alloys of varied composition and performance may fall within the same general category. That outcome alone complicates communication about the makeup and characteristics of an alloy between technician and alloy manufacturer, technician and technician, or even technician and dentist. As a result another classification method is needed to organize and to distinguish the wide array of dental casting alloys.

An alternative classification system

To address the technical limitations of the ADA classification, an alternative system for classifying ceramic alloys was first devised in 1986[4] and revised in 1992[8] (Fig 3-3). In this system, alloys are separated into two major types (ie, noble and base metal), arranged by system, and subdivided into constituent groups, if required. As a result, alloys are classified based on their composition and the levels of content of their major constituents.

Composition

The name of the major component in an alloy is listed first, followed by the next most abundant component. Key trace or minor alloying elements that distinguish the performance or the properties of alloys in the same system (eg, beryllium, copper, cobalt, silver, and gold) are used to identify subcategories as groups.

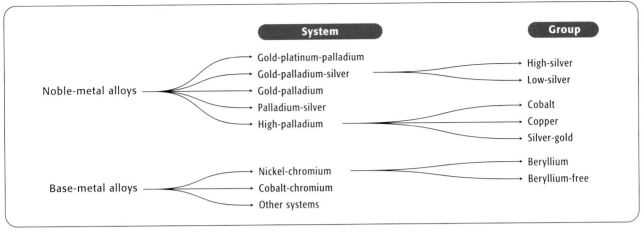

Fig 3-3 Composition-based classification system for metal-ceramic alloys.

Levels of content

Gold-based alloys containing less than 70% gold are often referred to as "low-gold alloys," despite the fact that the total gold content may actually account for the majority of the alloy's composition (greater than 50%). Obviously, the designation *low* is confusing when alloys with 10% and 69% of the same element are grouped together, although they may differ markedly in actual composition and handling characteristics. To avoid potential misinterpretations, the designations *low, medium, and high* are given the following values in this classification system to describe the level of the principal constituent on which an alloy is based.[4]

- Low—0% to 33%
- Medium—34% to 66%
- High—67% to 100%

This simple division of the total composition percentage of an alloy into thirds permits categorization in a more recognizable and understandable format. Employing three equal groups encourages the use of more meaningful terminology and discourages the use of vague identifiers such as "palladium-rich" in a palladium-based alloy or references to the "gold level" in a gold-based metal. An exception comes in describing and comparing the level of secondary or tertiary elements in alloys with a similar general composition. The gold-palladium-silver system is a good example because it contains products with varying amounts of silver. Metals in this category are based on gold and have a gold content in the medium range (39% to 55%). Yet because silver is such an important constituent, it is helpful to recognize its two subgroups, *high-silver* or *low-silver*.

> A classification based on systems and groups not only provides adequate criteria to categorize all available alloys, it also facilitates communication between the dental laboratory technician and the prescribing clinician.[4]

Contemporary classification

New metal-ceramic alloys of varied composition continue to be introduced to the market. A classification based on systems and groups not only provides adequate criteria to categorize alloys, it also facilitates communication between the dental laboratory technician and the prescribing clinician.[4] In contrast, the ADA classification remains essential for differentiating base metals from high-noble and noble casting alloys as well as for enabling clinicians to file for appropriate reimbursement from dental insurance companies (see Table 3-1). Beyond these, some other classification system is needed.

Unfortunately, both the ADA classification and the composition-based classification fail to distinguish between *white* (actually gray in color) and *yellow* gold-based alloys. This limitation can be addressed by a modified ADA classification system using a color identifier (ie, white or yellow) as a distinguishing feature within each of the three main categories (Table 3-2). It is important to note that clinicians and dental laboratories using high-noble yellow alloys are purchasing products with gold content equal to or greater than 90%. Alloys with extremely high gold levels differ in cost from yellow and white high-noble and noble alloys.

Likewise, the composition-based classification for ceramic alloys has been modified to reflect contemporary usage (Fig 3-4). This more contemporary classification system not only recognizes the categories used in the ADA classification, but also uses composition and color (ie, yellow versus white) to distinguish metal-ceramic alloys. Alloy color is easy to identify by the physical appearance of the ingots. Manufacturers often include alloy color in their

Table 3-2	Modified ADA classification for dental alloys	
Classification	**Color**	**Content (%) requirement***
High-noble	Yellow	Noble metal > 90 and gold > 90
	White	Noble metal > 60 and gold > 40
Noble	White	Noble metal ≥ 25†
	Yellow‡	Noble metal ≥ 25†
Predominantly base	White	Noble metal < 25
	Yellow‡	Noble metal < 25

*Noble metals include gold, platinum, palladium.
†There is no upper limit to the high-noble content in alloys with less than 40% gold.
‡Certain yellow-colored noble crown-and-bridge (nonceramic) alloys are included in the noble and predominantly base metal categories.

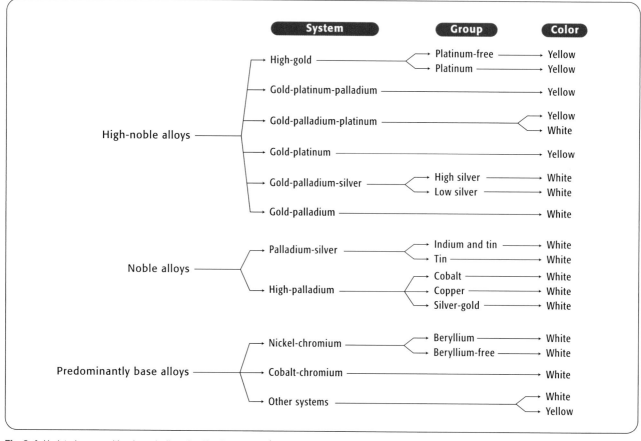

Fig 3-4 Updated composition-based alloy classification system.[4] Please note that there are yellow-colored base metal crown-and-bridge alloys that are accepted by the ADA, such as copper-based NPG and NPG+2 (Aalba Dent).

product brochures, even though past dental classifications for metal-ceramic alloys have typically failed to capture this distinction.

The addition of the separate high-gold system in this contemporary composition-based classification is driven by the reemergence of a category best described as having a very high-gold content (greater than 90% gold) and a bright or rich yellow hue. High-gold–content metal-ceramic alloys have been available for decades, yet this particular category has attracted renewed interest by virtue of its biocompatibility and esthetic qualities. Manufacturers promote the very high noble–metal content and warm appearance (yellow hue) of substructures cast from these high-gold–content metal-ceramic alloys (Table 3-3).

Table 3-3 Percentage composition of representative metal-ceramic alloys*

High-Noble Alloys

High-gold	Au	Pd	Pt	Ag	Sn	In		Other	Color
Aztec (Jensen)	99.9	–	–	–	–	+		–	Yellow
UltraCrown PG (Dentsply)	99.8	–	–	+	+	+		Mn	Yellow
Goldtech Bio 2000 (Argen)	99.7	–	–	–	–	0.2		Zn	Yellow
Bio-98+ (Talladium)	98.42	–	1.0	–	–	–		–	Yellow
Argedent 98 (Argen)	97.7	–	1.99	–	–	+		Ir, Zn	Yellow
Brite Gold (Ivoclar Vivadent)	96.3	–	2.6	–	< 1	< 1		Cu, Ir	Yellow
Gold-platinum-palladium	**Au**	**Pd**	**Pt**	**Ag**	**Sn**	**In**		**Other**	**Color**
JP-II (Jensen)	87	4.5	7	–	+	+		Fe, Re	Yellow
Aquarius Hard (Ivoclar Vivadent)	86.1	2.6	8.5	–	–	1.4		Fe, Li, Ru, Ta	Yellow
Degudent H (Dentsply)	84.5	5	8	–	–	2.5		Ta	Yellow
700SL (Leach & Dillon)	84	6	7	1.5	–	1		–	Yellow
Y2 (Ivoclar Vivadent)	82	4.5	8	3.5	< 1	< 1		–	Yellow
Gold-palladium-platinum	**Au**	**Pd**	**Pt**	**Ag**	**Sn**	**In**		**Other**	**Color**
Jelenko O[†] (Jelenko)	87.5	6	4.5	1	0.4	0.3		–	Yellow
Argedent 87 (Argen)	87.42	5.9	4.5	1	+	+		Ir, Fe	Yellow
SMG-3 (Dentsply)	81	11	6	–	+	–		Re	White
Sagittarius (Ivoclar Vivadent)	75	16.8	2	2	2	2		Cu, Fe	White
Overture (Jensen)	74.5	15.2	3	5	+	–		Re, Ru	White
Gold-platinum	**Au**	**Pd**	**Pt**	**Ag**	**Sn**	**In**	**Rh**	**Other**	**Color**
Classic-IV (Jensen)	88	–	9.5	< 1	–	+	–	Fe, Re	Yellow
Argedent Bio Yellow PF (Argen)	86.5	–	10.4	–	–	+	+	Ir, Mn, Ta	Yellow
Degudent G (Dentsply)	86	–	10.4	–	–	+	< 2	Ta	Yellow
Gold-palladium-silver	**Au**	**Pd**	**Pt**	**Ag**	**Sn**	**In**		**Other**	**Color**
Will-Ceram W[†] (Ivoclar Vivadent)	54	26.5	–	15.5	< 5	< 5		–	White
Argedent 52 (Argen)	52.5	26.9	–	16	2	2.5		Ru	White
Cameo[†] (Jelenko)	52.5	27	–	16	2	2.5		–	White
W-5 (Ivoclar Vivadent)	52.2	26	< 1	17.1	2.7	< 1		Ir, Re	White
Ceramco White (Dentsply)	50.3	30.2	–	14.4	+	+		Ru	White
JPW (Jensen)	49	31.5	–	15	+	–		Re	White
Special White (Dentsply)	45	40	–	6.5	3	4		Ga, Ru	White

Gold-palladium	Au	Pd	Pt	Ag	Sn	In	Co	Cu	Ga	Other	Color
Olympia[†] (Jelenko)	51.5	38.4	–	–	–	8.5	–	–	1.5	–	White
Eclipse (Dentsply)	52	37.5	–	–	+	+	–	–	–	Re, Zn	White
Argedent 52 SF (Argen)	51.5	38.4	–	–	–	8.5	–	–	1.4	Ir	White
Deva 4 (Dentsply)	51.1	38.5	–	–	–	9	–	–	< 2	–	White
JP-1 (Jensen)	51.5	38.5	–	–	+	–	–	–	+	Ru	White
Lodestar (Ivoclar Vivadent)	51.5	38.5	–	–	< 1	8.5	–	–	1.5	Re, Ru	White
Will-Ceram W-3[†] (Ivoclar Vivadent)	48.5	39.5	–	–	< 1	10.6	–	–	< 1	–	White

*Exact alloy formulations are considered proprietary information and are not always available for publication. Many of these alloys also contain trace amounts of other base metals that serve as grain refiners (eg, ruthenium), oxide scavengers (eg, boron, silicon), and strengtheners (eg, iron), to mention just a few.
[†]Rated *acceptable* by the ADA Acceptance Program.
+ Elements present in unspecified amounts.
– Elements not identified as being present.

(table continued)

Table 3-3 (cont)

Noble Metal Alloys

Palladium-silver	Au	Pd	Pt	Ag	Sn	In	Co	Cu	Ga	Zn	Other	Color
Superior (Jensen)	–	62.5	–	24.5	+	+	–	–	–	+	Re, Ru	White
Argelite 61 (Argen)	–	60.55	–	28.1	2.5	6.6	–	–	2.1	–	Ru	White
Jelstar† (Jelenko)	–	60	–	28	6	6	–	–	–	–	–	White
Lunar (Dentsply)	–	60	–	29.5	+	+	–	–	+	+	Ir	White
Palladius-Ag (Vident)	–	60	–	27	7	5	–	–	–	1	–	White
Pors On (Dentsply)	–	58	–	30	6	4	–	–	–	–	–	White
Pors On Lite (Dentsply)	–	61.4	–	26	+	+	–	–	–	+	Ru	White
Applause (Dentsply)	–	54.5	–	35	+	–	–	–	–	+	Ir	White
Will-Ceram W1† (Ivoclar Vivadent)	–	53.5	–	37.7	8.5	<1	–	–	–	–	Ru	White
JP-5 (Jensen)	–	53.5	–	37.5	+	–	–	–	–	+	Ru, Re	White
Degustar GA-2 (Dentsply)	2	52	–	36	+	+	–	–	–	+	Ru	White

High palladium

High palladium–copper	Au	Pd	Pt	Ag	Sn	In	Co	Cu	Ga	Other	Color
Palladium V (Vident)	–	79	–	–	–	–	–	9.5	9	Ge (0.5)	White
Spartan Plus (Ivoclar Vivadent)	2	78.8	–	–	–	–	–	10	9	Ir	White
Option (Dentsply)	2	78.8	–	–	–	–	–	10	+	B, Ir	White
Stability (Jensen)	2	77	–	–	–	+	–	+	+	Ru, Zn	White

High palladium–silver-gold	Au	Pd	Pt	Ag	Sn	In	Co	Cu	Ga	Other	Color
IPS d.SIGN 84 (Ivoclar Vivadent)	9	75.2	–	3	–	6.5	–	–	6	Li, Re, Ru	White
Integrity (Jensen)	6	75	–	7	–	+	–	–	+	Ru, Re	White
Argelite 75+6 (Argen)	6	75	–	6.5	–	6.0	–	–	6.0	Ru	White
Protocol (Ivoclar Vivadent)	6	75.2	–	6.5	<1.0	6.0	–	–	6.0	Ru	White
300SL (Leach & Dillon)	6	75	–	6.6	–	~6.4	–	–	6.0	–	White
Ovation (Dentsply)	3	69.8	–	9.7	+	+	–	–	+	Ru, Zn	White

Predominantly Base Metal Alloys

Nickel-chromium

Nickel-chromium-beryllium	Ni	Co	Cr	Be	Al	Mo	Ti	Ru	V	Other	Color
Tech Star (Leach & Dillon)	78	–	13	1.8	–	5	–	–	–	–	White
Argeloy NP (Argen)	76	–	14	1.9	2.0	6.0	–	–	–	+	White
Rexillium III† (Jeneric/Pentron)	76	0.25	13.5	1.8	2.5	5.25	0.25	–	–	–	White

Nickel-chromium beryllium-free	Ni	Co	Cr	Be	Al	Mo	Nb	W	Fe	Cb	Other	Color
Argeloy NP (Be-Free) (Argen)	54	–	22	–	–	9.0	4.0	–	4.0	–	Ta (4.0)	White
Pisces Plus (Ivoclar Vivadent)	61.5	–	22	–	2.3	–	–	11.2	–	–	Si (2.6)	White
Duceranium U (Dentsply)	59	+	21.5	–	–	4.5	–	–	+	–	C, Mn, Si	White

Cobalt-chromium	Ni	Co	Cr	Be	Al	Mo	Si	Ru	W	Other	Color
IPS d.SIGN 30 (Ivoclar Vivadent)	–	60.2	30.1	–	<1	0.6	0.9	–	–	B, Fe, GA (3.9), Nb (3.2)	White
Argeloy NP Special (Argen)	–	59.5	31.5	–	–	5.0	2.0	–	–	~2, Mn (1.0)	White

Cobalt-palladium	Pd	Co	Cr	Be	Al	Mo	Si	Ru	Ga	W	B	Li	Color
Callisto CP (Ivoclar Vivadent)	28.2	56.0	10.0	–	<1.0	–	<1.0	–	2.0	3.0	<1.0	<1.0	White

†Rated *acceptable* by the ADA Acceptance Program.
+ Elements present in unspecified amounts; – Elements not identified as being present.

Evolving alloy formulations and classification conflicts

If commodity prices of precious metals increase significantly or remain above historical averages for protracted periods of time, new categories of alloys likely will be introduced. It is easy to label new alloys using either the ADA or the modified ADA classification systems, but changes to the composition-based classification systems will also be needed, particularly if new formulations offer greater economy with comparable physical properties, handling characteristics, and biocompatibility. Obviously, sustained growth and longevity will determine if new products necessitate refinements to any classification system.

It is probable that a product would be classified differently in various classification systems. One example is the alloy Callisto CP (Ivoclar Vivadent). Although the major constituent is cobalt (56%), the alloy contains 28.2% of a noble metal, palladium, and 10% chromium. Therefore, Calisto CP can be classified as a noble alloy under the ADA and modified ADA classification system. However, under composition-based classifications, the alloy falls in the base metal or predominantly base metal (white) alloy category under a new cobalt-based system (ie, cobalt-palladium).

Challenges in classifying alloys such as Callisto CP highlight the major differences between the different classification methods. The simplicity of the ADA classification allows it to categorize diverse products using noble element content as the principal factor. Composition-based classifications examine the entire alloy content and rely on the major constituents to determine how to differentiate a product from others on the market.

New formulations that may be introduced certainly merit our attention. Their biocompatibility, physical properties, and handling characteristics (eg, castability, metal finishing, bond to porcelain, polishability, and preceramic and postceramic soldering) should be assessed along with their potential costs. The Callisto CP alloy, for example, blurs the lines among physical properties for different alloy systems. It has a white color and low density (9.0 g/cm³) like that of a base metal alloy, but its other properties are similar to high-noble and noble metal-ceramic alloys. This product is included in Tables 3-3 and 3-4 to facilitate comparison of its composition and physical properties with those of other alloys.

Scientific reports on biocompatibility and data on clinical performance and long-term success will determine the place of new entries in the metal-ceramic alloy market.

Descriptions of Metal-Ceramic Alloys

A brief description of the alloy systems and groups is provided as an overview of the numerous categories in which alloys can be placed.[4,8,9] The reader is advised that these characterizations contain generalizations that are common to many, but not all, members of each category. New formulations and minor variations of existing alloys make it difficult to keep up with many of the changes that occur in this field. Yet most of the broader features, advantages, and disadvantages of each category are likely to hold true for new products and make it possible for them to be placed in a given system or group.

The desired physical, mechanical, and thermal properties of an alloy are affected by more than the type of metals it contains. For example, physical properties can be influenced by the level of purity of the ingredients and by manufacturing procedures, as well as by the sequence in which the different elements are added during the melt to create that alloy. Thus, it is difficult to compare the performance of metal-ceramic alloys with only slight variations in minor alloying elements, even though their composition might appear quite similar.

To be classified as *high-noble or noble,* an alloy should contain a substantial quantity of platinum-group elements and/or gold. If these elements are absent or if they are present in only small quantities, then the alloy's major constituents presumably are base elements, and it is classified as a *base metal* or *predominately base metal.* Trace amounts of a platinum-group element (eg, ruthenium in cobalt-chromium alloys) do not warrant labeling the entire alloy as noble if the major component clearly is a base metal (eg, cobalt). Table 3-3 lists representative alloys from the different categories with their composition (see appendix C for percentage compositions of historical metal-ceramic alloys).

Use of alloy color for classification

The inclusion of an alloy's color in the modified ADA classification permits the differentiation of high-noble yellow and high-noble white ceramic alloys (see Table 3-2). In the absence of such a distinction, both the yellow and white alloys are lumped under the broad designation *high-noble.* Yet the composition of alloys in this category, along with their physical appearance and processing requirements, can differ significantly and potentially have important clinical implications. In general, the high-noble yellow alloys can contain as much as 99.9% gold. They produce a light oxide layer and provide a warm yellow hue to the underlying metal

Table 3-4 Physical properties of representative metal-ceramic alloys

Product	Density (g/cm³)	Hardness (VHN)	Elongation (%-hard)	Yield strength*	Melting range (°C)	CTE (500°C)	Presolder / Postsolder
High-Noble Alloys							
High-gold							
Aztec (Jensen)†	19.3	22	45	~3,500	1,063	15.3	CPS / 650
Bio-98+ (Talladium)	19.2	38	52	20,225	1,035–1,078	15.7	#1060 / #201
UltraCrown PG (Densply)	19.2	40	30	5,800	1,050–1,060	15.0	Bio-Pre / 650
Goldtech Bio 2000 (Argen)	19.2	35	50	2,000	1,030–1,070	15.5	Goldtech / —
Argedent 98 (Argen)	18.9	45	40	12,300	1,045–1,090	14.7 / 15.0	— / —
Brite Gold (Ivoclar Vivadent)	19.0	115	15	23,200	1,030–1,070	14.8	HGPKF 1015 Y / 650, 615, LFWG
Gold-platinum-palladium							
JP-II (Jensen)	18.5	155	17	50,700	1,085–1,200	14.2	Spirit / 615
Aquarius Hard (Ivoclar Vivadent)	18.5	230	13	66,000	1,050–1,145	14.8	HGPKF 1015 Y / 650, 615, LFWG
Degudent H (Dentsply)	18.1	220	3	87,000	1,100–1,210	14.2	YPG / Degulor 2
Gold-palladium-platinum							
Argedent 87 (Argen)	18.5	185	5	65,000	1,150–1,180	14.5 / 14.7	YSF / 650, 720
SMG-3 (Dentsply)	17.4	240	5	101,000	1,160–1,270	13.9	SMG-3, Ceramco White / 650, 615
Sagittarius (Ivoclar Vivadent)	16.4	280	10	84,100	1,130–1,255	14.0	SHFWC / 615, LFWG, 585
Overture (Jensen)	16.6	230	9	72,500	1,165–1,260	14.0	PWS / 1400
Gold-platinum							
Classic-IV (Jensen)	19	175	11	55,800	1,055–1,155	14.2	CPS / 650
Argedent Bio Yellow PF (Argen)	18.6	250	5	96,400	1,040–1,130	14.5	YSF / 720
Degudent G (Dentsply)	19	195	9	68,000	1,045–1,140	14.5	Degudent G-1 / Degulor 2
Gold-palladium-silver							
Will-Ceram W (Ivoclar Vivadent)	13.8	240	21	65,900	1,230–1,280	14.2	HFWC / 615, LFWG, 585
Argedent 52 (Argen)	14.2	225	10	85,000	1,205–1,260	14.2	W, WSF, WG / LO, 500
W-5 (Ivoclar Vivadent)	13.8	255	20	73,200	1,185–1,230	14.0	SHFWC / LFWG
Ceramco White (Dentsply)	14.5	220	10	61,600	1,260–1,285	14.4	Ceramco White, YPG / Regular White
JPW (Jensen)	13.6	260	12	80,600	1,105–1,275	14.0	Spirit / 1400
Special White (Dentsply)	14.4	260	10	89,900	1,160–1,260	14.1	YPG, WPG/ Regular White, Degulor 2
Gold-palladium							
Eclipse (Dentsply)	13.8	254	23	83,400	1,160–1,265	13.8	SMG-3 / 650, 615
Argedent 52SF (Argen)	14.5	230	20	82,000	1,275–1,300	13.9 / 14.1	WSF / LO, 500
Deva 4 (Dentsply)	14.5	234	18	79,000	1,235–1,315	13.5	Ceramco White, WPG / Regular White, Degulor 2
JP-1 (Jensen)	14	240	25	73,000	1,135–1,215	13.8	Spirit / 1400
Lodestar (Ivoclar Vivadent)	13.7	330	20	71,700	1,275–1,300	14.1	HFWC / 615, LFWG, 585 Fine
Olympia (Jelenko)	13.7	255	20	80,000	1,220–1,350	13.9	Jelenko Olympia Pre Solder / Jelenko 750 Solder
Will-Ceram W-3 (Ivoclar Vivadent)	13.8	255	17	71,700	1,235–1300	13.9	HFWC / 615, LFWG, 585

(table continued)

Table 3-4 *(cont)*

Product	Density (g/cm³)	Hardness (VHN)	Elongation (%-hard)	Yield strength*	Melting range (°C)	CTE (500°C)	Presolder / Postsolder
Noble Metal Alloys							
Palladium-silver							
Superior (Jensen)	11	220	35	69,000	1,190–1,275	14.2	PWS / 1400
Argelite 61 (Argen)	11.2	310	13	107,600	1,130–1,275	14.5 / 14.7	W, P / LO, 500
Lunar (Dentsply)	11	244	35	64,000	1,180–1,290	14.7	SMG-YW / 650, 615
Pors On Lite (Dentsply)	11.3	250	16	85,600	1,170–1,280	14.5	YPG / Degulor 2
Applause (Dentsply)	10.8	240	10	85,600	1,180–1,260	15.1	SMG-YW, White 2 Pre / 650, 615
Will-Ceram W1 (Ivoclar Vivadent)	11.1	285	11	70,240	1,185–1,270	15.2	HFWC / 615, LFWG, 585
JP-5 (Jensen)	11	250	16	74,500	1,180–1,245	14.9	PWS / 1400
Degustar GA-2 (Dentsply)	11.3	250	10	81,200	1,150–1,230	14.8	YPG / Regular White
High palladium							
High palladium–copper							
Option (Dentsply)	10.6	425	23	130,500	1,100–1,190	14.3	Degulor 2 / 615
Spartan Plus (Ivoclar Vivadent)	10.7	310	20	115,300	1,180–1,210	14.3	Spartan / SHFWC
Stability (Jensen)	10.7	300	20	103,230	1,110–1,210	13.5	Spirit / 1400
High palladium–silver-gold							
IPS d.SIGN 84 (Ivoclar Vivadent)	11.3	310	29	71,800	1,140–1,335	13.8	SHFWC / 615, LFWG, 585
Integrity (Jensen)	10.9	250	30	79,200	1,120–1,300	13.8	Spirit / 1400
Argelite 75+6 (Argen)	11.4	265	30	87,000	1,145–1,240	14.3 / 14.5	W, WSF / LO, 500
Protocol (Ivoclar Vivadent)	11	235	34	72,400	1,270–1,310	13.8	Spartan, HFWC / 615, LFWG, 585
Ovation (Dentsply)	10.7	255	16	92,000	1,155–1,285	14.0	SMG-YW / 650
Predominantly Base Metal Alloys							
Nickel-chromium							
Nickel-chromium-beryllium							
Argeloy NP (Argen)	7.8	240	12–15	80,000	1,230–1,290	14.0 / 14.4	P, NP, Flux-N-Sol / LO, R
Nickel-chromium beryllium-free							
Argeloy NP (Be-Free) (Argen)	8.6	240	6–7	52,000	1,220–1,230	14.1 / 14.4	P, NP, Flux-N-Sol / LO, R
Pisces Plus (Ivoclar Vivadent)	8.4	280	10	86,900	1,255–1,330	14.1	Super Solder / LFWG
Duceranium U (Dentsply)	8.5	200	17	48,600	1,320–1,330	14.1	SMG-YW / 650
Cobalt-chromium							
IPS d.SIGN 30 (Ivoclar Vivadent)	7.8	385	6.0	75,300	1,145–1,165	14.5	SHFWC, HFWG / LFWG
Argeloy NP Special (Argen)	8.8	280	9.0	65,000	1,240–1,350	14.3 / 14.8	P, NP, Flux-N-Sol / LO, R
Cobalt-palladium							
Callisto CP (Ivoclar Vivadent)	9.0	365	9.0	88,473 (610 MPa)	1,100–1,350	14.2	HGPKF 1030 Y / 585

*Yield strength given for psi at 0.2% offset.
†Only initial temperature given.
CTE = coefficient of thermal expansion
VHN = Vickers Hardness Number

substructure that, compared to the high-noble white alloys, is believed to pose less of a challenge for opaque masking and developing natural-looking esthetics. Moreover, visible metal with a yellow hue is more apt to harmonize with gingival tissue than is exposed white metal, which appears dark and unattractive. However, there are more high-noble white alloys than there are high-noble yellow alloys.

It is important to recognize that the high-noble yellow alloys tend to be higher in density, lower in hardness, and easier to melt and cast, but they require delicate handling in preparation of the porcelain-bearing surface. Some alloys in this category should be limited in use to single units (with complete porcelain coverage) and to short three-unit fixed partial dentures in select cases. As with all products, it is especially important to review the manufacturers' instructions prior to use to avoid potential processing errors.

Alloys in the noble category also may appear yellow or white depending on the particular systems and percentage of gold relative to other noble elements. As a rule, most fall into the noble white category, whereas a large number of noble crown-and-bridge alloys containing gold retain a yellow hue (ie, noble yellow).

The vast majority of metals based on nickel and chromium in the base metal and predominantly base metal classifications are white. However, the copper-based product NPG+2 (Aalba Dent) is an example of a predominately base metal crown-and-bridge alloy that is yellow.

High-noble metal alloys

The high-noble metal alloys, highlighted in the following three sections, contain more than 60% noble metal and at least 40% gold.

High-gold system

Alloys that fall into this category are characterized by an extremely high content of gold (90.0% to 99.9%) that gives castings a rich yellow hue (Table 3-5). Such products have gold as the principal constituent and contain a few minor alloying elements; some, but not all, include up to 2% platinum.

High-gold alloys are soft and weak, but they are also dense relative to other high-noble and noble alloys. Therefore, substructures must be designed for complete veneering by dental porcelain and require delicate handling during metal finishing. Single-unit castings are preferred over fixed partial dentures because of an inherent lack of strength.

These alloys are classified as *high-noble* (ADA) or as *high-noble yellow* (modified ADA).

Gold-platinum-palladium system

Although one of the oldest systems, gold-platinum-palladium alloys (white and yellow) are not used widely today because of their high cost. The composition range of gold-platinum-palladium alloys varies considerably (see Table 3-5). Alloys with a palladium level greater than that of the platinum are designated as *gold-palladium-platinum metals*. Alloys in which palladium has been completely eliminated are referred to as *gold-platinum alloys*.

These alloys are classified as *high-noble (ADA)* or as *high-noble yellow* or *high-noble white* (modified ADA).

Gold-palladium-silver system

These alloys were developed to overcome the major limitations (ie, poor sag resistance, low hardness, and high cost) of the gold-platinum-palladium system. Two subgroups are identified as the *high-silver group* and the *low-silver group* (see Table 3-5). Because both subgroups are gold based, they handle like gold-platinum-palladium metals and possess many of their general advantages and disadvantages. These alloys are available in white or yellow gold.

These alloys are classified as *high-noble* (ADA) or as *high-noble yellow* or *high-noble white* (modified ADA).

Gold-palladium system

The gold-palladium system was developed to overcome the two major problems (ie, porcelain discoloration and a high CTE) associated with the gold-palladium-silver and palladium-silver alloys (see Table 3-5). These white-colored alloys are popular among users of both high-noble and noble metal-ceramic alloys. However, they are not thermally compatible with some high-expansion dental porcelain systems. One of the more popular alloy formulations is 51.5% gold, 38.5% palladium, and 5% gallium, with trace amounts of indium and tin.

It has been reported that oxidation of gold-palladium castings leads to the formation of gallium oxide on the casting surface, which, it is believed, chemically reacts with porcelain in the creation of a porcelain-metal bond.[10] The gallium oxide is unaffected by the postoxidation hydrofluoric acid treatment recommended by the alloy manufacturer.[10]

Gold-palladium alloys represent an excellent alternative to high-gold alloys because of their improved physical properties; however, they are expensive due to their noble metal content.

These alloys are classified as *high-noble* (ADA) or as *high-noble white* (modified ADA).

Table 3-5 Advantages and disadvantages of specific metal-ceramic alloy systems

Systems	Advantages	Disadvantages
High-gold		
	Yellow hue	Must be completely veneered by porcelain
	Biocompatible	Expensive
	Excellent castability	Poor sag resistance (ie, unsuited for long-span FPDs)
		Delicate finishing technique
		Low hardness
		High density
		Best suited for single crowns
Gold-platinum-palladium*		
	Excellent castability	Poor sag resistance (ie, unsuited for long-span FPDs)
	Excellent porcelain bonding	Low hardness
	Easy to adjust and finish	Expensive
	High nobility level	High density
	Excellent corrosion and tarnish resistance	
	Biocompatible	
	Some are yellow	
	Not technique sensitive	
	Burnishable	
Gold-palladium-silver		
High-silver group		
	Less expensive than Au-Pt-Pd alloys	Possible porcelain discoloration
	Improved rigidity and sag resistance	High CTE
	High nobility level	High cost
	Tarnish and corrosion resistant	
Low-silver group		
	Less expensive than Au-Pt-Pd alloys	High cost
	Porcelain discoloration less likely than high-silver group	Possibility of porcelain discoloration remains
	Improved sag resistance	High CTE
	High-noble metal content	
	Tarnish and corrosion resistant	
Gold-palladium		
	Excellent castability	Not thermally compatible with high-expansion porcelains
	Good bond strength	High cost
	Corrosion and tarnish resistant	
	Improved hardness	
	Improved sag resistance	
	Lower density	
Palladium-silver†		
	Low cost	Possible porcelain discoloration
	Low density	Prone to gas absorption
	Good castability with torch casting	Castability problems with induction casting
	Good porcelain bonding	Should not be cast in a carbon crucible
	Bunishability	Regular purging of the porcelain furnace
	Low hardness	May form internal oxides
	Excellent sag resistance	High CTE
	Moderate nobility level	Noncarbon phosphate-bonded investments
	Good tarnish and corrosion resistance	
	High yield strength	
	High modulus of elasticity	
	Suitable for long-span FPDs	

*Platinum content must exceed that of palladium.
†These compositional variants better represent palladium-silver alloy systems than the general description of 60% palladium and 40% silver.
FPD = fixed partial denture; CTE = coefficient of thermal expansion; Au = gold; Pt = platinum; Pd = palladium

(table continued)

Table 3-5 *(cont)*

Systems	Advantages	Disadvantages
High-palladium		
High-palladium–cobalt[‡]		
	Low cost	Only compatible with higher-expansion porcelains
	Good sag resistance	More prone to overheating than high-palladium–copper alloys
	Low density	Thick, dark-colored oxide layer that may blue porcelain
	Some melt and cast easily	Prone to gas absorption
	Good polishability	Little information on long-term clinical success
	Easier to presolder than high-Pd–Cu alloys	
High-palladium–copper[§]		
	Good castability	Thick, dark-colored oxide layer
	Lower cost than gold-based alloys	Discoloration (gray) of some porcelains
	Low density	Visual evaluation necessary to determine whether proper adherent oxide was formed
	Tarnish and corrosion resistant	Should not be cast in a carbon crucible
	Compatible with many porcelains	Prone to gas absorption
	Some are available in 1-dwt ingots	Subject to thermal creep (marginal opening)
		May be unsuitable for long-span FPDs
		Little information on long-term clinical success
		Polishing difficulty
		Presoldering difficulty
		High hardness (may wear opposing teeth)
High-palladium–silver-gold		
	Low cost	A relatively new alloy group
	Low density	No data on long-term performance
	Improved sag resistance	Prone to gas absorption
	Light-colored oxide layer	Should not be cast in a carbon crucible
Nickel-chromium		
Nickel-chromium-beryllium		
	Low cost	Cannot use with nickel-sensitive patients
	Low density	Beryllium exposure potentially harmful to technicians and patients
	High sag resistance	Difficult to properly melt and cast
	Can produce thin castings	Bond failure more common in the oxide layer
	Poor thermal conductor	High hardness (may wear opposing teeth)
	Can be etched	Difficult to solder
		Ingots do not pool
		Difficult to cut through cemented castings
Nickel-chromium beryllium-free[‖]		
	Do not contain beryllium	Cannot use with nickel-sensitive patients
	Low cost	Cannot be etched
	Low density	May not cast as well as Ni-Cr-Be alloys
		Forms more oxides than Ni-Cr-Be alloys
Cobalt-chromium		
	Nickel-free composition	More difficult to process than nickel-based alloys
	Beryllium-free composition	High hardness (may wear opposing teeth)
	Poor thermal conductor	Forms more oxides than nickel-based alloys
	Low density	No information on long-term clinical success
	Low cost	

[‡]In response to the initial popularity of the high-palladium–copper alloys containing 79% palladium and 2% gold, some manufacturers marketed a high-palladium–cobalt alloy with the small addition of gold.

[§]Some manufacturers produce high-palladium–copper alloys with small quantities (1% to 3%) of gold and/or platinum.

[‖]These nickel-based alloys share many of the advantages and disadvantages listed for the of the nickel-chromium-beryllium alloys.

Pd = palladium; Cu = copper; FPD = fixed partial denture; Ni = nickel; Cr = chromium; Be = beryllium

Noble-metal alloys

Alloys within the noble metal category *must* contain at least 25% noble elements (there is no upper limit) and *can* include metals with less than 40% gold that cannot be classified as *high-noble*.

Palladium-silver system

This was the first gold-free system introduced in the United States (1974) that contained a noble metal (palladium). Palladium-silver alloys continue to offer an economic alternative to expensive gold-based metals (ie, gold-platinum-palladium and gold-palladium-silver) and possess excellent physical properties (see Table 3-5). Unfortunately, palladium-silver alloys are one of the least appreciated and most maligned groups of metal-ceramic alloys.[4,7,8]

A classic generalization of alloys in this system is that they contain roughly 60% palladium, up to 40% silver, and additions of indium and tin. In reality, some manufacturers market two types of palladium-silver alloy. One has 55% to 60% palladium, 28% to 30% silver, plus indium, tin, and other trace elements to make up the balance. The other variation of palladium-silver alloy contains 50% to 55% palladium, 35% to 40% silver, plus tin and other trace elements, but little or no indium. Palladium-silver alloys with less palladium and more silver are slightly less expensive then their counterparts with a higher palladium level. In addition, the palladium-silver alloys generally are cheaper than other noble, gold-free "alternative" alloys, such as the various types of high-palladium alloys.

Differences in composition influence physical characteristics of these alloys. The higher palladium formulations, containing both indium and tin, generally produce a bluish violet oxide.[4] In contrast, the lower palladium/higher silver alloys with tin but no indium produce a transparent tin oxide (SnO_2).[4] One study noted the formation of external palladium-silver nodules and internal oxidation just below the metal surface with no oxidation of the nodules.[11] Some investigators found indium and tin at the alloy surface, with indium diffusing into the porcelain veneer.[12] Yamamoto indicated that tin oxide actually improves chemical bonding and wettability.[13]

One of the most often cited disadvantages of the palladium-silver alloys is their tendency to discolor, or "green," dental porcelain. If discoloration does occur, it is not always manifest as a true "greening" of the dental porcelain; a color change is most likely to present itself as a yellow or light brown surface discoloration.[14] At least three theories have been offered to explain porcelain discoloration by silver.[14]

Silver-sodium exchange theory

It is hypothesized that during the cooling phase, an exchange takes place in which silver, from silver vapors, replaces sodium in the dental porcelain, resulting in what is more aptly described as a yellow or brown discoloration rather than a true green color. The cause of the discoloration has been attributed to an interaction between silver in the alloy and sodium in the porcelain that produces a colloidal precipitate.[6] This silver-sodium exchange continues in porcelain that is prone to discoloration until the porcelain furnace is purged with carbon to remove all traces of silver.[4]

Bulk-transfer theory

According to the bulk-transfer theory, silver migrates into the porcelain at the porcelain-metal interface, diffuses to the surface, and discolors the porcelain through an unknown chemical process.

Surface diffusion theory

Like the silver-sodium exchange theory, this hypothesis contends that silver diffuses to the metal surface and discolors the surface of the porcelain. The most likely explanation for the discoloration of porcelain by silver rests with the silver-sodium exchange theory and may also involve some surface diffusion. This explanation is supported by the observation that discoloration, when it occurs, is most likely to appear as a surface phenomenon with more intense coloration at the porcelain-metal junction (Fig 3-5).[14] Contrary to popular belief, the mere presence of silver does not necessarily mean that a ceramic veneer will become discolored. Certain porcelains are formulated specifically for silver-containing alloys. In other words, adverse porcelain color changes can be circumvented by using one of several chemically compatible dental porcelain systems.[4,14] However, little published data are available to support claims of equal levels of resistance to discoloration from silver by different brands of dental porcelain, so laboratory testing is recommended (Fig 3-6).[14]

Over the years, descriptions of palladium-silver alloys have focused on their castability, potential to discolor porcelain, and tendency to form subsurface porosity, and were not always accurately reported in the literature.[4] Naylor pointed out this mischaracterization in 1986.[4] In Goodacre's extensive review of the literature on palladium-silver alloys published several years later, he also described how these alloys had been characterized inaccurately.[7] For example, casting problems attributed to palladium-silver metal-ceramic alloys were actually based on studies of silver-palladium crown-and-bridge metals.[4,7,15] Subsurface porosity associated with one palladium-silver alloy occurred only when the

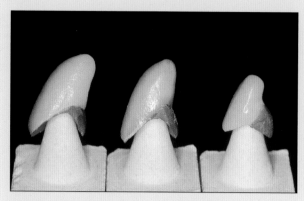

Fig 3-5a Three different brands of dental porcelain fired on copings made from the same palladium-silver alloy. The two nongreening porcelains *(left and right)* maintained their resistance to discoloration by silver after five body bakes, whereas the conventional porcelain *(middle)* took on a substantial yellow discoloration (particularly at the porcelain-metal junction) after just two firings.

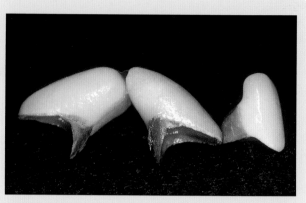

Fig 3-5b When the discolored porcelain surface *(middle)* was ground, it revealed a nondiscolored interior, suggesting that the silver-porcelain reaction is a surface phenomenon. The two restorations with nondiscoloring dental porcelains *(left and right)* did not discolor after multiple firings.

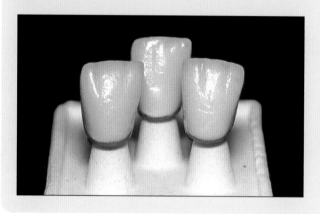

Fig 3-6 Metal-ceramic restorations fabricated on a palladium-silver alloy *(left and right)* and a nickel-chromium-beryllium alloy *(middle)*. The conventional porcelain *(left)* and a reportedly nongreening porcelain *(right)* both discolored on the palladium-silver alloy. As would be expected, a recognized nongreening porcelain *(middle)* did not discolor on the nickel-chromium-beryllium alloy.

alloy was induction cast, not torch cast, and may have been caused by overheating of the metal.[4,7] Laboratory technicians who pair these silver-containing alloys with a chemically compatible metal-ceramic porcelain and use proper casting methods should be able to produce well-fitting and esthetic restorations.

These alloys are classified as *noble* (ADA) or as *noble white* (modified ADA).

High-palladium system

When this system was introduced, initial compositions included a group containing cobalt and another containing copper (see Table 3-5).[16] Of these two formulations of high-

palladium alloys, the copper group was more popular. However, the most commercially successful high-palladium products had an advertised composition of 79% palladium and 2% gold.[4,17] Some manufacturers claimed that a 1% to 2% addition of a noble metal (eg, gold, platinum) improved the grain structure of a high-palladium alloy,[18] but that view is not widely held because of a lack of undisputed evidence.

Both the high-palladium–cobalt and high-palladium–copper alloys failed to acquire sustained market share because of their dark oxide, poor high-temperature strength (copper group), and marginal creep (copper group). In an effort to overcome these shortcomings, a second generation high-palladium system containing small amounts of silver and gold was developed (see Table 3-5). The advantages of the high-palladium–silver-gold alloys include their lower cost (compared with gold-based alloys), reported improvement in high-temperature strength, and formation of a lighter surface oxide layer.[16]

The issue of internal oxidation noted in palladium-silver alloys surfaced again in a 1996 study of high-palladium alloys.[19] Of the four products evaluated, internal oxidation was noted with three: high-palladium–copper-gallium-indium, high-palladium–silver-indium-tin, and high-palladium–silver-indium-gold.

These alloys are classified as *noble* (ADA) or as *noble white* (modified ADA).

Predominantly base metal alloys

Two recognized base metal alloy systems are in use today: one based on nickel and the other based on cobalt. Both alloy systems contain chromium as the second largest constituent. Chromium is responsible for *passivation*, the formation of a thin, invisible surface oxide layer on the alloy that is believed to prevent further reaction of the metal with its environment.[1,9] All other base metal alloys are minor systems (eg, Callisto CP in cobalt-palladium system). The biologic implications of using alloys containing nickel, beryllium, and chromium are addressed later in this chapter.

Nickel-chromium system

These metal-ceramic alloys offer such economy that they also can be used as crown-and-bridge alloys for complete metal crowns and fixed partial dentures.[9] The major constituents are nickel and chromium, with a wide array of minor alloying elements. This system contains two major groups: those that contain beryllium and those that are beryllium-free (see Table 3-5). Of the two, the nickel-chromium-beryllium alloys are generally regarded as possessing superior properties and have been more popular.[20,21] Among other benefits, beryllium increases fluidity, improves castability, aids in the formation of a stable bond with porcelain, and lessens the tendency for these alloys to form a thick oxide at high temperatures.[22] The small weight percentage of beryllium (1.8% to 2.0%) in nickel-chromium-beryllium alloys is somewhat misleading because this element has a low atomic weight and density. In fact, the volume percentage of beryllium is greater than the atomic weight would suggest because beryllium ions are very small.[23]

The nickel-based alloys that were introduced in the late 1960s were the forerunners of this system; however, conclusions drawn from research of more than a decade ago may be less relevant to the products in today's market.

Early problems with castability and fit have largely been overcome by improvements in the alloy formulations and by a better understanding of the proper ways to sprue, invest, and cast these low-density metals. The nickel-chromium system is in widespread use and dominates a substantial portion of the base metal market. Products in this category should be referred to as *nickel-chromium* or *nickel-chromium-beryllium* alloys, and not as *nickel-chrome* alloys.

These alloys are classified as *predominantly base* (ADA) or as *predominantly base white* (modified ADA).

Cobalt-chromium system

Like the nickel-chromium system, the cobalt-based alloys have been marketed as porcelain alloys that also can be used to fabricate economic all-metal restorations (see Table 3-5). Because the major constituent is cobalt, not chromium, these metals are appropriately described as *cobalt-chromium* alloys rather than as *chrome-cobalt* or *chromium-cobalt* alloys. There has been some reference to a possible subdivision of the cobalt-based system into two groups—ruthenium and ruthenium-free alloys. Whether sufficient differences exist to warrant such a separation is unclear. However, it is important to note that, although cobalt-chromium alloys are being promoted as porcelain alloys, they are not regarded with the same favor and level of success as the nickel-chromium-beryllium alloys. Nonetheless, cobalt-chromium alloys are being advertised as non-nickel, nonberyllium, and nonprecious alternative alloys to attract consumers of base metal products who are concerned about the biocompatibility of nickel and beryllium.[22,24–26]

These alloys are classified as *predominantly base* (ADA) or as *predominantly base white* (modified ADA).

Other systems

This category includes titanium alloys and minor systems that appear on the market but are not generally sold by major alloy manufacturers. Improvements in titanium alloys continue, and research is ongoing to overcome the unique demands of technical processing.

The vast majority of base metal alloys are classified as white (although actually gray in appearance), but there are some crown-and-bridge base metal alloys with a yellow hue, such as NPG+2, a copper-based (78.7%) alloy containing aluminum, nickel, iron, zinc, manganese, and 2.0% gold.

These alloys are classified as *predominantly base* (ADA) or as *predominantly base white* or *predominantly base yellow* (modified ADA).

Other Important Features of Metal-Ceramic Alloys

Aside from a basic understanding of the composition and classification systems, the following items also relate to metal-ceramic alloys.

Alloy packaging and contents disclosure

Not all manufacturers include sufficient product information on alloy packages to permit easy identification. However, major manufacturers disclose most, if not all, elements in their casting alloys in product literature and on company websites. More technical information is now available online than ever before. It is important that dentists and dental technicians be aware of the composition of the materials they use and include that information in patient dental records and on laboratory work authorizations.

> For a stable porcelain bond, the CTE of the metal should be slightly greater than that of the dental porcelain if the ceramic veneer is to be held under compression.

Ingot identification

High-noble and noble alloys typically have some form of ingot identification such as alloy shape or manufacturer name. On the other hand, not all base metal alloys are recognizable either by name or shape (Fig 3-7). Ingot identification is especially important for consumers who maintain an inventory of different alloys.

Alloy composition vs alloy performance

Composition is one consideration when selecting an acceptable alloy, but it should not be the sole criterion. The fact that two alloys have the same percentage composition for the major constituents is no guarantee that they will perform similarly. If an alloy has a history of proven success with a specific dental porcelain, there is no assurance that a lesser-priced product of similar makeup will provide comparable performance.

Small changes to the minor alloying elements, major differences in the purity of raw materials, or variations in the alloy manufacturing process (eg, quality control, in-house refining of ingredients) are features the consumer cannot assess from alloy packaging.

Alloy composition vs density

As shown by the composition of the representative alloys in Tables 3-3 and 3-4, the density of metal-ceramic alloys can range from as little as 7.8 g/cm^3 for base metal alloys to as much as 19.3 g/cm^3 for high-noble alloys. Pure gold has a density of 19.32 g/cm^3, compared with 8.91 g/cm^3 for nickel.[27] In practical terms, the lower-density alloys are lighter in weight, so more castings can be produced per ounce than from a high-gold–content high-noble alloy.

When two metal-ceramic substructures cast in the same color metal are compared visually, it is not always possible to differentiate between a restoration cast in a high-noble or noble alloy and one cast in a base metal alloy. However, the differences in density are readily apparent if one casting is held in each hand; such a test permits rapid identification of the high-noble metal by its greater weight. The high-noble casting will feel much heavier, yet the two castings would appear equivalent. For the dental laboratory, this translates into more castings per troy ounce for the lighter-density alloy and fewer castings per troy ounce for the higher-density metal, ie, a higher material cost.

Casting alloy–dental porcelain compatibility

With so many alloys on the market today, it is unwise to assume that a given dental porcelain can be used with any alloy. Moreover, success with a single-unit metal-ceramic crown is no guarantee of suitable pairing in a fixed partial denture. Occasionally, a metal and a dental porcelain lack a predictable level of compatibility, and the porcelain veneer may craze, fracture, or unexpectedly pop off the metal surface (see Fig 3-2). Unfortunately, not all casting alloy–dental porcelain mismatches are readily identifiable, so consult with your porcelain manufacturer before considering alloy substitutions.

As indicated in chapter 2, the CTE of most metal-ceramic alloys is in the 13.5 to 15.5 ×10^{-6}/°C range (see Table 3-4). For a stable porcelain bond, the CTE of the metal should be slightly *greater* than that of the dental porcelain if the ceramic veneer is to be held under compression.[4,6]

Roles of constituent elements

The following is an alphabetic listing of elements that may be included in a porcelain alloy. It is important to remember that

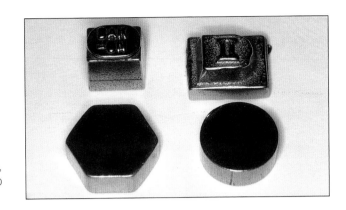

Fig 3-7 Some base metal ingots can be identified by product name *(top left)*, unique shape *(bottom left)*, or both *(top right)*, whereas other ingots have no recognizable markings as to alloy type or manufacturer *(bottom right)*.

the function of a particular element in an alloy can vary among alloy systems (Table 3-6).

Aluminum (Al)

Aluminum is added to lower the melting range of nickel-based alloys. Aluminum is a hardening agent and influences oxide formation. With the cobalt-chromium alloys used for metal-ceramic restorations, aluminum is one of the elements that is etched from the alloy's surface to create micromechanical retention for resin-bonded prosthesis (commonly referred to as *Maryland bridges*).

Beryllium (Be)

Like aluminum, beryllium lowers the melting range of nickel-based alloys. It also increases fluidity, improves castability and polishability, acts as a hardener, helps to control oxide formation, and aids in the formation of a more reliable bond[28] with porcelain. The etching of nickel-chromium-beryllium alloys removes a nickel-beryllium phase to create the micromechanical retention so important to the etched-metal resin-bonded prosthesis. Questions have been raised as to potential health risks associated with beryllium-containing alloys to both technicians and patients.[29] In its free state, beryllium is highly toxic[30] and has been proven to migrate toward the surface of a casting.[24,31] Beryllium has a lower atomic weight (9.012) and density (1.848 g/cm^3) than nickel (58.71 and 8.902 g/cm^3, respectively).

Boron (B)

Boron is a deoxidizer. In nickel-based alloys, it acts as a hardening agent, reduces ductility, and decreases the surface tension of the molten alloy, thereby improving castability. The nickel-chromium beryllium-free alloys that contain

boron pool on melting, while the nickel-chromium-beryllium alloys do not pool.

Chromium (Cr)

Chromium increases hardness and contributes to corrosion resistance by the passivation it imparts to nickel- and cobalt-based alloys.

Cobalt (Co)

Cobalt-based metals are an alternative to the nickel-based alloys, but they generally are more difficult to process. Cobalt was included in some high-palladium alloys (high-palladium–cobalt) to increase their CTE and to act as a strengthener.

Copper (Cu)

Copper serves as a hardening and strengthening agent. It lowers the melting range and gives platinum-, palladium-, silver-, and gold-based alloys a heat-treating capability. Copper helps form an oxide for porcelain bonding, lowers the density slightly, and enhances passivity in the high-palladium–copper alloys.

Gallium (Ga)

Gallium is added to silver-free alloys to compensate for the decreased CTE created by the removal of silver. (Concerns over silver's potential to discolor dental porcelain have greatly limited its use in ceramic alloys.). Gallium is also believed to enhance alloy-porcelain adherence in gold-palladium alloys containing both indium and gallium.[10] This element has a low melting point (29.8°C), oxidizes readily, and is a precious metal.

51

| Table 3-6 | Roles of constituent elements in metal-ceramic alloys |

	Ag	Al	Au	B	Be	Cr	Co	Cu	Fe	Ga	In	Ir	Mn
Affinity for hydrogen, oxygen, and carbon												■	
Affinity for oxygen	■										■[12]		
Burnishability, improves			■										
Castability, improves				■[1]	■								
CTE, raises	■					■[2]				■[3]			
CTE like gold													
Color, gives yellow hue			■					■[5]					
Color, whitens alloys	■	■			■								
Corrosion/tarnish, increases	■[6]												
Corrosion/tarnish resistant			■										■
Cost, decreases	■												
Cost, increases			■										
Density, raises			■										
Deoxidizer													
Ductility, increases			■										
Ductility, reduces				■									
Etched from alloy by acid			■		■								
Fluidity, improves	■										■		
Grain refiner												■[8]	
Hardener		■		■[4]	■	■		■	■[9]				■[10]
Health risk (potential)			?		■								
Heat treatment (helps with)									■[11]				
Melting range, lowers	■	■[4]			■[4]			■			■		
Melting range, raises			■										
Noble element[12]			■									■	
Oxide formation, for porcelain bonding		■			■	■			■[7]		■		
Oxide scavenger											■		■[10]
Passivates						■[13]		■[14]					
Polishability, improves					■								
Precious element[15]	■		■		■						■		
Sag resistance, improves													
Strength, improves							■	■			■		
Tarnish resistance, enhances			■							■[16]	■		
Workability, improves			■										

Gold (Au)

Gold provides a high level of corrosion and tarnish resistance and improves workability and burnishability. It increases an alloy's density and cost and slightly increases its melting range. Gold imparts a very pleasing yellow hue to an alloy (if present in sufficient quantity); however, that yellow color can be offset by the addition of sufficient quantities of white metals (eg, palladium, silver). Gold is both a precious and a noble metal.

Indium (In)

Indium serves many functions in gold-based alloys: it lowers melting range and density, improves fluidity, and has a strengthening effect. Indium is less volatile than other oxide-

Mo	Ni	Pd	Pt	Ru	Si	Sn	Ti	Zn	
		■							Affinity for hydrogen, oxygen, and carbon
							■12		Affinity for oxygen
									Burnishability, improves
							■	■	Castability, improves
■4									CTE, raises
	■								CTE like gold
									Color, gives yellow hue
	■	■	■						Color, whitens alloys
									Corrosion/tarnish, increases
■	■	■	■	■					Corrosion/tarnish resistant
									Cost, decreases
			■						Cost, increases
			■						Density, raises
								■	Deoxidizer
									Ductility, increases
									Ductility, reduces
									Etched from alloy by acid
									Fluidity, improves
				■8					Grain refiner
		■	■		■	■	■	■	Hardener
	■								Health risk (potential)
									Heat treatment (helps with)
						■		■	Melting range, lowers
		■	■				■		Melting range, raises
		■	■	■					Noble element12
						■	■	■	Oxide formation, for porcelain bonding
					■			■	Oxide scavenger
									Passivates
									Polishability, improves
		■	■	■					Precious element15
		■							Sag resistance, improves
		■	■						Strength, improves
		■	■	■					Tarnish resistance, enhances
									Workability, improves

1Lowers surface tension.
2For high-palladium alloys.
3In silver-free alloys.
4In nickel-based alloys.
5In some base metal crown-and-bridge alloys.
6In the presence of sulfur.
7In non–gold-based alloys.
8For gold- and palladium-based alloys.
9In gold-based alloys.
10In nickel- and cobalt-based alloys.
11In gold-, silver-, and palladium-based alloys.
12Counters silver's affinity for oxygen.
13In nickel- and chromium-based alloys.
14In high-palladium-copper alloys.
15Osmium and rhodium not listed
16In high-silver alloys.

scavenging agents and protects molten alloys. It is added to non–gold-based alloy systems to aid the formation of an oxide layer for porcelain bonding. Alloys with a high silver content rely on indium to enhance tarnish resistance. In gold-palladium alloys, indium may enhance porcelain-metal adherence.10 Indium is a precious metal.

Iridium (Ir)

Iridium is a grain refiner for gold- and palladium-based alloys. It improves the mechanical properties and tarnish resistance of an alloy. Iridium is a member of the platinum group, so it is both a noble and a precious metal.

Iron (Fe)

Iron is added to some gold-based porcelain systems for hardening and oxide production. It is included in a few base metal alloys as well.

Manganese (Mn)

Manganese is an oxide scavenger and a hardening agent in nickel- and cobalt-based alloys.

Molybdenum (Mo)

Molybdenum improves corrosion resistance, influences oxide production, and helps in adjusting the CTE of nickel-based alloys.

Nickel (Ni)

Nickel has been selected as a base for porcelain alloys because its CTE approximates that of gold and it provides resistance to corrosion. Unfortunately, nickel is a sensitizer, a contact allergen, and a known carcinogen. In the United States, estimates of nickel sensitivity range from 9.0% to 31.9% among women and from 0.9% to 20.7% among men.[26,32,33]

Palladium (Pd)

Palladium increases strength, hardness (with copper), and resistance to corrosion and tarnishing in gold-based alloys. Palladium also elevates an alloy's melting range and improves its sag resistance. It has a strong whitening effect, so an alloy with 90% gold and only 10% palladium is a white-colored metal. Palladium possesses a high affinity for hydrogen, oxygen, and carbon. It slightly lowers the density of the gold-based alloy, but has little similar effect on silver-based metals. As a member of the platinum group, palladium is both a noble and a precious metal.

Platinum (Pt)

Platinum increases the strength, melting range, and hardness of gold-based alloys while improving their corrosion, tarnish, and sag resistance. It whitens alloys and, because of its high density, increases the density of non–gold-based metals. Platinum is a member of the platinum group, so it is both a noble and a precious metal.

Ruthenium (Ru)

Ruthenium acts as a grain refiner for gold- and palladium-based alloys to improve their mechanical properties and tarnish resistance (much like iridium). Ruthenium is a member of the platinum group, so it is both a noble and a precious metal.

Silicon (Si)

Silicon serves primarily as an oxide scavenger to prevent the oxidation of other elements during the melt. Like manganese, silicon also acts as a hardening agent.

Silver (Ag)

Silver lowers melting range, improves fluidity, and helps to control the CTE in gold- and palladium-based alloys. Silver's CTE ($19.2 \times 10^{-6}/°C$) is considerably higher than that of gold ($14.4 \times 10^{-6}/°C$)[27] and palladium ($11.8 \times 10^{-6}/°C$).[5] Silver-containing metal-ceramic alloys have been known to induce discoloration (yellow, brown, or green) with some dental porcelains. Silver possesses a high affinity for oxygen absorption, which can lead to casting porosity and/or gassing. However, the addition of small amounts of zinc or indium to gold- and silver-based alloys helps to control this absorption. Silver also corrodes and tarnishes in the presence of sulfur. Although silver is a precious element, it is not universally regarded as noble when used in the oral cavity.[2,3]

Tin (Sn)

Tin is a hardening agent that lowers the melting range of an alloy and assists in oxide production for porcelain bonding in gold- and palladium-based alloys. Tin is one of the key trace elements needed for oxidation of the palladium-silver alloys. It is capable of forming a "transparent" tin oxide layer on the porcelain-bearing surface,[4] which improves chemical bonding and wettability.[13]

Titanium (Ti)

Like aluminum and beryllium, titanium lowers melting range and improves castability. Titanium also acts as a hardener and influences oxide formation at high temperatures.

Zinc (Zn)

Zinc is valuable in lowering the melting range of an alloy and in acting as a deoxidizer, or scavenger, in combination with other oxides. Zinc improves the castability of an alloy, and when combined with palladium, increases hardness.

Biocompatibility

Collectively, the volume of information in published reports, journal articles, and anecdotal evidence on the subject of the efficacy and biocompatibility (or safety) of dental alloys is substantial and spreads across multiple disciplines. In an effort to address these and related issues of biocompatibility, select references have been chosen to highlight several noteworthy findings. Individuals interested in exploring the subject of alloy biocompatibility in more detail are encouraged to read the references and review the cited reports in those publications as well.

Noble metals

Biocompatibility issues are not limited to base metals and their alloys but extend to noble elements as well. As a result the subject of biocompatibility is multifaceted, so the identification of specific elements or alloys as responsible for changes in the human body retains some speculation and is subject to interpretation or misinterpretation. Furthermore, symptoms and diseases attributed to occupational exposure to specific metals can be affected by *confounding variables* found in the dental laboratory environment (eg, smoking, direct skin contact, inhalation and ingestion of lab dust).

Gold

Although regarded as the "gold" standard and best biocompatible element, gold-based alloys have been implicated in some cases of allergic response by a dental patient, but such reactions are rare. In a 1983 article in the *Journal of the American Dental Association,*[34] a case was reported in which a 36-year-old woman developed a burning sensation in her tongue, buccal mucosa, and gingiva surrounding a gold-based fixed partial denture. Within days, pruritis and erythematous lesions appeared, which resolved when the fixed partial denture was replaced. Upon further evaluation and sensitivity testing, the authors concluded that the patient was allergic to gold. To their knowledge, there were only seven previously reported cases involving such reactions to gold-containing restorations. Surprisingly, the patient received a new metal-ceramic fixed partial denture with porcelain occlusal surfaces made with a base metal alloy of unspecified composition.

Another article reported that a 55-year-old man developed a "painful buccal and lingual ulceration" on the right side after receiving a "cast-gold jacket crown" on the mandibular right first premolar, a mandibular removable par-

tial denture with stainless steel clasps, and a maxillary acrylic resin complete denture.[35] When evaluated further, the patient was found to have a strong reaction to the 1% gold trichloride patch test. The gold crown was removed, and after 1 week the lesions reportedly began to resolve. The authors' diagnosis based on the clinical reaction and histologic response was that of contact sensitivity to dental gold and specifically to "the chloride salt of gold." Not only did the patient's condition improve when the gold crown was removed, but a longstanding dermatitis localized under a gold signet ring also resolved. The authors suggested that the gold ring was the sensitizing agent.

Palladium

Another study evaluated 200 patients of whom 17 had a history of allergic reactions and were patch tested. Nine of these subjects were found to be allergic to one or more of the following metals: nickel, palladium, copper, and chromium.[36] While local intraoral reactions of stomatitis occurred in patients with positive reactions to nickel skin testing, no similar correlation was found with palladium. The link between palladium and oral mucosal changes was not definitive in this report.

Base metals

Most base metal are stable in the oral environment because of passivation that produces oxide layers on their exterior surface as a barrier to corrosion and the leaching of elements[37]; exceptions include beryllium and nickel, which leach and are potential causative agents of adverse biologic responses. The Summary of the 1985 ADA Association Report on the risks of base metal alloys stated, "the dental profession may be overgeneralizing the relative safety of nickel alloys because of the lack of allergy-induced intraoral lesions observed in private practices."[22] In the ADA Association Report[38] of 2003, the ADA Council on Scientific Affairs recommended "that—where possible—practitioners use alloys that do not contain beryllium in the fabrication of dental prostheses."

Beryllium

This element is not only a component of base metal alloys for metal-ceramic restorations but also can be found in alloys used to fabricate frameworks for removable partial dentures. As stated previously, up to 1.8 weight percentage of an alloy may be beryllium. This low weight percentage must be put into perspective because, given beryllium's small atomic size, its actual volume percentage ranges from

10%[23,24] to 12%.[28] Furthermore, even higher concentrations of beryllium (35%) and nickel (31%) ions have been detected on the external surface of specimens stored in human saliva at different pH levels.[24]

What is perhaps of greater importance is that beryllium and nickel are dynamic and migrate to the external surface rather than maintain a static state in a casting. As the surface concentration increases, beryllium is lost from the surface in an acidic environment and potentially can migrate into saliva and soft tissue.[24] Furthermore, it has been shown that the presence of nickel enhances the release of beryllium, and vice versa, due to a potentiating effect.[24] A laboratory study simulating 1 year of mastication also found that nickel and beryllium were released from cast nickel-chromium-beryllium crowns as a result of dissolution and wear. Occlusal wear increased the concentration of these elements two to three times that noted from dissolution alone.[39]

Beryllium ingestion should be viewed as a potential problem because the extent to which beryllium is transported in the human body is not known. It is possible that beryllium may have a cumulative effect on chronic exposure because beryllium is unlikely to be cleared by the human body.[24]

Nickel

For decades nickel-based alloys, with and without beryllium, have been used to produce a wide variety of fixed and removable partial denture prostheses. However, reports from multiple disciplines, including articles in the trade press, have increased awareness among clinicians and the general public that elemental nickel is a toxic material responsible for nickel hypersensitivity. Consequently, nickel-containing alloys should not be used for patients with a known history of nickel-sensitivity.[40] The potential threat of nickel sensitivity in patients had been thought to affect only about 9.0% of women and 0.9% of men,[25] and these low values were repeatedly cited in the literature. However, a 1953 study of 3,287 people in Sweden found that 9.4% of the women and 7.9% of the men had positive reactions to a 5% nickel sulfate patch test.[22] Even higher numbers were reported in a 1984 investigation of 403 patients, where 31.9% of the women and 20.7% of the men tested positive for nickel sensitivity.[24] In this same group, 81.1% of patients with a history of allergy to jewelry were considered hypersensitive to nickel. One laboratory study found that simple tasks such as toothbrushing can aid the release of elements in dental casting alloys, resulting in a dramatic 30-fold increase in nickel concentration from a nickel-based alloy.[41]

Allergic responses

Patients may experience certain types of adverse responses as a result of contact with or handling of certain metals—nickel-chromium-beryllium alloys in particular. Several examples of potential risks are described in this section.

Intraoral and localized responses

A number of different types of localized responses are known to occur in dental patients with undiagnosed nickel hypersensitivity. Kalkwarf reported on a woman who experienced gingival inflammation around six maxillary anterior metal-ceramic crowns made with a nickel-based alloy.[25] Lamster et al noted that it is not simply soft tissues that are affected; they described cases involving rapid alveolar bone loss around base metal alloy crowns in two women, which suggests a Type IV hypersensitivity.[29] In addition, the link between nickel sensitivity and gingival inflammation and bone loss surrounding teeth restored with nickel-chromium-beryllium metal-ceramic crowns also has been documented in a male patient.[42] Some authors noted that most patients tolerate such restorations well but urged caution in case selection,[25,29] while others recommended that nickel-chromium alloys "should be avoided."[42]

Intraoral and remote responses

Adverse reactions need not be limited to the surround gingival tissues and underlying osseous foundation but may also manifest in the mouth diffusely as burning sensations, pruritis, or erythematous lesions,[32] and progress to painful ulcerations.[35] Patients with removable partial dentures made from nickel-containing alloys may experience a metallic taste accompanied by inflamed tissues. Of note is the case of a generalized adverse response by palatal tissues in a male patient wearing a nickel-based removable partial denture; the actual outline of the prosthesis' major connector was visible on the patient's palatal tissues (Fig 3-8).

Systemic responses

According to the 1985 ADA Association Report on base metal alloys, some patients with nickel-based alloys in their mouth experience itching at the site of their nickel patch test—a manifestation of a remote, extraoral response.[22] This outcome was reported in one clinical case in which the authors suggested that a link existed between the placement of nickel-based crowns and immunoglobulin A (IgA) nephropathy, a common form of glomerulonephritis.[43] The authors concluded that this was a case of nickel-induced sensitization, and the crowns were removed. The patient's nephropathy improved with medical treatment, and it remained to be seen if the improvement was due to removal of the nickel-containing restorations, medical treatment, or spontaneous remission.

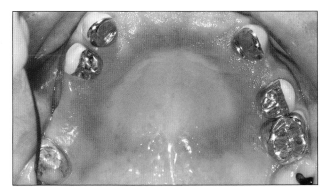

Fig 3-8 This male patient presented with painfully inflamed tissues in the palate and edentulous ridges that were in direct contact with his nickel-chromium-beryllium removable partial denture. Use of an acrylic resin interim prosthesis allowed the inflammation to resolve while a new metal framework was fabricated in a cobalt-chromium alloy.

| Box 3-1 | Work practices to reduce the risks of occupational exposure |

- Use high-noble and noble alloys.
- Wear recommended personal protective equipment such as a respirator mask, safety glasses with side shields, hearing protection, and a laboratory coat.
- Cast in a separate, well-ventilated area.
- Perform grinding procedures at a workstation with controlled suction (to retrieve noble and precious metals).

Opposing views

There are those who contend that nickel-containing alloys, when used according to "established techniques," are not associated with increased cancer risk and do not pose a hypersensitivity threat either to patients or to members of the dental team.[44] One study tested patients using a nickel-containing alloy for removable partial dentures and found no manifestations of nickel hypersensitivity either locally (at the point of contact) or remotely.[45] An earlier study observed 10 patients with a history of skin reactions to nickel. Over periods of 12 to 40 months, the investigators found no adverse responses, either generalized or localized, in the mouth and no adverse histologic changes.[46]

However, in another instance, a cobalt-chromium removable partial denture was diagnosed as a contributing factor to a severe allergic reaction in a young woman.[47] In this case report, the authors noted that cobalt-chromium alloys contain sufficient amounts of nickel to induce allergic responses in sensitive individuals.

Occupational Exposure

Dental laboratory technicians potentially have direct physical contact with nickel-containing alloys, and some individuals risk developing contact dermatitis. Without adequate physical protection, they also run the risk of ingesting fine metal particles, inhaling metallic dust during finishing procedures, and breathing vapors during casting that could lead to impaired health.[48] The occupational risks assumed by dental laboratory technicians exposed to nickel, beryllium, and laboratory dust merit discussion as does the issue of unreported cases of potential adverse reactions.

Although the 1984 ADA association report stated that "no cases have been reported from contact with dental materials containing beryllium,"[49] claims have appeared in published sources since that time.[48] A few examples illustrate the diversity and scope of these reports for both nickel and beryllium.

In 2002 the US Department of Labor published a bulletin[50] that provides an overview of the occupational risk to technicians posed by beryllium exposure and offers recommendations to reduce the risks for developing chronic beryllium disease. In addition, dental laboratory technicians and clinicians actively engaged in metal-ceramic laboratory procedures can protect themselves in several ways (Box 3-1): by using high-noble and noble alloys; by wearing recommended personal protective equipment; by casting in a separate, well-ventilated area; and by performing grinding procedures at a workstation with controlled suction (to retrieve noble and precious metals).

Nickel

Patients who practice body piercing are at increased risk of allergic reactions to nickel.[51] Laboratory personnel who engage in body piercing and who handle nickel-containing alloys also may increase their risk of developing some form of allergic reaction.

Beryllium

Dental technicians who grind nickel-containing alloys can reduce their occupational exposure to beryllium and their risk of developing acute and chronic beryllium disease by working under proper ventilation and by following good safety practices.[48,52] A 1998 case report cited exposure to beryllium and aluminum as possible causes of pulmonary granulomatosis in one dental laboratory technician.[53]

A self-reported case of acute beryllium poisoning by a dental laboratory technician appeared in a trade publication via a letter to the editor in which the author described his exposure, symptoms, medical assessment, diagnosis, and subsequent survey of his laboratory.[54] Concerns over possible subclinical and clinical chronic beryllium disease exist not only among industrial beryllium workers but also extend to dental laboratory workers who handle beryllium-containing alloys.[55]

Laboratory dust

The risk to laboratory personnel of developing an occupationally related respiratory disease has been associated with inhalation of dental laboratory dust containing particles of silica from porcelain grinding, as well as aluminum, nickel, beryllium, and chromium particles from casting, metal finishing, and polishing.[56,57]

> Dental laboratories that use high-noble, noble metal, and even predominately base metal alloys containing valuable elements should have a protocol for precious metal reclamation.

Unreported cases

Despite the apparent link between exposure to nickel and beryllium and adverse health effects, what remains unclear is the level of unreported cases of symptoms and disease related to handling certain dental casting alloys. It is now known that the sensitivity levels for nickel among men and women are higher than initially believed due to increased contact with certain metals.[24,26] Until the tracking and reporting of adverse effects improves, uncertainty will continue to surround the question of whether or not a link exists between medical- and dental-related health issues and occupational exposures to nickel- and beryllium-containing alloys.

Precious metal reclamation

Dental laboratories that use high-noble, noble, and even predominately base metal alloys containing valuable ele-

ments should have a protocol for precious metal reclamation. One of the simplest ways to recover noble and precious metals is to vacuum each technician's lab coat and work area where metal is cast, finished, and polished. A light-weight, portable vacuum cleaner, such as the Hippo Portable Hand-Held Vacuum (1.5 hp; Shop-Vac) can be used to collect dust produced from metal finishing and polishing as well as slag generated from casting. Collection bags can be sent on a regular basis to a gold refinery for processing.

Summary

The fact that no single classification system is adequate to categorize and describe all metal-ceramic casting alloys underscores the complexity of this subject. Yet with an understanding of the modified ADA classification differentiating between yellow and white high-noble alloys, as well as the composition-based classification methods, you should be better able to distinguish between the wide range of compositions of ceramic alloys. The descriptions of the different types of alloys, the roles played by their various constituents, and the complexity of the subject of biocompatibility should further your understanding of alloy selection, performance, and limitations. Readers interested in more information on biocompatibility can search the dental and medical literature to gain perspective on potential risks that may or may not exist in their workplace.

With this background, you are now ready to address the issues of proper substructure design presented in chapter 4.

References

1. Craig RG. Restorative Dental Materials, ed 12. St Louis: Mosby, 2006.

2. Phillips RL. Skinner's Science of Dental Materials, ed 8. Philadelphia: Saunders, 1982.

3. Classification system for cast alloys. Council on Dental Materials, Instruments, and Equipment. J Am Dent Assoc 1984;109:766.

4. Naylor WP. Non-Gold Base Dental Casting Alloys. Vol II: Porcelain-fused-to-metal alloys [ADA173766]. Brooks AFB, TX: School of Aerospace Medicine, 1986.

5. Anusavice KJ. Phillips' Science of Dental Materials, ed 11. Philadelphia: Saunders, 2003.

6. McLean JW. The Science and Art of Dental Ceramics, Vol I: The nature of dental ceramics and their clinical use. Chicago: Quintessence, 1979:68–69.

7. Goodacre CJ. Palladium-silver alloys: A review of the literature. J Prosthet Dent 1989;62:34–37.
Goodacre describes palladium-silver alloys as "comparable or superior to other noble metal ceramic alloys."

8. Naylor WP. Introduction to Metal Ceramic Technology. Chicago: Quintessence, 1992.

9. Bertolotti RL. Selection of alloys for today's crown and fixed partial denture restorations. J Am Dent Assoc 1984;108:959–966.
In 1984, there were no long-term data on biocompatibility risks of nickel and beryllium.

10. Sarkar NK, Verret M, Eyer CS, Jeansonne EE. Role of gallium in alloy-porcelain bonding. J Prosthet Dent 1985;53:190–194.
Hydrofluoric acid removes indium leaving surface gallium oxide for porcelain bonding.

11. Mackert JR Jr, Ringle RD, Fairhurst CW. High-temperature behavior of a Pd-Ag alloy for porcelain. J Dent Res 1983;62:1229–1235.

12. Payan J, Moya GE, Meyer JM, Moya F. Changes in physical and chemical properties of a dental palladium-silver alloy during metal-porcelain bonding. J Oral Rehabil 1986;13:329–338.

13. Yamamoto M. Metal-Ceramics: Principles and Methods of Makoto Yamamoto. Chicago: Quintessence, 1985.
Refer to chapter 1 for summary.

14. Naylor WP. A practical laboratory test for detecting porcelain discoloration in silver-containing metal ceramic alloys. QDT Yearbook 1990/1991;13:83–90.

15. Nitkin DA, Asgar K. Evaluation of alternative alloys to type III gold for use in fixed prosthodontics. J Am Dent Assoc 1976;93:622–629.
Authors evaluated silver-palladium alloys and not palladium-silver alloys, as is often reported.

16. Tuccillo JJ. Palladium alloys . . . Today's choice for PFM restorations. Trends Tech Contemp Dent Lab 1987;4(9):14, 31.

17. van der Zel JM, Vrijhoef MM. Early experiences with high palladium dental ceramic alloys. Quintessence Dent Technol 1985;9:291–296.

18. Hausselt JH. Benefits of a fine grain structure in dental alloys. Trends Tech Contemp Dent Lab 1984;1(6):31–35.

19. Vermilyea SG, Cai Z, Brantley WA, Mitchell JC. Metallurgical structure and microhardness of four new palladium-based alloys. J Prosthodont 1996;5:288–294.

20. Tuccillo JJ, Cascone PJ. The evolution of porcelain-fused-to-metal (PFM) alloy systems. In: McLean JW (ed). Dental Ceramics: Proceedings of the First International Symposium on Ceramics. Chicago: Quintessence, 1983:347–370.

21. Christensen GJ. The use of porcelain-fused-to-metal restorations in current dental practice: A survey. J Prosthet Dent 1986;56:1–3.
Refer to chapter 1 for summary.

22. Report on base metal alloys for crown and bridge applications: Benefits and risks. Council on Dental Materials, Instruments, and Equipment. J Am Dent Assoc 1985;111:479–483.

23. Moffa JP. Biocompatibility of nickel based dental alloys. CDAJ 1984;12(10):45–51.
Beryllium's small atomic size means 0.8% atomic weight is equivalent to 10 atomic percent.

24. Covington JS, McBride MA, Slagle WF, Disney AL. Quantization of nickel and beryllium leakage from base metal casting alloys. J Prosthet Dent 1985;54:127–136.

Nickel and beryllium migrate to the alloy surface and enhance the release of one another.

25. Kalkwarf KL. Allergic gingival reaction to esthetic crowns. Quintessence Int Dent Dig 1984;15:741–745.

26. Morris HF. Veterans Administration Cooperative Studies Project No. 147. Part IV: Biocompatibility of base metal alloys. J Prosthet Dent 1987;58:1–5.
With reports that 0.8% to 20.7% of men and 9.0% to 31.9% of women are nickel sensitive, this article includes five recommendations for users of nickel-based alloys.

27. Powers JM, Sakaguchi RL. Craig's Restorative Dental Materials, ed 12. St Louis: Mosby, 2006:361.

28. Asgar K. Casting metals in dentistry: Past—Present—Future. Adv Dent Res 1988;2(1):33–43.

29. Lamster IB, Kalfus DI, Steigerwald PJ, Chasens AI. Rapid loss of alveolar bone associated with nonprecious alloy crowns in two patients with nickel hypersensitivity. J Periodontol 1987;58:486–492.

30. van Noort R. Introduction to Dental Materials, ed 3. London: Mosby, 2007.

31. al-Hiyasat AS, Bashabsheh OM, Darmani H. Elements released from dental casting alloys and their cytotoxic effects. Int J Prosthodont 2002;15(5):473–478.
Laboratory tests reveal that more elements are released from copper- and nickel-containing base metal alloys (leading to greater toxicity) than from high-noble alloys.

32. Moffa JP. Biological effects of nickel-containing dental alloys. Council on Dental Materials, Instruments, and Equipment. J Am Dent Assoc 1982;104:501–505.
The relatively low values of 9.0% of women and 0.9% of men having a positive response to nickel-sensitivity testing were cited in the literature for many years.

33. Blanco-Dalmau L, Carrasquillo-Alberty H, Silva-Parra J. A study of nickel allergy. J Prosthet Dent 1984;52(1):116–119.

34. Shepard FE, Moon PC, Grant GC, Fretwell LD. Allergic contact stomatitis from a gold alloy-fixed partial denture. J Am Dent Assoc 1983;106:198–199.

35. Wiesenfeld D, Ferguson MM, Forsyth A, MacDonald DG. Allergy to dental gold. Oral Surg Oral Med Oral Pathol 1984;57(2):158–160.

36. van Loon LA, van Elsas PW, van Joost T, Davidson CL. Contact stomatitis and dermatitis to nickel and palladium. Contact Dermatitis 1984;11:294–297.

37. Biocompatibility of dental alloys. J Am Dent Assoc 2002;133:759.

38. ADA Council on Scientific Affairs. Proper use of beryllium-containing alloys. J Am Dent Assoc 2003;134:476–478.

39. Tai Y, De Long R, Goodkind RJ, Douglas WH. Leaching of nickel, chromium, and beryllium ions from base metal alloy in an artificial oral environment. J Prosthet Dent 1992;68:692–697.

40. Moffa JP, Beck WD, Hoke AW. Allergic response to nickel containing dental alloys [abstract 107]. J Dent Res 1977;56(special issue):B78.

41. Wataha JC, Lockwood PE, Frazier KB, Khajotia SS. Effect of toothbrushing on elemental release from dental casting alloys. J Prosthodont 1999;8(3):245–251.
High-noble and noble alloys are more resistant to elemental release than are base metal alloys.

42. Bruce GJ, Hall WB. Nickel hypersensitivity-related periodontitis. Compend Contin Educ Dent 1995;16(2):178, 180–184, 186.

43. Strauss FG, Eggleston DW. IgA nephropathy associated with dental nickel alloy sensitization. Am J Nephrol 1985;5:395–397.

44. Setcos JC, Babaei-Mahani A, Silvio LD, Mjör IA, Wilson NH. The safety of nickel containing dental alloys. Dent Mater 2006;22(12):1163–1168.

45. Jones TK, Hansen CA, Singer MT, Kessler HP. Dental implications of nickel hypersensitivity. J Prosthet Dent 1986;56(4):507–509.
Authors report that 20% of women were positive to the nickel patch test, as compared to 2% of men.

46. Spiechowicz E, Glantz PO, Axell T, Chmielewski W. Oral exposure to a nickel-containing dental alloy of persons with hypersensitive skin reactions to nickel. Contact Dermatitis 1984;10:206–211.

47. Brendlinger DL, Tarsitano JJ. Generalized dermatitis due to sensitivity to a chrome cobalt removable partial denture. J Am Dent Assoc 1970;81:392–394.
Cobalt-chromium alloys may contain enough nickel to instigate allergic response in nickel-sensitive patients.

48. Kotloff RM, Richman PS, Greenacre JK, Rossman MD. Chronic beryllium disease in a dental laboratory technician. Am Rev Respir Dis 1993;147:205–207.
Authors contend that technicians with chronic beryllium disease may be misdiagnosed with scarcoidosis.

49. Workshop: Biocompatibility of metals in dentistry. National Institute of Dental Research. J Am Dent Assoc 1984;109:469–471.
Recommendations include additional research on nickel, beryllium, and chromium as "potential carcinogens."

50. US Department of Labor: Occupational Safety & Health Administration. Preventing Adverse Health Effects from Exposure to Beryllium in Dental Laboratories. HIB 02-04-19 (rev. 05-14-02). Available at: www.osha.gov/dts/hib/hib_data/hib020419.html. Accessed at 29 August 2008.

51. Copeland SD, DeBey S, Hutchison D. Nickel allergies: Implications for practice. Dermatol Nurs 2007;19:267–268, 288.

52. Rom WN, Lockey JE, Lee JS, et al. Pneumoconiosis and exposures of dental laboratory technicians. Am J Public Health 1984;74(11):1252–1257.

53. Brancaleone P, Weynand B, De Vuyst P, Stanescu D, Pieters T. Lung granulomatosis in a dental technician. Am J Ind Med 1998;34:628–631.

54. Jensen B. Beryllium poisoning [letter to the editor]. Dent Lab Rev 1982;Oct:6, 8.
Jensen attributes beryllium poisoning to a nickel-chromium-beryllium alloy used in a porcelain course.

55. Carey J. Beryllium exposure: The "unrecognized epidemic." The metal can be toxic to the workers who handle it. Where has OSHA been? BusinessWeek 2 May 2005:40–42.
Ten of 271 OSHA inspectors were "sensitized" to beryllium, and 31% of sensitive individuals developed chronic beryllium disease.

56. Bernstein M, Pairon JC, Morabia A, Gaudichet A, Janson X, Brochard P. Non-fibrous dust load and smoking in dental technicians: A study using bronchoalveolar lavage. Occup Environ Med 1994;51(1):23–27.
Bronchoalveolar lavage is recommended to evaluate laboratory dust inhalation.

57. Kim TS, Kim HA, Heo Y, Park Y, Park CY, Roh YM. Level of silica in the respirable dust inhaled by dental technicians with demonstration of respirable symptoms. Ind Health 2002;40(3):260–265.

Essentials of Metal-Ceramic Substructure Design

At first glance, the process of designing and fabricating the substructure of a metal-ceramic restoration may appear complex. Yet once the functions and basic principles of framework design are understood, the task can be carried out efficiently and with relative ease.

By some estimates, improper substructure design is responsible for a majority of the porcelain-to-metal bond failures.[1] Frequently, this particular phase in the production of the metal-ceramic restoration is given little attention, or is poorly understood. Some design flaws eventually are masked by the porcelain veneers. Other design errors may go unnoticed, either until problems appear in the latter stages of laboratory production or the brittle porcelain veneer fails in service. Only then do these substructure design problems become apparent, but by that time the only options available are to remake a restoration in the laboratory or replace the defective restoration clinically. Such remakes are not only inconvenient for patients but also costly to the dental laboratory owner as well as to the clinician. Time taken to understand the essentials of proper substructure design is time well spent, especially if it can improve the longevity of the final prosthesis.

> Time taken to understand the essentials of proper substructure design is time well spent, especially if it can improve the longevity of the final prosthesis.

Functions of the Metal-Ceramic Substructure

As noted in chapter 2, conventional feldspathic low-fusing dental porcelains, when used alone, do not have the strength needed for long-term clinical viability.[2] To address this need, specially formulated ceramic alloys (see chapter 3) were developed that, when cast in the appropriate configuration, provide a foundation to support a uniform veneer of dental porcelain.[3–5] To appreciate how critical substructure design is to the long-term success of a metal-ceramic restoration, one need only examine all its various functions. For all practical purposes, a substructure has at least four primary functions and five secondary functions.

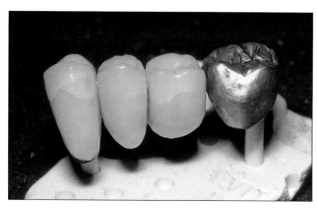

Fig 4-1 Crack formation in the porcelain veneer of all three units is evidence of stress, which was attributed to poor substructure design—specifically, too much freestanding porcelain.

Primary functions

 1. **A metal substructure provides the fit of the restoration to the prepared tooth.**

   The substructure is principally responsible for the fit of the restoration. Fit should be evaluated in terms of both *seat* (incisal/occlusal gap or internal adaptation) and *seal* (marginal opening). Though a great deal of attention is often focused on the level of marginal integrity of a restoration (seal), equal attention should be given to the internal adaptation of the metal to the prepared tooth to ensure that the casting is well fitted (seated). A restoration that binds against tooth structure may generate stresses that can be transferred to the porcelain-metal bond, inhibit complete seating, and prevent a good seat and seal of the restoration. Conversely, an overexpanded casting invariably relies more heavily on the luting cement for its retention than on good internal adaptation and may be more prone to dislodgement and failure. A properly formed metal-ceramic substructure should have what is called a *passive* fit and provide both proper internal adaptation (seat) and excellent marginal integrity (seal).

2. **A metal substructure produces surface oxides that bond chemically to dental porcelain.**

   A properly oxidized substrate enhances the attachment of porcelain to metal. This critical bond between the two key components of the metal-ceramic restoration is discussed in greater detail in chapter 6. However, an improperly designed or poorly contoured coping may permit the formation of stress concentrations as the

fired porcelain cools to room temperature. In turn, these stresses in the porcelain may not manifest themselves initially, but they can appear later and possibly lead to crack formation and bond failure (Fig 4-1).

3. **A metal substructure serves as a rigid foundation to which the brittle porcelain is attached for increased strength and support.**

   The metal substrate serves as a rigid supporting foundation that dental porcelain alone cannot provide for itself. To perform this function properly, however, the substructure must be thick enough to resist flexure or deformation when placed into function. In other words, the metal substructure should be as thick as necessary for strength and rigidity and yet not so thick as to compromise esthetics by adding unnecessary bulk to the restoration. Metal-ceramic alloys differ widely in composition and physical properties. Generally, the minimum thickness of finished metal for the porcelain-bearing areas of a single-unit metal coping ranges from 0.3 to 0.5 mm, depending on the type of alloy used.[5,6] Certain base metal alloys have sufficiently high yield strengths to permit finishing below the recommended 0.3-mm level,[7] but any attempts to reduce the metal below this level should be made with caution to avoid inadvertent perforation.

4. **A metal substructure restores a tooth's proper emergence profile.**

   The substructure should be designed to restore missing tooth structure and give the restoration a proper *emergence profile*.[1] The metal foundation of the metal-ceramic system restores tooth contour to its original form and function. In fact, certain substructure designs involve restoration of the original tooth form in metal with only the esthetically critical areas receiving a veneer of porcelain.

> Simply stated, the metal substructure should be as thick as needed for strength and rigidity, yet as thin as possible so as not to compromise esthetics by adding unnecessary bulk to the restoration.

Secondary functions

1. Generally, metal occlusal and lingual articulating surfaces are less destructive of the enamel of opposing natural teeth (depending on the type of casting alloy selected) than is dental porcelain.

2. Restorations with minimal occlusal clearance have greater potential for success when fabricated with a metal substructure (and occlusion) than do those fabricated with all-ceramic materials.

3. The occluding surfaces can be easily adjusted and repolished intraorally.

4. Metal axial walls can support the extracoronal components of a removable partial denture.

5. The axial surfaces can house attachments (precision and semiprecision) for fixed or removable partial dentures.

The metal substructure should be designed to restore lost tooth structure and to support a uniform ceramic veneer. To achieve this uniformity, the substructure must replace, in part, the tooth form lost during preparation or as a result of dental caries or trauma. The ideal thickness of porcelain varies in different areas of the restoration. For example, in the gingival third, 1.0 mm is considered ideal; the balance of the thickness would be metal (0.3 to 0.5 mm). To enhance translucency, vitality, and proper tooth contour, on the other hand, the desired dimension of porcelain at the incisal or occlusal third ranges from 1.5 to 2.0 mm, depending on the level of characterization in the natural tooth to be reproduced. A 2.0-mm occlusal dimension also is necessary to permit the

> To minimize the potential for cracking, fracture, and restoration failure, the amount of freestanding porcelain (porcelain unsupported by the metal substructure) should not exceed 2.0 mm as a general rule.

development of primary and secondary anatomy with the pits and fissures at depths sufficient to replicate a natural tooth and avoid unnecessary exposure of opaque porcelain or metal.

To minimize the potential for cracking, fracture, and restoration failure, the amount of freestanding porcelain (porcelain unsupported by the metal substructure) should not exceed 2.0 mm as a general rule (see Fig 4-1). According to one theory, the porcelain veneer is under compression for the first 2.0 mm of thickness—that is, from the metal-porcelain "interface to the region about 2 mm external to it."[3] Beyond this 2.0-mm distance is a so-called neutral zone with an area of tension for dimensions greater than 2.0 mm.[3] Porcelain is strongest under compression and weakest under tension, making the 2.0-mm thickness level an appropriate maximum dimension for porcelain unsupported by metal.

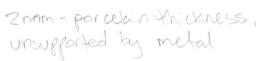
2mm - porcelain thickness, unsupported by metal

Principles of Substructure Design

Design rationales

When you understand the basic functions of the substructure, you are better prepared to appreciate the logic that you will need to apply in designing the metal framework for individual cases. While there are some established basic designs from which to choose for restoring teeth in different clinical situations, each case is unique.[8] The ability to select the most appropriate design modifications for different situations comes with time and experience. One method that has proven helpful uses an algorithmic approach to help you narrow your focus to the major design considerations that must be addressed in every case. In this method, the same five questions are asked for each case, whereas the answers vary from patient to patient.

To illustrate how easy it can be to use this question-and-answer format for substructure design, let's exam-ine each question individually. Follow the sequence as you proceed with the creation of a wax substructure. This technique illustrates how important it is to address the principles posed by each question.

1. Will the occlusal contacts be restored in metal or porcelain?

   This information should appear on the laboratory work authorization (prescription) submitted with the case by the prescribing dentist. However, if the occlusal design is not evident, you should contact the clinician for clarification before proceeding with the case.

Rationale:

Esthetics often drives this decision, particularly when there is a desire to minimize metal display and maximize the amount of porcelain coverage. Nonetheless, before recreating the occluding surfaces in metal or porcelain, you should assess the occlusion and determine whether

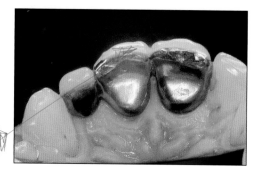

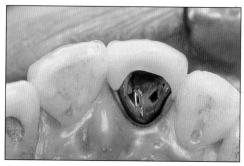

Fig 4-2a In this clinical situation, the lingual metal was extended too close to the incisal edge of the maxillary right and left central incisors and blocked light transmission. This was a poor choice of substructure design because it allowed the patient to occlude on and over the porcelain-metal junction, thus burnishing the metal and fracturing the porcelain veneer at the incisal edge.

Fig 4-2b This well-designed metal substructure permits light occlusal contact on metal in the gingival third along with proper light transmission at the incisal edge and in the interproximal areas. (Ceramics by Mr Larry Costin).

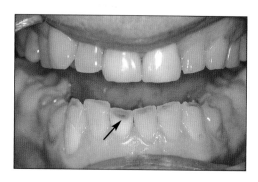

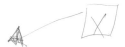

Fig 4-3 Dental porcelain, which has a high Knoop hardness value, can lead to the destruction of opposing natural teeth and other restorative materials. Note the severe wear *(arrow)* of these mandibular central incisors, which oppose central incisors restored with metal-ceramic crowns.

the following criteria have been met. Bear in mind that occlusal contacts can be created and maintained with greater precision in metal than in porcelain.[9]

First, analyze the amount of tooth reduction needed by evaluating the intra- and interarch clearance. Occlusion in metal requires less tooth removal (1.0 to 1.5 mm) and is appropriate in cases with minimal clearance. On the other hand, and in fairness to the dental laboratory technician, approximately 2.0 mm of occlusal reduction is necessary to restore posterior teeth in porcelain (so that the natural anatomy and esthetics can be re-created). Incisal reduction ranges from 1.5 to 2.0 mm for anterior teeth in order to permit light transmission and restore incisal translucency. It is possible to establish occlusion in metal on the lingual surface without compromising either incisal or interproximal esthetics (Fig 4-2).

Metal surfaces can easily be adjusted and repolished at chairside without any adverse effect on the restoration. However, removing the glaze from a metal-ceramic restoration during intraoral adjustments weakens the porcelain greatly; its transverse strength is reduced by one-half when compared with an intact glazed surface.[10]

Therefore, from a practical perspective, dentists with the facilities and equipment to reglaze porcelain as an in-office procedure might favor restoration designs that have a porcelain occlusion. Dentists without this capability should consider returning a case to the dental laboratory for reglazing and repolishing when extensive occlusal adjustments are required. Therefore, it is strongly recommended that clinicians who routinely provide metal-ceramic restorations invest in a glazing furnace.

In general, metal is less abrasive to opposing natural teeth than is dental porcelain (Fig 4-3). Certainly, the different types of casting alloys also vary in hardness and the potential to wear enamel or other restorative materials (eg, cast gold crowns, dental amalgam, or composite resin restorations) (Table 4-1). Nonetheless, the feldspathic porcelain materials are harder and potentially more abrasive than the metal-ceramic alloys to which they are bonded. These physical differences translate into a greater potential for porcelain to abrade any material it may oppose.

The potential for wear is particularly critical when a porcelain occlusal surface has been adjusted to the

Table 4-1 Comparative hardness values (means) for human enamel, dental ceramics, and casting alloys

Material	Knoop hardness No. (KHN)	Vickers hardness No. (VHN)
Human enamel[11]	340–431	—
Human dentin[11]	70	—
Human cementum[11]	40	—
Composite resin (hybrid)[10,11]	55	—
Dental amalgam[10,11]	90	—
Porcelain	560	—
Castable glass-ceramic[12]		
Cerammed surface	505	—
Shaded surface	447	—
Polished parent material	369	—
Gold-palladium alloy		
Lodestar (Ivoclar Vivadent)	—	330
Olympia (Jelenko)	—	235
Palladium-silver alloy		
Will-Ceram W1 (Ivoclar Vivadent)	—	285
High-palladium–copper alloy		
Option (Dentsply)	—	425
High-palladium–silver-gold alloy		
Integrity (Jensen)	—	250
Protocol (Ivoclar Vivadent)	—	235
Nickel-chromium alloy		
Argeloy NP (Argen)	—	240
Cobalt-chromium		
IPS d.SIGN 30 (Ivoclar Vivadent)	—	385

— Opaque porcelain: cannot be polished or glazed (handwritten)

point where the glaze has been broken or the opaque layer exposed. Invariably, overadjustment of the porcelain can be traced to inadequate tooth preparation—that is, failure to provide the 2.0 mm of clearance needed for the recommended thickness of metal and porcelain. An exposed opaque porcelain surface is rough and cannot be polished or glazed, and it poses a greater threat of damaging the opposing dentition or restoration under function. Such an outcome should be considered in designing a substructure.

Suggestion:

Evaluate both the interarch reduction and the intra-arch reduction (ie, tooth preparation). In the laboratory, assessment of clearance space usually is conducted by occluding the working cast with an opposing cast to visualize only the amount of interarch clearance available. Unfortunately, this single step does not reveal all you need to know. It is also important to gauge the amount of space needed for restorative materials (metal and porcelain) *within* the arch. The intra-arch space is assessed by visual comparison of the marginal ridge and occlusal height to the adjacent teeth or restorations.

In some cases, the amount of interarch clearance between a preparation and the opposing tooth or teeth is more than adequate, but the amount of intra-arch reduction is less than the desired 2.0 mm. In these cases, the anatomy of the occlusal surface may have to be shallower than anticipated to ensure that the final restoration is in the proper horizontal plane. *(Shallower — handwritten)*

2. Are the centric occlusal contacts 1.5 to 2.0 mm from the porcelain-metal junction?

If occlusal contacts are placed directly on or close to the porcelain-metal junction, the porcelain is more likely to chip or fracture at that point of contact (Fig 4-4).

Important (handwritten)

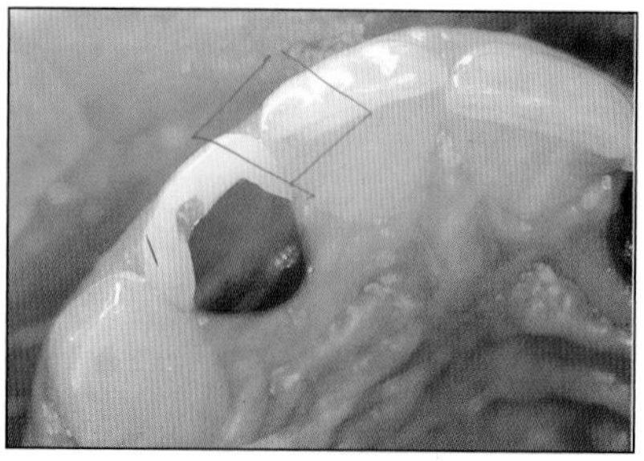

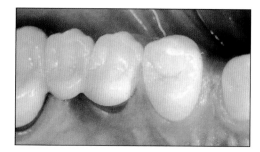

Fig 4-4 The porcelain incisal edge of this maxillary right lateral incisor was chipped as a result of improper substructure design. The patient occluded on the porcelain-metal junction during lateral mandibular movements.

Fig 4-5 The metal framework of this fixed partial denture provided inadequate support, leading to a fracture of the mesial marginal ridge.

Rationale:

Porcelain is strongest under compression and weakest under tension, so situations that induce tensile stresses in the ceramic during function are more apt to promote bond failures. For example, occlusal contacts that occur on[9] or travel across the porcelain-metal junction during function may generate a high level of these tensile stresses or cause areas of thin porcelain to fracture. Likewise, if the occlusal contact is on metal that has been thinned excessively, the metal may flex under function, and that flexure too may contribute to bond failure.

Therefore, you should establish the occlusal contact in either metal or porcelain, but not both. A substructure should be designed so that the functional incisal or occlusal contacts are located at least 1.5 mm[13] and perhaps as much as 2.0 mm[14] from the metal-porcelain junction. Be particularly careful to avoid situations involving excursive jaw movements across the porcelain-metal junction whenever possible.

Suggestion:

To adhere to this guideline for the location of occlusal contacts, a restoration should be waxed to full contour and evaluated in centric occlusion, right and left lateral excursions, and protrusive movement. Wax patterns can be dusted with powdered wax or marked with thin articulating medium such as AccuFilm II (Parkell) to identify the location of occlusal contacts.

3. Are the interproximal contacts to be restored in metal or porcelain?

   The interproximal contacts of anterior teeth, and at least the mesial contacts of posterior teeth, are frequently restored in porcelain. Obviously, a substructure design with porcelain interproximal contact areas would be more esthetic, particularly in the anterior region.

Rationale:

It is important to provide proper metal support to a porcelain marginal ridge in the substructure design to prevent possible fracture (Fig 4-5). However, the distal interproximal contacts of posterior teeth may be restored in either metal or porcelain because these areas are not as critical esthetically. Technically, it is easier to add to or re-create porcelain interproximal contact areas than it is to restore lost contours in metal through postceramic soldering. Postsoldering itself is not technically difficult, but the process is time consuming and subjects the porcelain to a risk of damage or contamination.

Suggestion:

Design the interproximal contacts in porcelain not only for esthetic reasons but also to maintain proper facial, lingual, and gingival embrasure spaces.

4. Are the cusp tips (or incisal edges) adequately supported by the metal substructure with no more than 2.0 mm of unsupported porcelain?

   As noted earlier, the ultimate goal of any substructure is to support a uniform thickness (1.0 mm minimum, 2.0 mm maximum) of the porcelain veneer.[3,5,15]

Rationale:

If the maximum thickness is exceeded, the ceramic layer may no longer be properly supported; this could result in a catastrophic failure at the cusp tip or incisal edge (see Fig 4-2a). Remember, dental porcelain is stronger under compression than it is under tension or shear forces. Figure 4-6a illustrates the type of failure that can occur when a substructure with a common design flaw is subjected to the type of forces produced by a hard bolus of food during mastication. The metal substructure fails to support the porcelain when it is exposed to occlusal forces, and the maxillary buccal, or shear, cusp is stressed

Maxillary

X

buccal

correct

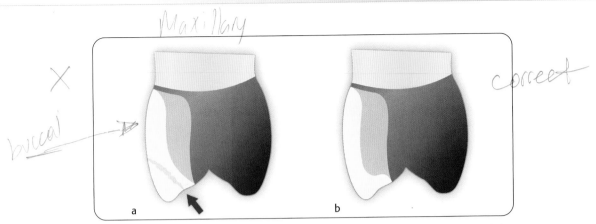

Fig 4-6 *(a)* The application of a force *(arrow)* to the buccal cusp of a crown with this substructure design can result in a shear fracture. *(b)* With proper buccal cusp support, the same forces put the porcelain under more compression than shear forces.

to the point of fracture. As a result, the porcelain that forms the buccal cusp is subjected to a shearing force that could possibly fracture the unsupported area. In contrast, the ceramic veneer illustrated in Fig 4-6b is supported when subjected to the same occlusal load. With a properly designed substructure, the porcelain is placed under compression, enabling the restoration to better withstand any potentially damaging forces of occlusion.

This design principle also applies to the preparation of substrates for both maxillary and mandibular posterior restorations.

Suggestion:
Waxing a restoration to full contour requires more time than does a simple wax-dipping technique. Yet, with a full-contoured wax pattern, the cutback for the ceramic veneer can be planned to ensure that the freestanding porcelain does not exceed the recommended 2.0-mm maximum in any area. Of course, experienced waxers undoubtedly can employ any number of techniques and still produce an appropriately designed wax substructure.

5. Is the substructure of adequate thickness to provide a rigid, inflexible foundation for the porcelain veneer? Areas of the metal substructure to be veneered with porcelain must be at least 0.3 mm thick. Some authors argue that with base metal alloys, the coping can be reduced to 0.2 mm or less and still maintain adequate strength to support the porcelain veneer.[7] Nonetheless, when you consider all of the challenges you would face to finish metal to a 0.1-mm thickness, the potential advantage may be insignificant.[3] Moreover, many of these alloys produce dark oxides that require increased thickness of opaque porcelain to adequately mask the oxide layer.

Rationale:
As noted in chapter 3, the physical properties of metal-ceramic alloys vary significantly, but even with base metal alloys a minimum thickness in the porcelain-bearing areas of 0.2 mm is needed to ensure rigidity (see Table 3-4). High-noble alloys, especially those with a very high gold content, should have a minimum thickness of 0.3 mm; there is no maximum. For example, when a major portion of a tooth has been lost to dental caries, fracture, or a previous restoration, the metal substructure may be 2.0 mm or even 3.0 mm thick. Such a dimension is required to reestablish the lost tooth form and ensure a uniform thickness of porcelain in the completed restoration.

Additional demands are placed on the connector areas of fixed partial dentures. The simplest rule for connector design is to create as large a surface area as possible without impinging on gingival tissues or interfering with esthetics.[16] A connector that lacks sufficient bulk in either a labiolingual or an incisogingival dimension is apt to flex under function.[16]

The design principles for metal-ceramic pontics and connectors are discussed later in this chapter. An understanding of these basic principles is imperative for designing substructures that will endure the variety of clinical situations encountered.

Suggestion:
Regardless of the type of alloy you select, leave a minimum thickness of wax in the porcelain-bearing area to ensure that the wax pattern can be cast completely and provide a rigid substructure. Be sure to allow for a slight loss of volume of alloy simply from the metal-finishing procedures.

facial porcelain connector

Allow slight loss of alloy from metal finishing

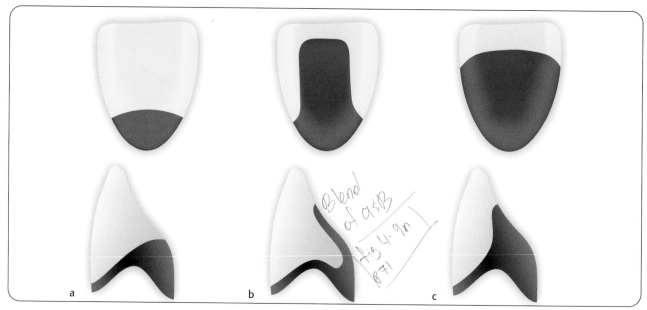

Fig 4-7 There are several design options for restorations of maxillary anterior teeth. *(a)* When esthetics are paramount and there is adequate tooth structure, the lingual surface may be veneered in porcelain. *(b)* A metal lingual surface also may be modified so that the marginal ridges are in porcelain for maximum light transmission, yet the principal functional area is restored in metal. *(c)* The lingual surface may be restored in metal. Of course, variations of these basic three designs also are possible.

Single-Unit Restorations

Procedures for maxillary anterior substructure designs

In restorations for maxillary anterior teeth, more emphasis is typically placed on esthetics than on any other single requirement. Occasionally, this creates a conflict for technicians and clinicians. Realistically, not all cases lend themselves to ideal substructure design. Therefore, you must be prepared for instances in which you have to decide whether to rigidly follow design principles at the expense of esthetics, or attempt to achieve maximum esthetics at the expense of an ideal design and potentially risk mechanical failure of the restoration.

> The extent to which the lingual surface is restored by porcelain or metal is dictated by two factors: the location of occlusal contacts (if present) and the amount of clearance (tooth reduction) with the opposing dentition.

The three basic design options for maxillary incisors are illustrated in Fig 4-7. The major differences between them are the shape and the height of the lingual surface. Of course, combinations of these designs are used often. However, the extent to which the lingual surface is restored by porcelain or metal is dictated by two factors: (1) the location of occlusal contacts (if present), and (2) the amount of clearance (tooth reduction) with the opposing dentition.

Location of occlusal contacts

If the mandibular anterior teeth contact the lingual surfaces of the maxillary anterior teeth in centric occlusion, articulating film can be used to identify the location of those contact areas. When centric occlusal contacts are located in the incisal half of the restoration (Fig 4-8), the ceramic veneer may be extended over the incisal edge of the maxillary teeth for occlusion in porcelain. If these occlusal contacts are located in the gingival half of the restoration (see Fig 4-8c), it is better to restore the anterior teeth in metal rather than porcelain.

According to the concept of *mutually protected articulation* (also known as *canine-protected articulation* or *organic articulation*), when the anterior teeth are in centric occlusion, they are out of contact by approximately 25 µm, or two thicknesses of 12.7-µm (0.005-inch) shimstock.[17] The design of the lingual aspect of the metal-ceramic substructure should then be based on the clinician's preference of restorative materials (metal versus porcelain) and the amount of clearance available.

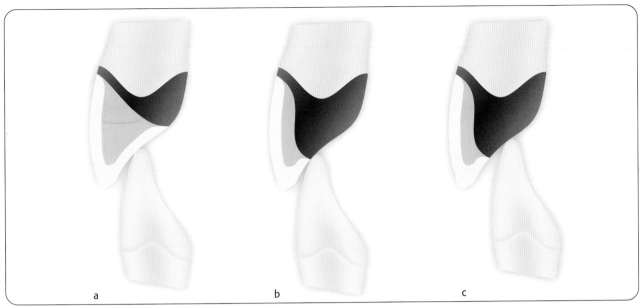

Fig 4-8 *(a)* When the anterior teeth contact in the incisal region, it is often necessary to consider a design with porcelain on the lingual surface to avoid function on or over the porcelain-metal junction. *(b)* Do not design the substructure so that contact occurs at the porcelain-metal junction. *(c)* When the anterior teeth occlude in the gingival half of the maxillary teeth or when the lingual tooth reduction is less than 1.0 mm, it is better to design the substructure with the occlusion in metal than in porcelain.

Amount of clearance (tooth reduction)

One of the advantages of restoring the lingual surface of anterior teeth with metal is that the maximum amount of tooth reduction needed ranges from 0.7 to 1.0 mm depending on the location of the porcelain-metal junction, whereas dental porcelain would require at least 1.0 mm of tooth reduction to accommodate the recommended thicknesses for both the metal substrate and the ceramic veneer. It is technically possible to fabricate the lingual surface in metal with less than 0.7 mm of lingual tooth reduction, but such a situation is not ideal for all types of metal-ceramic alloys, and it may limit your ability to reproduce the desired depths of natural lingual anatomy in the final restoration.

Regardless of the location of the occlusal contacts or the amount of tooth reduction, contacts located at or near the porcelain-metal junction during closure and in excursive movements should be avoided (see Fig 4-4). If possible, porcelain should overlap the incisal edges of the coping onto the lingual surface to reproduce the appearance of natural incisal translucency. This overlap can be as little as 2.0 mm; however, a substructure that does not include this design feature may lead to failure in anterior restorations.

> According to the concept of *mutually protected articulation* (also known as *canine-protected articulation* or *organic articulation*), the anterior teeth are out of contact by approximately 25 μm, or two thicknesses of shimstock, in centric occlusion.

Wax pattern fabrication for anterior copings

Wax pattern fabrication need not be challenging. By following a few simple procedures, satisfactory substructures can be waxed as a matter of routine.

Maxillary anterior substructures with a metal lingual surface

The first step in creating a substructure is to obtain a wax coping that is free of defects and well adapted to the die. Discard patterns with voids in the intaglio (interior) surface; such discrepancies indicate insufficient adaptation of the wax to the die and translate into poor fit. Wax patterns that are not well adapted also may unnecessarily increase the contour of the final restorations. A discrepancy of only 0.2 to 0.3 mm, for example, can have a significant adverse effect on the esthetic results of a metal-ceramic restoration.

The master die can be dipped into wax to cover the entire prepared surface, or alternatively, wax can be applied directly to the die in large increments with the use of a hot wax spatula. Using either technique, you must visually inspect the internal surface of the coping after proper

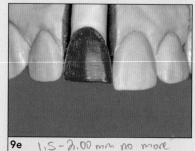
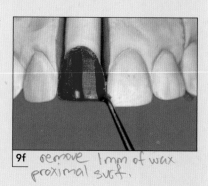

Fig 4-9a The tooth to be restored is waxed to its full and correct anatomic contour. This is probably the most frequently ignored step in the entire waxing procedure. Do not rely on "eyeballing" the contours of the wax pattern as the means to achieve the proper design. Technicians who appreciate the importance of proper contour are more likely to rely on the full-contour waxing technique than on free-hand waxing. In fact, many highly skilled technicians insist on waxing to full contour even for "simple" single-unit restorations. As with so many procedures in dentistry, the technicians most in need of an established procedure, such as waxing to full contour, are the ones least likely to recognize their own limitations and the benefits of this technique.

Fig 4-9b Using the full-contour wax pattern, determine the location of the patient's centric and excursive occlusal contacts, then scribe a line for the position of the porcelain-metal junction at least 1.5 mm and as much as 2.0 mm from the closest occlusal contact. Mark the wax pattern just lingual to the interproximal contact areas to indicate the most *labial* position of the metal interproximally if the contact areas are to be restored in porcelain.

Fig 4-9c Next, scribe a line 0.5 to 1.0 mm above the marginal finish line across the labial surface and a second line 1.5 mm from the incisal edge across the labial surface.

Fig 4-9d Remove the die and wax pattern from the master cast. Connect the lines drawn for the porcelain-metal junction on the lingual surface with the interproximal lines. You should end up with a continuous outline for the areas of the wax pattern that are to be cut back.

Fig 4-9e Reduce the incisal edge by at least 1.5 mm to provide sufficient space to re-create the appearance of natural translucency but by no more than 2.0 mm to avoid excessive unsupported porcelain. Carefully evaluate the wax pattern from the facial, incisal, and lingual aspects.

Fig 4-9f The wax pattern is now ready to be cut back. The objective of the cutback procedure is to remove a minimum uniform thickness of approximately 1.0 mm of wax from all proximal surfaces of the substructure that will be covered in porcelain. To facilitate the cutback, begin by making a 1.0-mm-deep cut in the midfacial region of the wax pattern. Follow with cuts of the same depth at both the mesial and the distal line angles.

cooling to confirm that the wax is well adapted and free of voids before proceeding to the next step (Figs 4-9 to 4-11). It is helpful to use a binocular microscope or magnifying loupes in the evaluation process to assess fine detail and detect discrepancies. You also may find it easier to identify defects in the intaglio surface of patterns using a light-colored wax (eg, yellow, green, red) rather than a dark-colored wax (eg, blue, dark green).

Metal lingual restoration

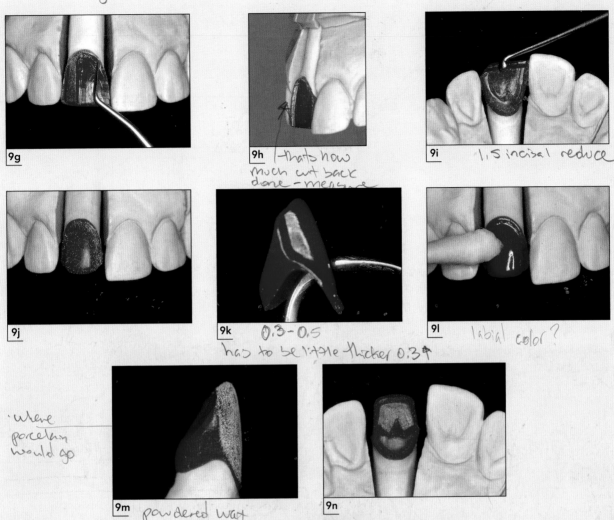

9g

9h — that's how much cut back done - measure

9i   1.5 incisal reduce

9j

9k   0.3-0.5
has to be little thicker 0.3+

9l   labial color?

• where porcelain would go

9m   powdered wax

9n

Fig 4-9g Remove all of the wax between two of the depth cuts, remaining within the outline of the porcelain-metal junction.

Fig 4-9h With half of the facial surface still intact, examine the profile of the cutback to ensure that a uniform thickness of wax has been removed.

Fig 4-9i Use a discoid carver or similarly shaped instrument to refine the porcelain-metal junction on the labial and lingual surfaces. The shape of the instrument will create a sharp external finish line and a rounded internal line angle.

Fig 4-9j Evaluate the cutback on the master cast for proper extension and adequate clearance by viewing it from all angles—labial, lingual, and incisal.

Fig 4-9k Using the rounded tips of the Iwanson wax caliper, measure the thickness of the wax pattern. The porcelain-bearing area of the wax pattern should measure from 0.3 to 0.5 mm, depending on the type of alloy that will be used and the requirements of the particular case. Leave sufficient wax to ensure that the pattern can be cast completely and metal finished to the desired final thickness.

Fig 4-9l Smooth any sharp line angles to produce rounded contours. A cotton swab moistened with debubblizer and warmed by a flame can be used for this procedure. If the substructure is to have a labial metal

collar, seal the margins before cutting back in this area. Leave a 0.3 to 0.5 mm height to the labial collar and allow metal finishing to reduce it to its final dimension. The height of the labial metal collar is determined by the length of the labial bevel, assuming a bevel is present on the preparation. However, when the tooth has been prepared with a very wide bevel, esthetic consideration may demand that the collar's final dimension be reduced to only 0.3 mm. (Several acceptable finish line designs are discussed later in this chapter).

Fig 4-9m Redefine the porcelain-metal junction until it is sharp, continuous, and well defined. The wax should form a 90-degree external line angle at the junction line. At this point, the full-contour waxing technique has accomplished two objectives considered vital to the success of the completed metal-ceramic restoration. First, and perhaps more important, is the formation of an even thickness of the cutback. Second is the formation of continuous and anatomically correct crown contours at the porcelain-metal junction.

Fig 4-9n The anterior substructure design illustrated in Fig 4-7b is a blend of designs 4-7a and 4-7c since it retains most of the metal on the lingual surface yet permits restoration of the interproximal areas in porcelain.

another way of cutbuck

△ 18 g wire on lingual   (Central)

under mag. or microscope

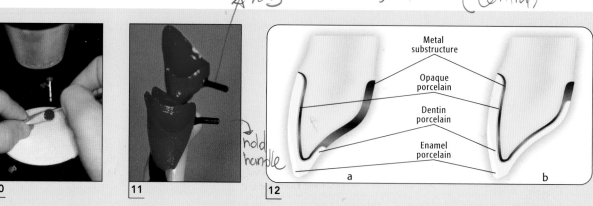

hold handle

| 10 | 11 | 12 |

Fig 4-10 Use some form of magnification (such as a microscope, shown here) whenever possible to critically evaluate your work, whether you are assessing the intaglio surface of a wax pattern, marginating a wax pattern, or attaching sprue formers. Contemporary microscopes with flexible arms are available to facilitate the inspection of laboratory work.

Fig 4-11 Two pieces of 18-gauge wax have been attached to the lingual collars of each retainer of this three-unit fixed partial denture; these should be luted *before* the wax sprue formers are attached to the wax

patterns. Invest the wax pattern as soon as possible after it has been completed and the margins finalized. Once cast, these metal extensions can be grasped without fear of damaging the delicate metal margins. This technique also can be used for single-unit metal-ceramic copings.

Fig 4-12 Prepare a substructure design like those shown in Fig 4-7. The basic difference between an anterior metal-ceramic restoration with a metal lingual surface *(a)* and one with a porcelain lingual surface *(b)* is the extent of the porcelain coverage and the height of the lingual metal collar.

everything smooth

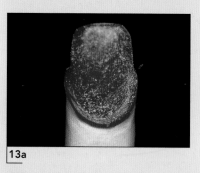 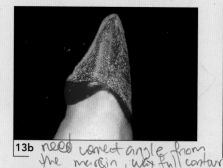 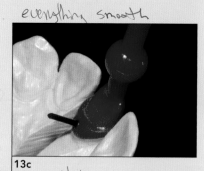

| 13a | 13b | 13c |

need correct angle from the margin, wax full contour, overbuild it

Fig 4-13a Cut back the facial surface of the wax pattern using the technique illustrated in Figs 4-9a to 4-9l, but extend the location of the porcelain-metal junction cervical to the occlusal contacts on the lingual surface.

Fig 4-13b Leave at least 2.0 mm of metal in the midlingual area to provide rigidity to the substructure, and then smooth the entire wax pat-

tern. The wider lingual collar can be tapered through the interproximal area to blend with the facial metal collar. In the absence of a facial metal collar, taper the lingual collar accordingly.

Fig 4-13c Lute an 18-gauge sprue former to the lingual collar to create a handle, and attach a wax sprue former to the wax pattern in preparation for investing.

Maxillary anterior substructures with a porcelain lingual surface

The technique for fabricating an anterior metal ceramic-crown substructure with the lingual surface restored in porcelain (Fig 4-12) is virtually the same as that presented in Figs 4-9 to 4-11. The major difference is the extent of the cutback; all other procedures are identical (Fig 4-13).

Maxillary posterior substructure design

The substructure for maxillary posterior teeth is constructed according to the design principles outlined previously. However, you often have more freedom in the final substructure

design because, generally speaking, esthetic requirements for posterior teeth may be less stringent. The basic design options are illustrated in Fig 4-14.

As in anterior restorations, the posterior crown is waxed to full contour with the desired occlusion. How the wax pattern is completed depends, of course, on whether the occlusal surface is to be restored in metal or porcelain. By waxing the restoration to full contour, the exact location of the occlusal contacts and the cusp-fossa contours can be established and evaluated. If the occlusal surface is to be maintained in metal, the occlusion should be finalized in the full-contoured wax pattern. If the final restoration is to have complete porcelain occlusal coverage, the occlusion is not finalized in wax but subsequently is developed in the porcelain veneer. Deter-

[handwritten: ← Same Principle →]

[handwritten: (Bi)]

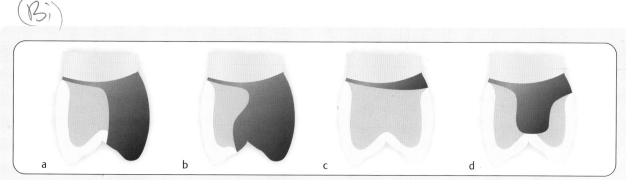

Fig 4-14 Four basic design options for maxillary posterior restorations: substructures with occlusal surfaces in metal and interproximal contacts in porcelain *(a)* or metal *(b)*, and substructures with porcelain occlusal surfaces without *(c)* or with *(d)* interproximal support in metal.

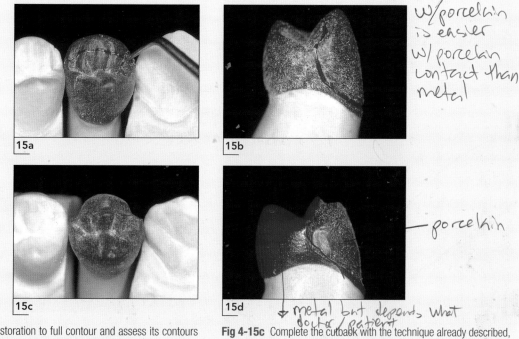

[handwritten: w/ porcelain is easier w/ porcelain contact than metal]

[handwritten: — porcelain]

[handwritten: → metal but depends what doctor / patient]

Fig 4-15a Wax the restoration to full contour and assess its contours from occlusal and facial views. Dust the pattern with powdered wax and locate the areas of occlusal contacts. Scribe a line on the inner incline of the buccal cusp from the distal to the mesial, 2.0 mm from any area of occlusal contact.

Fig 4-15b Scribe the gingival and interproximal lines for the proposed cutback. Remove the die and wax pattern from the master cast, and connect the occlusal and interproximal scribe lines for the cutback.

Fig 4-15c Complete the cutback with the technique already described, and then view the completed wax pattern from occlusal and facial views.

Fig 4-15d Carefully examine the cutback to make certain sufficient wax has been removed to ensure that the ceramic veneer will be uniform in all areas. If the interproximal contact area is to be restored in porcelain (see Fig 4-14a) rather than metal (see Fig 4-14b), extend the cutback of the porcelain-metal junction further lingually.

mining an appropriate occlusal relationship is vitally important because it will ensure a proper cutback as well as a uniform thickness of porcelain for the final restoration.

Regardless of which restorative material is chosen for the occlusal table, you should analyze the preparation clearance with the opposing teeth in centric occlusion and during all excursive movements. Check the right and left lateral excursions and protrusive (anterior) jaw movement. If a restoration with a porcelain occlusal surface is to have satisfactory esthetics and proper contours, a minimum of

1.5 mm of occlusal reduction is necessary, but 2.0 mm is preferred. Check the intra-arch reduction as well.

Maxillary posterior substructures with a metal occlusal surface

Whether because the esthetics are less critical or minimal tooth reduction is possible, some cases lend themselves to restoring the occlusal surface in metal (Fig 4-15). The technique is similar to that described for anterior restorations.

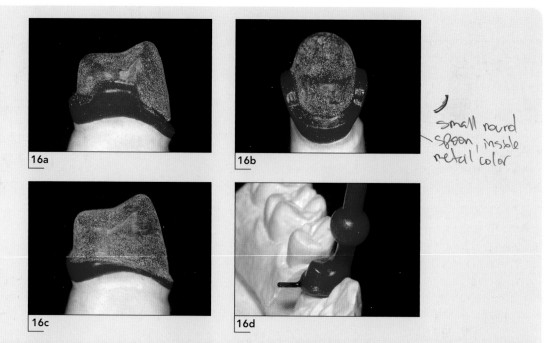

handwritten note: small round spoon, inside metal color

Figs 4-16a and 4-16b The extent of the wax cutback will depend on the occlusogingival height of the tooth being restored and the esthetic requirements for restoring the interproximal area. Support the marginal ridge by retaining metal in the interproximal (Fig 4-16a) and lingual (Fig 4-16b) areas.

Fig 4-16c Alternatively, cut back the interproximal area (see Fig 4-14c), creating a 2.0-mm lingual collar through the interproximal area to the facial metal collar.

Fig 4-16d Examine the completed wax pattern from all views (occlusal, lingual, and interproximal) to make certain the cutback is correct and the wax pattern is smooth. Lute an 18-gauge wax sprue former to the middle of the lingual collar to facilitate handling of the restoration once the substructure has been cast. Attach a wax sprue former to the completed pattern (as shown), and make certain the transition from sprue former to wax pattern is smooth and without irregularities.

Maxillary posterior substructures with a porcelain occlusal surface

Esthetics may necessitate the use of porcelain rather than metal in the design of occlusal surfaces. For these cases, the substructure will be much like that of an anterior restoration with a porcelain lingual surface (Fig 4-16). The principal requirement is sufficient tooth reduction for adequate interarch and intra-arch clearance to accommodate the thickness of the metal substructure and the porcelain veneer.

Again, you should wax the restoration to full contour to reproduce the proper axial contours. Then select the type of substructure most appropriate for the particular clinical case (see Figs 4-14c and 4-14d) and continue with the steps outlined in Fig 4-16.

Mandibular anterior substructure designs

When the mandibular anterior teeth are in a normal Class I occlusal relationship in terms of horizontal and vertical overlap, esthetic demands necessitate restoration of the incisal, labial, and interproximal surfaces in porcelain, with a small lingual metal collar, if present. In situations where lingual tooth reduction has been minimal, that surface may be readily restored with an adequate thickness of metal. However, overlapping of the porcelain onto the incisal-lingual surface is recommended for strength.

Mandibular posterior substructure designs

Mandibular posterior teeth are not always completely visible in normal function and speech; therefore, it may not be necessary to restore them with metal-ceramic restorations. From a strictly functional point of view, these teeth often can be adequately restored with complete metal crowns. Nevertheless, patient and clinician preferences vary enormously, and it is not uncommon to receive requests to restore mandibular first molars and, on occasion, mandibular second molars with metal-ceramic crowns with porcelain occlusal surfaces.

Figure 4-17 illustrates four substructure designs that have been used historically for the mandibular posterior region. These are only basic design configuration options, any one

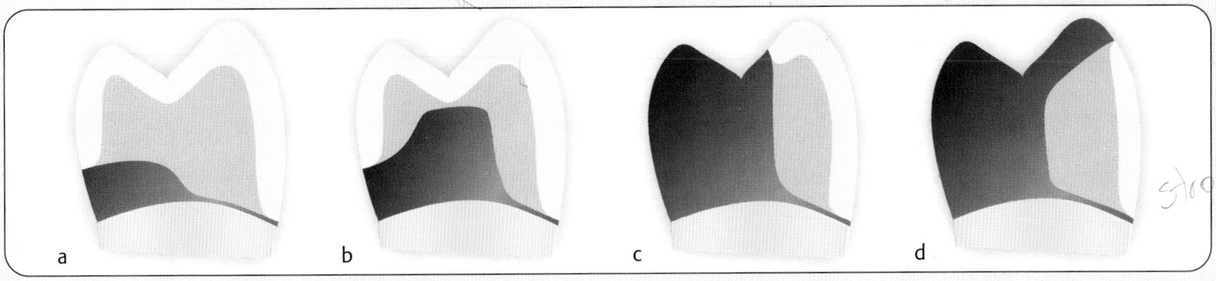

Mandibular posterior

stronger

Fig 4-17 Four basic substructure designs for the mandibular posterior teeth.

of which may be modified to meet the specific and unique occlusal and esthetic requirements of a particular patient. The results of one study found no differences in strength, as measured by load to failure, between the first three substructure designs (see Figs 4-17a to 4-17c).[18] However, the coping design with a metal occlusal and facial window (see Fig 4-17d) was found to be significantly stronger. Owing to the growing emphasis on esthetics, however, substructures with this design are uncommon despite the strength advantage provided by the metal coping.

Unfortunately, the complete porcelain occlusal design is often prescribed for an underprepared or otherwise poorly suited clinical situation. The net result is an overadjusted restoration or opposing tooth. In either case, the error is made at diagnosis and/or again at the time of tooth preparation by a failure to obtain the requisite 1.5 to 2.0 mm occlusal reduction.

Short clinical crowns, a not-uncommon characteristic of mandibular posterior teeth, are more ideally suited for restorations with metal occlusal surfaces. Bear in mind that restorations with complete porcelain coverage quickly become esthetically compromised when large areas of opaque or metal are exposed, or nearly exposed, as a result of extensive occlusal adjustment resulting from a lack of interocclusal space.

> Bear in mind that restorations with complete porcelain coverage quickly become esthetically compromised when large areas of opaque or metal are exposed, or nearly exposed, as a result of extensive occlusal adjustment resulting from a lack of interocclusal space.

addressed before a multiple-unit substructure is cast. For example, will the prosthesis be cast in one piece or in sections? If you choose to make a two-piece casting, you must also decide whether the framework will be presoldered or postsoldered. If you choose preceramic soldering, you must consider the location of the solder connector(s). Will the connector(s) be located interproximally or diagonally through a pontic? The very design of the substructure in the connector areas must allow for the location of possible solder joint(s).

All of these issues are important determinants in the fabrication of a fixed prosthesis; however, the basic concepts discussed here are applicable whether the substructure is cast as a single unit or as multiple units and soldered. More extensive discussion of connector and pontic design can be found in Riley,[16] Shillingburg et al,[17] and Yamamoto.[3]

Anterior fixed partial denture substructure design

Modified ridge lap pontic

Figure 4-18a illustrates a basic design for the anterior pontic, referred to as a *modified ridge lap pontic*.[6,13,19] This configuration is often favored in the replacement of missing anterior teeth because the labial extension of the pontic offers maximum esthetics and permits proper cleaning of the convex lingual and gingival contours of the prosthesis.[17] This well-designed pontic substructure promotes a uniform thickness of porcelain even in the gingival region, where the cervical third of the pontic is composed of porcelain, and the porcelain-metal junction is located well

Fixed Partial Dentures

The same basic principles and design considerations used in fabricating a single-unit metal coping can be applied in planning the substructure for a metal-ceramic fixed partial denture. However, several technical issues must be

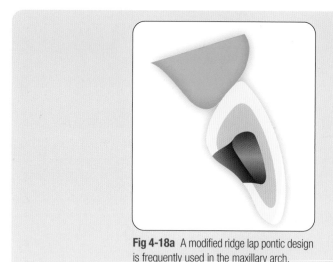

Fig 4-18a A modified ridge lap pontic design is frequently used in the maxillary arch.

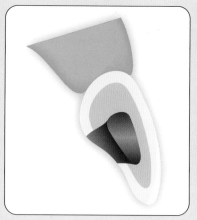

Fig 4-18b The ovate pontic design is popular for replacing maxillary anterior teeth.

away from the soft tissue of the edentulous ridge. Regardless of the amount of care taken during the finishing and polishing procedures, the junction of the porcelain and metal is a potential source of roughness and tissue irritation, yet it would obviously be esthetically unacceptable to extend the metal substructure onto the labial aspect of the gingival portion of the pontic. The logical alternative is to restore all tissue contact in porcelain. An additional advantage to this type of pontic design is that highly glazed porcelain has been shown to be more resistant to plaque accumulation than metal.[1,20]

The same general design considerations for the location of occlusal contacts and lingual contour with single-unit restorations would apply to the design of retainers for a fixed partial denture.

Ovate pontic

The ovate pontic (Fig 4-18b) has reemerged as a popular alternative to a modified ridge lap pontic to replace missing anterior teeth in the effort to retain the papillae and give the illusion that the pontic is emerging from the edentulous ridge.[21–24] To promote the practice of good oral hygiene by the patient, it is important to make sure that any porcelain in contact with tissue is highly polished and that the embrasures are properly shaped and opened for ready access.[25]

Procedures for an anterior fixed partial denture

An accurate full-contoured wax pattern is even more critical for a fixed partial denture than for a single-unit restoration. The occlusal scheme should be finalized in centric occlusion as well as in all excursions (left lateral, right lateral, and protrusive movements). The size and position of the pontic(s) need to be established in wax because it is far easier to make contour adjustments in wax than in either porcelain or metal. Moreover, the size and position of the interproximal connectors and their accompanying labial, incisal, and gingival embrasures can be evaluated. The following steps offer valuable guidance for proper anterior fixed partial denture design.

In framework design, it is important to understand that the degree of deformation of the metal is proportional to the cube of the length.[16] When the length of the fixed partial denture is doubled and the load remains constant, the degree of deflection reportedly increases by a factor of eight. Even more significant is that if the span (number of pontics) of the prosthesis is increased 3 times and the load remains constant, the degree of deflection increases by a factor of 27.[16] Consequently, an increase in the length of the span of a fixed partial denture has a profound effect on the stresses placed on the interproximal connectors. Moreover, significant consequences ensue when the proper connector dimensions are compromised. If the occluso-gingival thickness of a given connector is reduced by half, the resulting deflection will be 8 times as great. This is particularly important with long-span posterior fixed partial dentures.

Follow the steps outlined in Fig 4-19.

Posterior fixed partial denture substructure design

A posterior fixed partial denture substructure is fabricated essentially according to the same design principles that

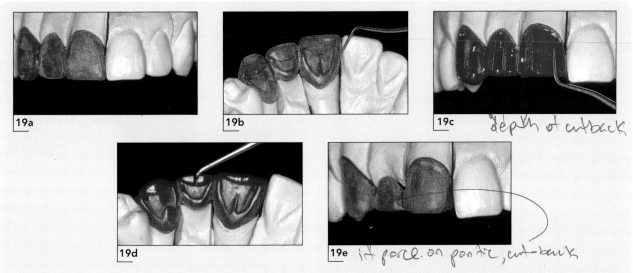

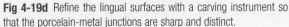

Fig 4-19a Carefully inspect the fixed partial denture waxed to full contour to ensure that it has the proper contours and outline form sought in a fixed restoration.

Fig 4-19b After the occlusion is marked, scribe a line on the lingual surfaces of the wax pattern to indicate the location of the porcelain-metal junction. Place a scribe line on the facial surface to indicate the boundary of the incisal cutback. Connect the facial and lingual scribe lines in the interproximal areas as done previously with the anterior single-unit restoration (see Fig 4-15b). Cut back the incisal edges.

Fig 4-19c Place three facial depth cuts in each unit. Carefully remove the wax in between each depth cut with a warmed instrument to complete the cutback on the facial surface.

Fig 4-19d Refine the lingual surfaces with a carving instrument so that the porcelain-metal junctions are sharp and distinct.

Fig 4-19e After the cutback, critique the substructure from the facial, incisal, and lingual views. Note the removal of 1.0 mm of wax from the tissue side of the pontic to permit that area to be restored in porcelain. You can now attach appropriate-sized sprue formers to the completed wax pattern, along with a 3.0- to 4.0-mm-long piece of 18-gauge wax to each retainer pattern, to facilitate handling of the cast substructure during porcelain application. Take care to avoid potential damage to the metal margins. The completed pattern can be luted to the connector (reservoir) bar of a prefabricated indirect wax sprue former (see chapter 5) and invested immediately.

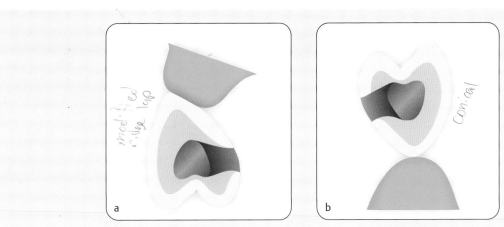

Fig 4-20 *(a)* A popular design to replace missing posterior teeth is the modified ridge lap pontic. *(b)* The conical configuration is an alternative design used with metal-ceramic restorations.

apply to single-unit posterior restorations. Two basic pontic designs are illustrated in Fig 4-20. As with the anterior fixed partial denture, the modified ridge lap pontic is the design most widely used to replace missing posterior teeth (see Fig 4-20a). An alternative option is the conical configuration (see Fig 4-20b), but this pontic design usually is restricted to less visible areas of mandibular posterior restorations. The steps are outlined in Fig 4-21.

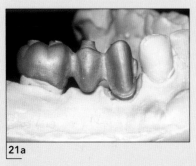
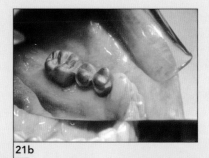
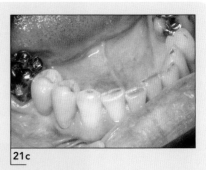

21a   21b   21c

Fig 4-21a Uniform cutback of the wax is reflected in this one-piece, three-unit fixed partial denture framework fitted to the solid (uncut) master cast.

Fig 4-21b The fit of the framework noted on the master cast is confirmed during a clinical try-in. The gingival area of the pontic is adjusted, if additional clearance is needed, to ensure that the proper

tissue-porcelain relationship can be created. A soft tissue cast can be used to replicate the edentulous area in this step.

Fig 4-21c The final restoration has a porcelain veneer that is esthetic and well supported by the underlying metal substructure. The tissue side of the pontic (not visible in this photo) had sufficient body porcelain thickness for esthetics and strength and was polished mechanically after glazing.

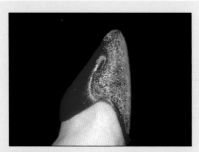

interprox in metal

Fig 4-22 If you wish to restore the interproximal contacts in metal, the porcelain-metal junction line will lie facial to the contact area, as illustrated in Fig 4-9j. Should you prefer to retain metal contacts but also want to maximize the extension of porcelain into the interproximal areas, you can create a scalloped effect by removing the wax *below* and *lingual to* the contact area.

Interprox in porcelain

Fig 4-23 To retain the lingual surface in metal while restoring the interproximal contacts in porcelain, simply move the porcelain-metal junction *lingual to* the contact area. When you choose a substructure with a porcelain lingual surface, the interproximal areas should be restored in porcelain.

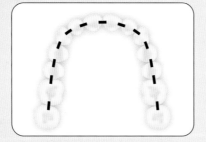

Fig 4-24a Location of interproximal contacts *(bold lines)* for the maxillary arch.

Fig 4-24b Location of interproximal contacts *(bold lines)* for the mandibular arch.

Designing the Interproximal Areas of Substructures

The third principle of substructure design involves determining the restorative material (ie, metal or porcelain) to be used in the interproximal contact areas. However, the designs for the anterior and posterior substructures provide only approximate

locations for the porcelain-metal junction in the interproximal areas (see Figs 4-9d, 4-9m, 4-15b, and 4-15d).

The design of the interproximal porcelain-metal junction in the final restoration depends on the location of the interproximal contact areas and whether these areas are to be restored in porcelain or metal (Figs 4-22 and 4-23). You should know the location of these interproximal contact areas for the maxillary (Fig 4-24a) and the mandibular

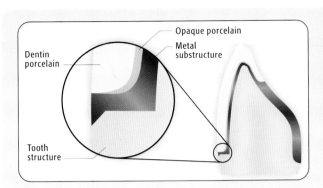

Fig 4-25 Ninety-degree (square shoulder) bevel finish line. Note that the collar of exposed metal should be at least as wide as the bevel itself.

tissue response

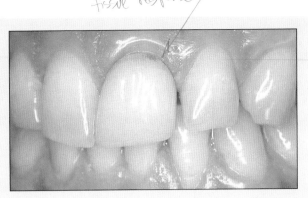

Fig 4-26 Note the adverse marginal tissue response (gingival inflammation and recession) at the facial margin on the maxillary left central incisor created by the poorly contoured restoration.

arches (Fig 4-24b).[26] Once you have identified the correct faciolingual location of the interproximal contact areas, decide if you want to retain that contact in metal or porcelain (see Fig 4-7a). If you opt to use porcelain, simply move the porcelain-metal junction until it is lingual to that area (see Fig 4-7b).

Margin Designs for Metal-Ceramic Restorations

The dentist should select the appropriate margin (shoulder) design at the time of tooth preparation so that he or she can prepare the proper finish line for the case. The design of the labial margin of a metal-ceramic restoration can be finalized during the waxing and margination of the wax pattern.

Finish line designs representative of those most commonly used, and the margins that are produced by each, are illustrated and described later in this chapter.

Ninety-degree (square shoulder) bevel finish line

The *90-degree bevel* finish line angle (Fig 4-25) is believed to provide internal buttressing of the shoulder margin.[27] If the shoulder is angled more than 90 degrees, the finish line design is then referred to as a *slant shoulder*.

Any finish line preparation that includes a bevel should be accompanied by a restoration with a collar of exposed metal at least as wide as the bevel itself. Obviously, this exposed metal collar can present an unacceptable esthetic result in some situations. When a bevel is present, attempts to cover

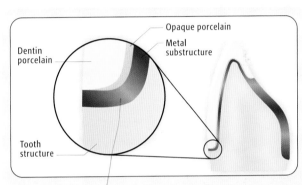

Fig 4-27 Rounded shoulder, or deep, chamfer finish line.

axial gingival-angle is rounded
Rounded shoulder/with or without bevel

all of the substructure with porcelain invariably result in an overcontoured restoration. Even slight overcontouring in the gingival 1.0 or 2.0 mm of a restoration usually creates an adverse marginal tissue response (Fig 4-26).

Rounded shoulder (deep chamfer) finish line

The *rounded shoulder*, or *deep chamfer*, finish line (Fig 4-27) is the same design as the 90-degree, or square shoulder, bevel finish line except that the internal (axial-gingival) line angle is rounded. The rounded shoulder finish line too can be prepared with or without a bevel. If the shoulder is slanted more than 90 degrees, it can also be called a *slant shoulder finish line*.

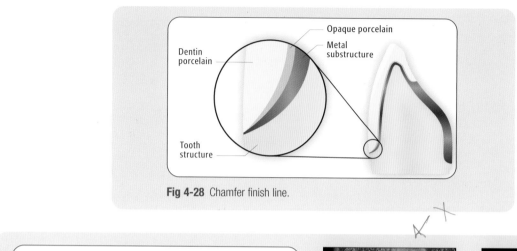

Fig 4-28 Chamfer finish line.

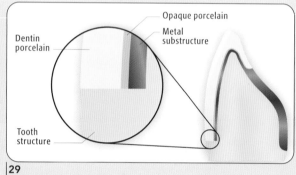

29

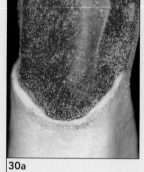

30a

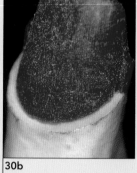

30b

Fig 4-29 Ninety-degree (square shoulder) finish line.

Fig 4-30a Incorrectly waxed substructure for a metal-ceramic crown with a porcelain margin. The exposed shoulder is too narrow and irregular.

Fig 4-30b When correctly designed, the coping will have a uniform exposed shoulder that extends well into the interproximal areas. Alternatively, some technicians prefer to wax and cast a complete substructure and then finish the metal to the desired substructure design.

Chamfer finish line

The *chamfer* finish line design (Fig 4-28) allows the technician to feather the metal at the labial margin so that only a minimal amount of exposed metal margin is visible in the completed crown. When meticulous attention is paid to waxing, metal finishing, and porcelain application, the result can be an esthetically acceptable restoration even in certain demanding clinical situations.

Ninety-degree (square shoulder) finish line

Although the labial margin in this metal-ceramic restoration design is constructed with porcelain, a properly designed substructure is nonetheless essential. The finish line for the labial surface should be a shoulder of approximately 1.0-mm width. The junction of the shoulder and the axial wall

of the preparation generally is a well-defined line angle of 90 degrees[3] (Fig 4-29) but can be managed if it is slightly rounded.

If this finish line design is to be used for a metal-ceramic crown with a porcelain margin, there are several opinions as to where the metal should terminate in relation to the shoulder.[3] Some prefer to stop the metal axially just short of the shoulder, leaving approximately 0.5 mm of the axial wall exposed. Others recommend extending the metal substructure so it terminates at the axial-gingival line angle of the shoulder itself.[28] Most often, the metal ends at the junction of the axial wall and the prepared shoulder (see Fig 4-29).

The same substructure design principle prevails here as in all other areas: The ultimate goal is to attain uniform thickness of porcelain at the labial margin (Fig 4-30). If the shoulder is wider than desired because of previous restorations, erosion, dental caries, or some other factor, that extra width should be replaced by the metal substructure rather than the porcelain margin.

A 0.7- to 1.0-mm-wide porcelain margin is considered ideal because it allows 0.2 mm for opaque porcelain and 0.5 to 0.8 mm for margin porcelain. Porcelain thicknesses greater than 1.0 mm with porcelain margin restorations should be avoided. When the shoulder width exceeds 1.0 mm by a significant amount, the porcelain margin is more difficult to fabricate.

Substructure Design Checklist

1. Do you have an accurate full-contoured wax pattern?
2. Are occlusal contacts located 1.5 to 2.0 mm from the porcelain-metal junction?
3. Is there a minimum metal thickness of 0.3 mm for porcelain-bearing areas? (Remember, there is no maximum thickness of metal.)
4. Are all surfaces to be veneered with porcelain smooth with rounded or convex contours? Have you removed all sharp line angles?
5. Does the porcelain-metal junction have a sharp, well-defined cavosurface but rounded internal line angles?
6. Has the substructure been designed to provide a porcelain veneer with a nearly uniform thickness with no areas of more than 2.0 mm of unsupported porcelain? (The veneer thickness may vary from 1.0 mm in the gingival third to a maximum of 1.5 to 2.0 mm at the incisal or occlusal surface).

Summary

It should now be apparent that the essentials of metal-ceramic substructure design are similar for a variety of restorations, from single-unit anterior and posterior crowns to anterior and posterior fixed partial dentures. Aside from a few minor modifications, the substructure for a porcelain margin restoration is prepared in essentially the same manner as any other metal-ceramic substructure.

Taking the time and care to plan and prepare a well-designed metal-ceramic substructure will in part ensure the longevity of the final prosthesis. Chapter 5 describes how to properly sprue, invest, and cast the finished waxed patterns.

References

1. Stein RS, Kuwata M. A dentist and a dental technologist analyze current ceramo-metal procedures. Dent Clin North Am 1977;21: 729–749.
   Authors feature substructure designs for single-unit and fixed partial denture metal-ceramic restorations, and covers topics ranging from decontamination (oxidation) to porcelain application to glazing restorations.

2. van Noort R. Introduction to Dental Materials, ed 3. London: Mosby, 2008.
   Refer to chapter 1 for summary.

3. Yamamoto M. Metal-Ceramics: Principles and Methods of Makoto Yamamoto. Chicago: Quintessence, 1985.
   Refer to chapter 1 for summary.

4. Mackert JR Jr, Butts MB, Fairhurst CW. The effect of the leucite transformation on dental porcelain expansion. Dent Mater 1986;2:32–36.
   Refer to chapter 1 for summary.

5. Naylor WP. Non-Gold Base Dental Casting Alloys. Vol II: Porcelain-fused-to-metal alloys [ADA173766]. Brooks AFB, TX: School of Aerospace Medicine, 1986.

6. Tamura K. Essentials of Dental Technology. Fowler JA (trans). Chicago: Quintessence, 1987.

7. Weiss PA. New design parameters: Utilizing the properties of nickel-chromium superalloys. Dent Clin North Am 1977;21:769–785.
   Classic article on base metal alloys, particularly the Ni-Cr-Be alloys, used for the metal-ceramic restoration. Covers a wide range of topics such as waxing, casting, metal finishing, and establishing a bond with dental porcelain.

8. Miller LL. Framework design in ceramo-metal restorations. Dent Clin North Am 1977;21:699–716.
   Excellent overview of metal-ceramic substructure design for both single units and fixed partial dentures with drawings and photographs and a well-written text.

9. Hobo S, Shillingburg HT Jr. Porcelain fused to metal: Tooth preparation and coping design. J Prosthet Dent 1973;30:28–36.
   Although historical by virtue of the date of publication, this article contains valuable information for tooth preparation and substructure design for single-unit restorations and fixed partial denture metal-ceramic restorations with substructure designs still used today.

10. Phillips RL. Skinner's Science of Dental Materials, ed 8. Philadelphia: Saunders, 1982.

11. Anusavice KJ. Phillips' Science of Dental Materials, ed 11. Philadelphia: Saunders, 2003.
    Refer to Table 13-1 on page 362 for Knoop hardness value.

12. Naylor WP, Munoz CA, Goodacre CJ, Swartz ML, Moore BK. The effect of surface treatment on the Knoop hardness of Dicor. Int J Prosthodont 1991;4:147–151.

13. Rosenstiel SF, Land MF, Fujimoto J. Contemporary Fixed Prosthodontics. St Louis: Mosby, 1988.

14. Dykema RW, Goodacre CJ, Phillips RW. Johnston's Modern Practice in Fixed Prosthodontics, ed 4. Philadelphia: Saunders, 1986.

15. Naylor WP. Introduction to Metal Ceramic Technology. Chicago: Quintessence, 1992.

16. Riley EJ. Ceramo-metal restoration. State of the science. Dent Clin North Am 1977;21:669–682.
Riley includes explanations for engineering principles related to fixed partial denture substructure design for metals, proper metal finishing, and the porcelain-to-metal bond.

17. Shillingburg HT, Hobo S, Whitsett LD. Fundamentals of Fixed Prosthodontics, ed 2. Chicago: Quintessence, 1981.

18. Lund PS, Barber BA. The effect of porcelain veneer extension on strength of metal ceramic crowns. Int J Prosthodont 1992;5: 237–243.
Authors compare the strength (as measured by vertical load to failure) of different substructure designs.

19. Malone WFP, Koth DL. Tylman's Theory and Practice of Fixed Prosthodontics. St Louis: Ishiyaku EuroAmerican, 1989.

20. Chan C, Weber H. Plaque retention on teeth restored with full-ceramic crowns: A comparative study. J Prosthet Dent 1986;56: 666–671.
Authors measured plaque accumulation on an all-ceramic crown (Cerestore), a metal-ceramic crown, a complete gold crown, an acrylic resin provisional crown, and an unrestored natural tooth using the Silness and Löe plaque index. The study found less plaque accumulation on ceramic surfaces compared to the other restorative materials tested.

21. Dewey KW, Zugsmith R. An experimental study of tissue reactions about porcelain roots. J Dent Res 1933;13:459–472.
In their dog studies, the authors found that shallow sockets with porcelain-tipped pontics were completely epithelialized while deep sockets were not. Note: The description "ovate" pontic was not found in this article.

22. Dylina TJ. Contour determination for ovate pontics. J Prosthet Dent 1999;82:136–142.
Dylina describes clinical and laboratory techniques for creating an anterior ovate pontic.

23. Johnson GK, Leary JM. Pontic design and localized ridge augmentation in fixed partial denture design. Dent Clin North Am 1992;36:591–605.
The authors credit KW Dewey and R Zugsmith with first reporting the use of the ovate pontic in their 1933 article, which includes an overview of maxillary anterior pontic designs: sanitary (spheroidal), ovate, saddle, ridge lap, and modified ridge-lap pontic designs.

24. Kois JC, Kan JY. Predictable peri-implant gingival aesthetics: Surgical and prosthodontic rationales. Pract Proced Aesthet Dent 2001;13:691-698, 700, 721–722.
Authors describe a case using an ovate pontic to preserve the gingival architecture until the definitive restoration was placed.

25. Wilson TG Jr, Kornman KS (eds). Fundamentals of Periodontics, ed 2. Chicago: Quintessence, 2003.
Use of the ovate pontic is increasing. Porcelain on the tissue side of an ovate pontic must be highly polished, and embrasures must permit access for proper oral hygiene.

26. Wheeler RC. Dental Anatomy, Physiology, and Occlusion, ed 5. Philadelphia: Saunders, 1974.

27. Preston JD. Rational approach to tooth preparation for ceramo-metal restorations. Dent Clin North Am 1977;21:683–698.
Preston discusses margin designs for the metal-ceramic restoration with and without a circumferential bevel.

28. Vryonis P. A simplified approach to the complete porcelain margin. J Prosthet Dent 1979;41:592–593.
Classic article describing a technique for a porcelain margin with opaque porcelain to the external line angle (exterior finish line). The metal substructure terminates at the axial-gingival line angle. Regular dentin porcelain is fired on the opaque porcelain. This technique preceded the development of high-fusing shoulder porcelains.

CHAPTER 5

Fundamentals of Spruing, Investing, and Casting

Success in the fabrication of metal-ceramic crowns and fixed partial dentures depends to a large extent on the ability to obtain high-quality castings that are not only designed properly but also fit properly. This chapter provides an overview of important topics related to the fundamental principles of spruing, investing, and casting. Emphasis is placed on the laboratory steps in the buttonless casting technique.

Terminology

While the practice of investing and casting wax patterns has been part of dentistry for quite some time, it is not uncommon for several key terms involved in these processes to be used interchangeably. The following definitions are presented to clarify the intended meanings of the terminology found in this chapter. Instead of an alphabetical list, the terms appear in a sequence that is intended to enhance your understanding of their meaning and proper use.

- **Sprue former** In its simplest application, a sprue former is a piece of round dental wax attached to a wax pattern at one end and a crucible former at the other end.[1] Patterns may be sprued directly (from the top of a crucible former straight to the pattern) or indirectly (circuitously from the crucible former to the pattern area). Small metal pins have been used in lieu of wax for direct spruing, and prefabricated wax and plastic sprue former patterns can be purchased for both methods.

- **Sprue way** Channel (void) in a mold created by the elimination of the wax or plastic sprue former network, regardless of whether the technique involves direct or indirect spruing.

- **Sprue** The portion of a metal casting that replicates the sprue former. (Note: Some use the word *sprue* to mean *sprue former*).

- **Direct spruing** A sprue former system that creates a channel from the opening of a mold directly to a pattern area.

- **Indirect spruing** A sprue former system that forms multiple channels in the mold that run circuitously, not directly, from the open end of the mold to the patterns.

- **Runner bar** The part of the indirect spruing system that supports multiple patterns. This bar creates a large sprue way that can retain a reservoir of molten alloy, allowing the pattern areas to solidify completely. A runner bar is sometimes referred to as a *reservoir bar* or a *connector bar*.

- **Reservoir** The portion of a sprue former (in wax) or sprue system (cast metal) that retains a large volume of wax or alloy, respectively. A straight sprue former with a round ball at one end is an example of direct spruing with a reservoir. With indirect spruing, a runner bar performs this role. An effective reservoir is expected to be the largest volume of metal cast and the area that solidifies last. A reservoir ball or runner bar can be a component in a spruing system but not actually function effectively as a reservoir if the thermodynamics inadvertently allow these areas to solidify early and a *button,* or other mass of alloy, solidifies last.

> All castings contain porosity in the area that solidifies last.

- **Crucible former** Round or oval base to which a sprue former or prefabricated sprue former pattern (wax or plastic and direct or indirect) is attached.
- **Wax gauge** Diameter of the wax used in a sprue former. Wax sprue formers are available in a number of different gauges (diameters) with the gauge number inversely related to the size of the wax. That is, the larger the gauge number, the smaller the diameter of the wax.
- **Wax gauge range** The gauge sizes used in dentistry generally range from 18 gauge (1.024 mm/0.0403 inch) to 4 gauge (5.2 mm/0.2048 inch).[2] Popular sizes include 4 gauge, 6 gauge (4.115 mm/0.1620 inch), 8 gauge (3.264 mm/0.1285 inch), 10 gauge (2.588 mm/0.1019 inch), and 12 gauge (2.053 mm/0.0808 inch).
- **Shrink-spot porosity** All castings contain porosity in the area that solidifies last. The main challenge in any casting process is to control the location of that porosity by choosing an appropriate spruing method, creating smooth transitions between components, establishing an appropriate sprue design, avoiding sharp internal angles in the mold, and casting with the correct volume of alloy. Too little or too much alloy can spell disaster for a casting regardless of the spruing design. Shrink-spot porosity also is referred to as *casting porosity, casting shrinkage,* and *solidification shrinkage.*

Spruing Techniques

A spruing system is merely a channel or series of channels in the set investment through which molten alloy flows to reach the wax pattern areas. Consequently, one of the first decisions to make before preparing a wax pattern for investing is which type of spruing system to employ. For best results, this decision should be made on a case-by-case basis to ensure that sufficient molten alloy will be made available to reproduce all of the invested units.

No single method of spruing is universally accepted as the technique of choice. On the contrary, opinions among dental technicians and recommendations by alloy manufacturers differ so widely that at times they may be in direct conflict with one another. For example, some manufacturers may suggest direct spruing whereas others may insist that only indirect spruing should be used with their alloys. To further complicate matters, even reports in the dental literature offer conflicting views of the subject. Nevertheless, it is extremely important to understand the general principles of spruing, including spruing methods (direct versus indirect), sprue placement (or location), sprue gauge (diameter), sprue length, reservoir location, constricted spruing, sprue composition (wax versus plastic), and the value of prefabricated wax sprue formers. This knowledge, linked with practical experience, will greatly improve your chances for successful casting results.

Spruing methods

Wax patterns can be sprued in one of two ways—directly or indirectly. Each method has its advantages and disadvantages, so you should understand the philosophy behind both techniques.

Direct spruing

As the name indicates, direct spruing involves the flow of molten metal straight (directly) from the casting crucible to the pattern area in the ring. This spruing method is not as complex as the indirect method and usually requires less time and effort.

In the direct spruing technique, one end of a straight sprue former is luted (attached) to the thickest part of the wax pattern, and the other end is secured to the crucible former.

Placing a ball reservoir between the pattern and the crucible former is a way to modify the sprue former. Alternatively, prefabricated direct wax sprue formers that include a reservoir also are available.[3–5] The purpose of a reservoir is to supply molten metal needed to fill the pattern areas completely. Despite the presence of a reservoir ball, the spruing method is still considered direct.

Direct spruing is used most frequently for single units (Fig 5-1) and for small, multiple-unit patterns. A weakness of direct spruing is the potential for *suck-back porosity,* which is manifested as a void at the junction of the restoration and the sprue[6] (Fig 5-2).

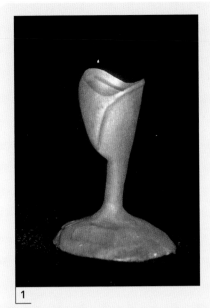

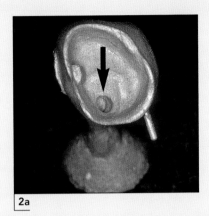

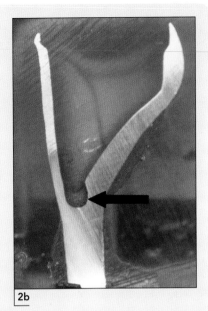

Fig 5-1 Casting produced using direct spruing. The straight sprue former can be modified with a ball reservoir, but the spruing method is still direct.

Fig 5-2a One problem associated with direct spruing is the increased likelihood of suck-back porosity at the pattern-sprue junction. Suck-back

porosity may not be detected externally but may be obvious on examination of the internal aspect *(arrow)* of the casting.

Fig 5-2b Suck-back porosity is apparent *(arrow)* in this cross-sectional view of a maxillary central incisor coping that was cast directly.

Indirect spruing

With indirect spruing, molten alloy does not flow straight from the casting crucible into the pattern area in the heated mold.[4,5,7] Instead, the casting alloy takes a circuitous (indirect) route before it reaches the pattern areas—hence the name *indirect* spruing (Fig 5-3).

Typically, pattern sprue formers are used to attach wax patterns to the superior surface of a round wax runner bar (typically 4 or 6 gauge). The void in the mold formed by the bar eventually is filled with molten alloy via the channels created by the two large ingate, or feeder, sprue formers (see Fig 5-3). The bar's large volume houses molten metal for a sufficient length of time to permit the pattern areas to fill with metal first and draw on this additional molten alloy as needed to complete the solidification process.[8] (This is why the runner bar is often referred to as a *reservoir bar*.) Again, because the molten metal cannot flow directly to the wax pattern areas, this method is referred to as *indirect spruing*.

> A weakness of direct spruing is the potential for suck-back porosity to occur at the junction of the restoration and the sprue.

It also has been shown that alloy composition influences the manner in which metal fills the mold. For example, a palladium-silver alloy fills the mold unidirectionally, whereas Type III gold fills the mold in a random or scattered fashion.[8]

Opinions differ as to the value of indirect spruing for a single crown or for multiple single units.[9,10] Although direct spruing can produce acceptable results, indirect spruing offers such advantages as greater predictability and reliability in casting plus enhanced control of casting porosity. Sprue formers of different lengths and diameters are available (Fig 5-4a). Prefabricated sprue formers not only make it possible to standardize a technique for greater consistency but also help eliminate errors in sprue design and standardize reservoir location as compared to direct spruing. Users of high-noble and noble alloys will find that the cast indirect sprue network can be sectioned into components of a size that can be reused (Fig 5-4b) far more readily than can accumulated buttons (description follows).

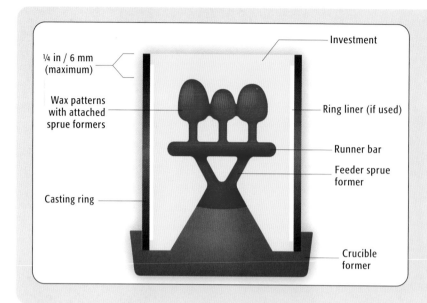

Fig 5-3 Illustration of indirect spruing. These general guidelines should be modified to meet the requirements of each case.

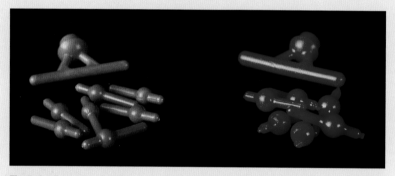

Fig 5-4a Examples of prefabricated direct sprue formers with a reservoir ball and indirect sprue formers (short and long) with runner bars of different gauges (Whip Mix).

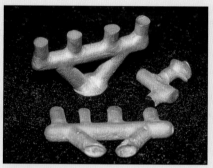

Fig 5-4b The cast indirect spruing network can be sectioned and reused more readily than can buttons of spent metal.

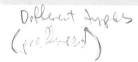

Understanding the Spruing Process

A multitude of factors must be considered before deciding if wax patterns are to be sprued directly or indirectly. The following section presents several key variables that lay the foundation for understanding the rationale for the *buttonless casting technique* and the laws of casting.

Sprue former placement

Ideally, the sprue former attached to the wax pattern (ie, the *pattern* sprue former as opposed to the *feeder* sprue for-

mer) should be luted to the thickest cross-sectional area of the pattern to allow the molten alloy to flow from regions of greater volume (thick areas) to regions of lesser volume (thin sections)[11] (Fig 5-5a). Placing the sprue former elsewhere might result in an incomplete casting if a thin section undergoes solidification before the mold has filled completely.

Of course, there are exceptions to every rule. With many anterior copings, this option is not available nor advisable because the patterns may be small and thin. In such instances, the most practical sprue former location is the midincisal area. The same logic should be used to locate an appropriate site on a molar coping that is to receive complete porcelain coverage. In any case, make certain the attachment of the sprue former to the wax pattern is smooth and uniform without sharp edges,[11,12] and flare this transi-

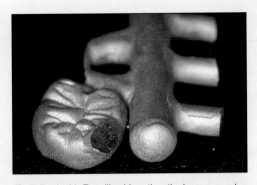

Fig 5-5a In this Type III gold casting, the large runner bar and the attached complete crowns (removed) were cast using a Tri-Wax sprue former (Ivoclar Vivadent). A runner bar of this size (4 gauge) is able to support large metal-ceramic pontics and retainers better than a smaller-diameter (6 gauge) runner bar. Note that the wax pattern was located off the runner bar by approximately 5 mm.

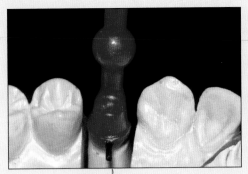

Fig 5-5b A smooth transition from sprue former to wax pattern prevents irregularities in the investment that could break off during casting.

18 gauge

tion from sprue former to wax pattern.[6] Avoid forming ridges that later may become irregularities in the investment, which potentially could break off during casting and contaminate the molten alloy (Fig 5-5b).

Sprue former gauge

A pattern sprue former of sufficient size (gauge) should be selected to supply the volume of alloy required by the patterns to be cast. The larger the gauge number, the smaller the diameter of the sprue former. Manufacturers invariably include sprue gauge recommendations for their alloys, but these suggestions are made without any direct knowledge of the size, geometry, thickness, and number of patterns to be cast. Therefore, it is the technician's responsibility to carefully assess the wax patterns, evaluate the particular requirements of each case, and select the appropriate gauge. When using direct spruing, select a sprue former with a reservoir ball. With indirect spruing, a runner bar should be chosen that is larger than the thickest cross-sectional area of the largest pattern. This requirement is especially critical for metal pontics and large molar retainers (see Fig 5-5a).

> Experience has shown that a 5-mm-long pattern sprue former is often sufficient to separate the wax patterns from the runner bar.

Pattern sprue former length

In the direct spruing method, the pattern sprue formers should be long enough to position the wax patterns outside the heat center of the investment and into a cold zone.[5,13,14] The length of the sprue formers will vary depending on the size of the wax pattern(s), the type and size of the crucible former, and the size (length) of the casting ring.

With indirect spruing, it is recommended that the patterns to be cast should be placed off the runner bar in a location just outside the thermal zone, or *heat center*, of the investment. Experience has shown that a 5-mm-long pattern sprue former is often sufficient to separate the wax patterns from the runner bar (see Fig 5-3).[3]

Incomplete castings may result if the wax patterns are positioned too far away from a runner bar because alloy may solidify in the sprue channel before the patterns have filled completely. Conversely, wax patterns placed on or very close to the runner bar may not undergo orderly solidification; consequently, the process may be compromised by the solidification of the runner bar itself. In other words, you could wind up with a dense, completely cast runner bar and incomplete restorations. Recognizing the need for balance in pattern placement between being too far from and too close to a runner bar comes with experience and thoughtful analysis of sprue former design, measured alloy use, and casting outcomes.

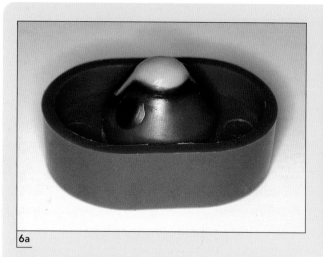
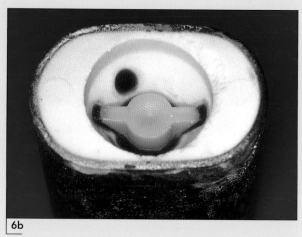

Fig 5-6 A wax orientation dot on the crucible former *(a)* will be picked up by the investment *(b)* and help you to locate the trailing edge of the wax pattern for casting.

Chill sets

Placement of a handle[12,15] or knob, as described by Yamamoto, on a wax pattern can make it easier to hold the metal castings during porcelain application.[16] The length of this handle can range from 2.0 mm[12] to 3.0 mm.[15] If no external handle or knob is placed on the wax pattern, the casting must be grasped over the marginal area—which might damage the margin—or internally with a diamond-tipped instrument, if the work can be removed. To avoid potential patient injury, the handles can be reduced and rounded for subsequent intraoral try-in of either the metal substructure or the bisque-baked porcelain.[16] Some believe these attachments also help the cast restorations cool quickly and properly during the solidification process and refer to them as *chill sets*.[3] According to the theory behind chill set use, molten alloy flows to fill the chill set area (which is closer to the external portion of the mold) where solidification occurs first, allowing the pattern to fill and solidify before the sprue.[3]

Orientation of a wax pattern

The casting of an otherwise properly sprued wax pattern can be jeopardized if the pattern is not correctly oriented in the casting ring. The sprue former must be attached to the thickest portion of the wax pattern. Do not create sharp 90-degree angles between the sprue former and the wax pattern nor position the pattern so the molten alloy has to flow backward in the open channel toward the ring entrance.

It is essential to take advantage of centrifugal and gravitational forces by positioning the wax patterns so the alloy is cast toward thinner sections, such as the margins. Therefore, position the waxed restorations so the margins of the patterns face the trailing edge in the casting ring. Place a wax dot on the crucible former (Fig 5-6) to serve as an orientation reference after the patterns have been invested. (This assumes the crucible former itself does not have any marking or orientation guide.)

Location of the reservoir

The reservoir portion of a spruing system—whether it is in the form of a 4- or 6-gauge large runner bar (indirect sprue former) or an 8-, 10-, or 12-gauge round ball (direct sprue former)—should be placed in the *heat center* of the ring[5,13,17,18] (Figs 5-7 to 5-10). Such positioning permits the reservoir to remain molten long enough to furnish metal to the patterns until each completely solidifies. Aside from being in the heat center, the reservoir should have the largest mass of any part in the spruing system. In other words, you do not want to cast a button if it can be avoided.

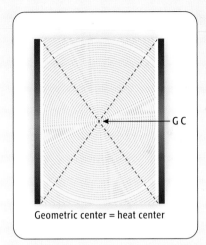

Geometric center = heat center

Fig 5-7 It may be incorrect to conclude that the geometric center (GC) and the heat center are one and the same.

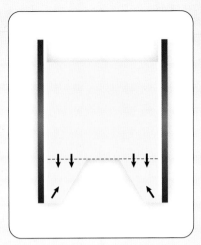

Fig 5-8 The investment surrounding the crucible former is less likely to contribute significantly to the heat center of the ring.

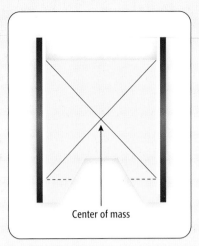

Center of mass

Fig 5-9 An area other than the geometric center of the ring may be the location of the ring's true thermal zone, or heat center, in an area referred to as the *center of mass* of the investment.

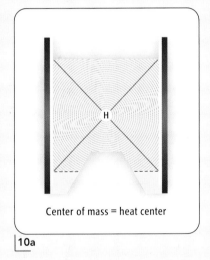

Center of mass = heat center

10a

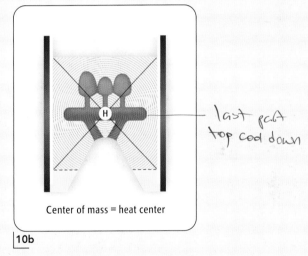

Center of mass = heat center

last part
top cool down

10b

Fig 5-10 The center of mass can be the heat center (H) of the ring *(a)* when it contains the largest mass of molten alloy *(b)*.

Buttonless Casting Technique

A *button* is solidified excess alloy that fills the mold in the area previously occupied by the upper portion of the crucible former. The goal of the *buttonless casting technique* is to cast everything *except* a button (Fig 5-11). If a button is present, or if the invested patterns are larger than the runner bar, these components compete with any reservoir as the largest mass of metal[19] and influence the location of the heat center in the casting ring.[5]

In contrast, with direct spruing where no reservoir ball is used, a button serves as the source of molten metal for the pattern during solidification. Therefore, the length of the pattern sprue former connecting the wax pattern to the button area is critical if the button is to serve as an effective reservoir. Should the pattern sprue former be too long, too short, or too narrow, there is greater likelihood of a miscast.

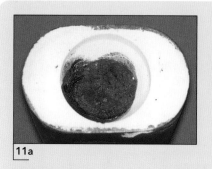
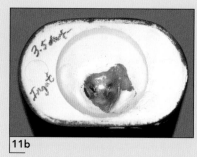
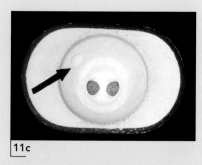

Fig 5-11 As one is able to better estimate the amount of alloy needed in the buttonless casting technique, the size of the cast button *(a)* will get smaller and smaller *(b)* until it is completely eliminated *(c)*. Note the small concavity *(arrow)* formed in the investment by the wax orientation dot.

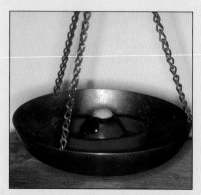
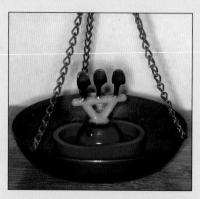
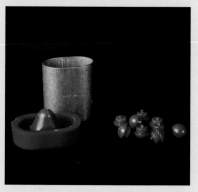

Fig 5-12a The opening in the crucible former is filled with wax and the orientation dot is placed. The crucible former is put on a scale and weighed. The weight of the crucible former is permanently recorded on the base with an indelible pen.

Fig 5-12b Wax buttons can be purchased to fill the opening in the top of the crucible former.

Fig 5-12c A prefabricated wax sprue former, with attached wax patterns, is placed in the crucible former, and the entire assembly is weighed.

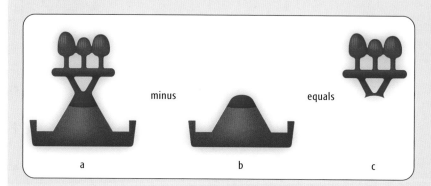

minus   equals

a   b   c

Fig 5-13 Illustration of the technique (shown in Figs 5-12a and 5-12c) used to arrive at the weight of the wax spruing system to be cast without a button according to the buttonless casting technique (shown in Fig 5-11c).

When using the buttonless casting technique, one of the best ways to ensure that no button is cast is to weigh the entire assembly of wax patterns and supporting sprue system. This can be accomplished by following four simple steps.

Step 1: Place a prefabricated "button" insert in the crucible former opening, or dome the crucible former by manually filling in the opening with wax, then weigh it on a digital scale (preferred) (Figs 5-12a and 5-12b).

Step 2: Attach the wax patterns to a prefabricated sprue former (preferred) or hand-fashioned spruing network. Insert the spruing system in the crucible former and secure it in place (Fig 5-12c).

Step 3: Weigh the entire assembly on the scale.

Step 4: Calculate the difference between the two measurements. That difference is the weight of wax above the top of the crucible former (ie, the sprue system) (Fig 5-13), which is the only part that should be cast in the buttonless casting technique.

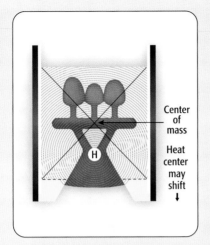

Fig 5-14 A large button can compete with the runner bar to function as the "reservoir" and cause the heat center (H) to shift toward the largest mass of metal (in this case, the button rather than the bar).

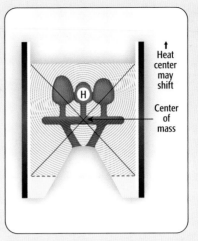

Fig 5-15 Likewise, the heat center (H) can shift upward toward large patterns when no button is cast and the restorations weigh more than the runner bar.

Too much alloy may produce a button that is larger than the runner bar. When this occurs, it can shift the heat center from the runner bar to the button itself (Fig 5-14). Likewise, if the wax patterns have a larger volume than that of the runner bar, or if the runner bar selected is too small for the restorations, the heat center may be shifted upward toward the wax pattern area (Fig 5-15). Expect *porosity* to occur in the area with the largest mass of metal that solidifies last. In Fig 5-14, that porosity is likely to occur in the button leaving a densely cast runner bar, but the wax patterns could be left incomplete. Conversely, the large pontic in Fig 5-15 is apt to solidify last and be the location of the porosity, leaving the runner bar dense and complete.

It is important to remember that correct placement of the runner bar in the mold and the use of an appropriate volume of alloy are critical to the buttonless casting technique. Adherence to these recommendations will help to ensure that the largest volume of alloy (the reservoir) will remain molten longest to furnish metal to the patterns until solidification is complete.

Constricted spruing

Tapering rather than flaring the sprue former at its point of attachment to the wax pattern is referred to as *constricted spruing*.[14] This taper is believed to permit the sprue former to serve as a true reservoir, thereby decreasing the likelihood of suck-back porosity.[4,7,13] In practical terms, the constriction may be helpful in the mold-filling process for low-density base metal alloys. However, one study showed that the use of a narrow-diameter (1.0 mm) sprue former for patterns cast in a nickel-chromium alloy had more defects than sprue formers of 2.0- and 3.0-mm diameters, even when vents were added.[20] As the density of the metal increases, constricted spruing is more apt to interfere with mold filling and lead to increased porosity,[6,21,22] as explained in the laws of casting.[5,18]

Therefore, it is recommended that you follow this general rule: the greater the alloy density, the larger the sprue-pattern access. High-density alloys tend to be sluggish compared to low-density metals. Keep in mind that some individuals will report success with constricted spruing for many alloy systems, regardless of density levels. This is not to say that both techniques will not work. However, the recommendation for the limited use of constricted spruing is intended to promote a technique more likely to offer consistent and highly reproducible results.

Sprue former composition: Wax vs plastic

It is not often emphasized, but the wax elimination technique for the spruing network should be different for wax and plastic sprue formers. Casting wax melts readily in the normal course of the wax elimination process, leaving little concern about the presence of carbon residues after heat soaking at the recommended maximum furnace temperature. In fact, casting waxes certified by the American Dental Association will not leave a residue of more than 0.1% of the specimen's original weight. There is no assurance, however, that all wax sprue formers perform equally well. Furthermore, plastic sprue formers do not burn out completely through the lower temperature range. In fact, plastic actually has a

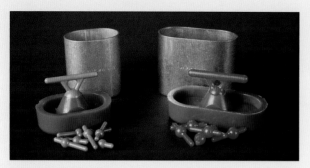

Fig 5-16 Examples of the different prefabricated wax sprue formers from the Ready Sprues system (KerrLab) and the Tri-Wax System (Ivoclar Vivadent). Note the variations in size for both the direct and indirect sprue formers.

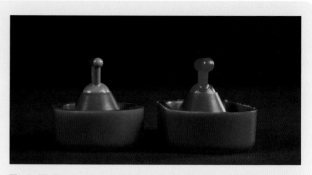

Fig 5-17 The prefabricated indirect Ready Sprues and Tri-Wax wax patterns may differ in gauge size, but they both position the runner bar in approximately the same vertical position in the crucible former and ring.

Table 5-1 Size, color, gauge, diameter, and length of direct and indirect prefabricated wax sprue formers

| Product (mfr) | Direct | | | | Indirect | | | | |
	Size	Color	Gauge	Diameter (mm)	Size	Color	Gauge	Diameter (mm)	Length (cm)
Ready Sprues	NA	NA	NA	NA	_	Yellow	~6	4.0	4.60
(KerrLab)					_	Green	~6	4.0	4.60
					_	Orange	~4	5.0	4.60
					_	Red	~4	5.0	5.50
Ringless Casting	Small	Blue	10	2.6	Small	Blue	6	4.1	4.30
System (Whip Mix)	Large	Red	8	3.3	Large	Red	4	5.2	4.30
Tri-Wax	Mini	Red	12	2.1					
(Ivoclar Vivadent)	Small	Red	10	2.6	Small	Red	6	4.1	3.75
	Large	Red	8	3.3	Large	Red	4	5.2	4.30

greater potential to leave carbon residue in the mold. Moreover, plastic tends to undergo greater expansion before softening than does wax. Should this expansion occur when the investment is in the green state, it can result in mold cracking. More important, if the pathway for the escape of molten wax is blocked by unmelted plastic, the wax may overheat (boil) and erode the inner surface of the mold. As a result, the castings may have a higher degree of surface roughness due to damage to the mold's interior surface; this is sometimes referred to as *mold wash*.

To overcome this problem, apply a thin layer of wax over the entire surface of a plastic sprue former to produce potential space and an escape mechanism for the melting wax patterns as the mold temperature increases. This procedure not only requires more time but also can increase the number of irregularities in the investment if the wax is not applied evenly and smoothly over the plastic components. With or without the application of a wax coating, a two-stage wax elimination process is recommended for plastic sprue formers,[17] beginning with a 30-minute heat soaking at 427°C (801°F) for the first stage, as recommended by Tombasco and Reilly.[23] At the end of this 30-minute heat soaking (single ring), reset the oven to the desired high temperature and continue wax elimination.

Prefabricated sprue formers

As mentioned previously, when carried out properly, spruing and investing can be made easier and yield more consistent results with the use of prefabricated wax sprue formers[5] (Figs 5-16 and 5-17). In particular, these ready-made wax formers have runner bars of various gauges to meet the needs of individual cases. Ready-made wax patterns offer a greater opportunity to obtain a predictable and time-saving method of spruing. More important, you also avoid having to construct a personal interpretation of an appropriate indirect sprue design. Table 5-1 lists some examples of prefabricated wax sprue formers.

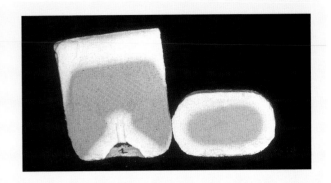

Fig 5-18 Carbon is still present in this carbon-containing investment even after wax elimination at 816°C (1,500°F) for 90 minutes. The resultant reducing atmosphere is helpful to gold-based alloys (reduces oxidation), but the residual carbon is a potential contaminant for palladium-, nickel-, and cobalt-based metal-ceramic alloys.

High-Heat Casting Investments

The elevated melting ranges of metal-ceramic alloys (see Table 3-4) exceed the recommended upper limits for heating gypsum-bonded investments (704°C/1,300°F) and require high-heat, phosphate-bonded investments or the silica-bonded investments that can be used with alloys heated up to 1,315°C (2,399°F). In addition, the alloys with a high melting range usually undergo more contraction during solidification than those with a lower melting range.[2] The two varieties of phosphate-bonded investments—carbon-containing and carbon-free (or noncarbon)—are more widely used than the silica-bonded materials.

Carbon-containing phosphate-bonded investments

A variety of carbon-containing, phosphate-bonded casting investments are available. These high-heat refractory materials are readily identifiable by their gray-black color, which is due to the presence of carbon even after wax elimination (Fig 5-18). Divestment is easier and castings typically are "cleaner," meaning they have little or no surface oxidation when retrieved from a carbon-containing investment.[2]

When mixed, these investments may appear coarse in texture compared to their gypsum-bonded investment counterparts. In lieu of distilled water, most phosphate-bonded investments require a mixture of a special liquid (colloidal silica) and distilled water. Concentrations of the special liquid may range from as little as 10% (for high-palladium alloys) to as much as 100% (for cobalt-chromium alloys). Used full strength, this liquid adds silica that thickens the mix and results in greater thermal expansion. Diluting the special liquid with distilled water has the opposite effect; that is, less colloidal silica reduces the amount of potential investment expansion.

Typically, investment manufacturers suggest a concentration of special liquid and distilled water as a starting point. It

should be understood that the special liquid–to-water ratio will have to be adjusted under the conditions of each laboratory until the desired level of investment expansion required of each alloy type has been achieved. Carbon-containing phosphate-bonded investments are generally recommended for gold-based metal-ceramic alloys and should not be used with palladium-, nickel-, or cobalt-based alloys. These alloy systems have the potential to absorb available carbon to form carbides and/or porosity (due to physical carbon inclusions). Some manufacturers believe that with the use of an appropriate wax elimination technique, no carbon should remain after heat soaking at the high temperature setting. They contend that there is more risk of carbon contamination when a torch is improperly adjusted than there is in a carbon-containing investment. However, a simple laboratory test will show that even after a 90-minute heat soaking at 816°C (1,500°F), a substantial amount of carbon appears to remain in the interior of a carbon-containing investment[24] (see Fig 5-18).

Noncarbon phosphate-bonded investments

The noncarbon phosphate-bonded investments are readily identifiable by their white color, both before and after they are mixed (see Fig 5-11). They were developed as a result of concerns for the potential interaction of carbon with the nickel- and cobalt-containing casting alloys, as well as the various palladium-based metals. Proponents of the carbon-free investments also prefer the added security of using a carbonless investment system and the avoidance of the prolonged high temperature wax elimination (871°C/1,600°F) required to eliminate all residual carbon.[24]

The noncarbon investments generally have a grainy texture like their carbon-containing counterparts. Exceptions include the fine-grained investments like Cera-Fina (Whip Mix) and similar products. These particular investments mix to a smooth, creamy consistency with ample working time (up to 10 minutes) (see Fig 5-11).

too much investment over wax pattern

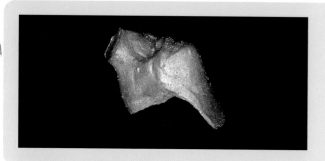

Fig 5-19 A rough casting with multiple nodules may be caused by a less-than-ideal alloy-investment pairing or a failure to evacuate the investment's gaseous by-products during mixing. Try another investment to determine if the problem is due to a lapse in technique, an issue with the investment, or an adverse alloy-investment interaction.

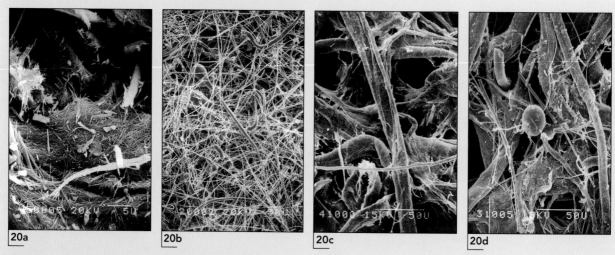

| 20a | 20b | 20c | 20d |

Fig 5-20 *(a)* Asbestos liner (original magnification ×500); *(b)* ceramic liner (original magnification ×150); *(c)* cellulose liner (original magnification ×500); *(d)* ceramic-cellulose combination liner (original magnification ×500).

Investment–casting alloy interaction

Variations can be seen in the performance of alloys with different investments.[12,25,26] It is possible that the problems attributed to a given metal are, in fact, caused by the investment. Excessive nodule formation and fins may occur more frequently with one brand of investment than another (Fig 5-19). Manufacturers often indicate that their alloys may be used with virtually any commercially available phosphate-bonded investment. That may not always be true, and studies support the view that alloy-investment pairing can influence results.[5,24–27] Therefore, it may be prudent to conduct laboratory tests for potential adverse alloy-investment interactions before making a large purchase of any new investment.[24]

Casting ring liners

Asbestos had been the material traditionally used for lining casting rings until its potential risk to the health of dental laboratory technicians was discovered.[28,29] Evidently, the asbestos

fiber bundles were found to produce hazardous-sized respirable particles capable of causing lung disease (Fig 5-20a).

Alternative nonasbestos ring liner materials fall into three categories: ceramic (aluminum silicate), cellulose (paper), and a ceramic-cellulose combination.[30] The microstructure of these materials varies (Figs 5-20b to 5-20d). Furthermore, the relative safety of ceramic ring liners remains uncertain because aluminum silicate also appears capable of producing hazardous-sized respirable particles.[30] These concerns can be eliminated by switching to a ringless casting system.

Investing Technique

Follow the same basic technique used to produce castings with crown-and-bridge alloys, but use high-heat phosphate-bonded investments instead of gypsum-bonded investments. Ask your alloy manufacturer for recommended investments, suggested liquid-to-powder ratios, and an initial special liquid concentration.

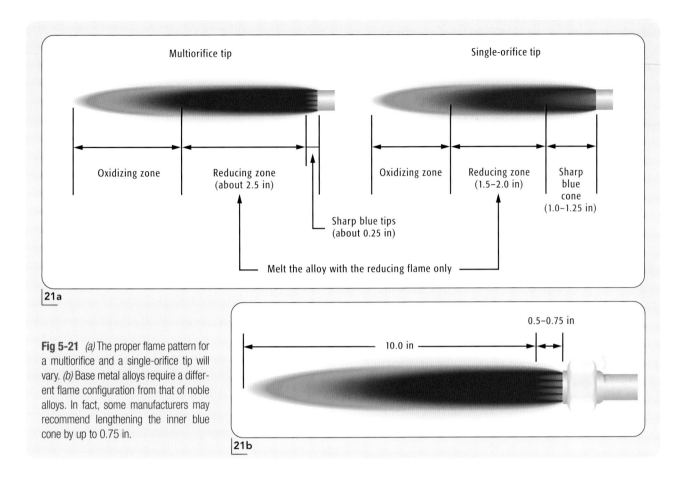

21a

Fig 5-21 *(a)* The proper flame pattern for a multiorifice and a single-orifice tip will vary. *(b)* Base metal alloys require a different flame configuration from that of noble alloys. In fact, some manufacturers may recommend lengthening the inner blue cone by up to 0.75 in.

21b

Wax elimination technique

The *wax elimination process*, which is commonly referred to as the *burnout technique*, varies for alloys of different compositions. High-temperature settings range up to 871°C (1,600°F) for base metal alloys and between 760°C (1,400°F) and 871°C (1,600°F) for noble and high-noble alloys. It is always advisable to refer to the instructions on an alloy package for the recommended temperature setting and wax elimination time for each specific metal. Also, check the investment manufacturer's suggested temperature rate of rise for the burnout furnace. It is important to adhere to the rate established for each type of investment.

Melting and Casting Techniques

Assuming that a case has been properly sprued and invested and that the wax elimination process has been completed, the next crucial steps involve melting and casting the metal-ceramic alloy. A poorly adjusted torch or improper casting method can ruin all of your efforts to this point. Given the importance of these procedures, the following additional topics are included to help you better understand the casting process.

Casting torch selection

There are two types of torch tips to choose from when selecting casting equipment: a multiorifice tip and a single-orifice tip[5] (Fig 5-21).

Multiorifice tip

Of the two types of tips, the multiorifice design is generally preferred for metal-ceramic alloys. Its main advantage is the distribution of heat over a wide area for more uniform heating of the alloy, which is particularly helpful in casting the high-fusing, base metal alloys.

Single-orifice tip

The single-orifice tip may concentrate more heat in one area, but the area of heat is smaller than that produced by the multiorifice tip (see Fig-21).

95

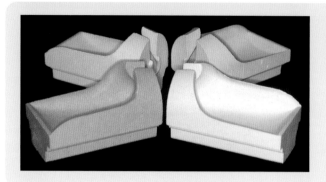

Fig 5-22 Zircon crucibles (KerrLab) are more durable than the quartz type. Color-coded crucibles permit assignment of different alloys to specific colors.

Choice of fuels

Three fuel sources could be used to melt metal-ceramic alloys[31]:

1. *Acetylene.* This colorless gas has a distinctive garlic-like odor. It will burn in air and can generate flame approaching 1,649°C (3,000°F). Unfortunately, acetylene is usually contaminated with carbon and other elements, so it should *not* be used to melt metal-ceramic alloys.
2. *Natural gas.* This fuel is the byproduct of the "natural" decomposition of organic matter in the ground. When mixed with air, the natural gas flame approaches a temperature of 1,204°C (2,200°F). Replacing air with oxygen enables natural gas to attain temperatures required to melt the high-fusing noble and base metal alloys. Natural gas is an acceptable fuel source, although it is not ideal. Inadequate pressure in gas lines, fluctuations in pressure levels, water contamination, and variations in composition among gas companies are some of the potential problems encountered by natural gas users. Nonetheless, natural gas is a widely used fuel.
3. *Propane.* The problems associated with natural gas are avoided entirely by using bottled propane gas. The constant, regulated mixture of pure, uncontaminated propane, when combined with oxygen, provides a clean, consistent burn that leads to a more ideal melt.

Casting equipment

The noble and base metal alloys can be cast either with a torch in a centrifugal casting machine or torchless in an induction casting machine. Irrespective of the type of equipment selected, the low-density base metal alloys typically require an additional winding of the casting arm in a centrifugal casting machine to ensure adequate casting pressure.

Casting crucibles

A variety of casting crucibles are available for different types of dental casting alloys:

High-heat crucibles

Crucibles made of zircon are capable of withstanding the temperatures required to melt metal-ceramic as well as crown-and-bridge alloys. Either a zircon or a quartz casting crucible is recommended for noble and base metal-ceramic alloys, but the zircon type generally is more durable. Zircon crucibles are available in a variety of colors (yellow, pink, blue, and white), so one color can be dedicated to a specific alloy to avoid potential contamination.

The following two types of casting crucibles should not be used to melt metal-ceramic alloys.

Clay crucibles

Clay crucibles are acceptable for melting gold-based crown-and-bridge alloys, but they have great potential to deteriorate when subjected to the high temperatures required to melt ceramic alloys and can possibly contaminate the melt.[32]

Carbon crucibles

Although carbon crucibles are suitable for gold-based alloys, exposure to such a ready source of carbon can lead to significant contamination of palladium-, nickel-, and cobalt-based metals. As mentioned previously, that contamination can result in carbide formation that can embrittle these alloys and/or cause porosity due to carbon inclusions.

After selecting the appropriate type of casting crucible, preheat it in the oven with the casting ring. Preheating the crucible prevents spalling (cracking) and helps to prolong the crucible's working life. Never cast different alloys in the same crucible because this will lead to alloy contamination. Instead, use color-coded crucibles (Fig 5-22) or carve the alloy name in each crucible for identification.

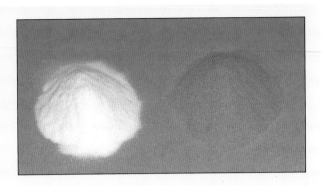

Fig 5-23 Pure aluminum oxide *(left)* is white and is less likely to contain contaminants than is a comparable all-purpose abrasive *(right)*.

Electric casting machines

Electric casting machines with carbon crucibles are appropriate for gold-based alloys, but they are not recommended for palladium-, nickel-, and cobalt-based alloys because of the potential for carbon contamination.

Compounds for airborne-particle abrasion

Commercially available abrasive compounds such as aluminum oxide (Al_2O_3), a general-purpose blasting compound, and glass beads can remove investment and surface oxides from a metal casting. A 50-μm grit, nonrecycled (white) aluminum oxide abrasive is commonly suggested for airabrading porcelain-bearing surfaces and dental porcelain[33] (Fig 5-23).

Aluminum oxides in colors other than white may contain impurities such as iron. Run a magnet through the material if you suspect it is contaminated.

Laws of Casting

Casting is both an art and a science governed by numerous rules, or "laws." Personal interpretation of these laws is demonstrated in a technician's approach to the procedure—that is, the *art* of casting. Integrating the theoretical principles supporting this art enables the user to blend science with art in dental technology. At times, casting problems can be attributed to poor casting technique and/or a failure to adhere to one or more of the basic principles (laws) of casting.

An important foundation of these laws is that *every* casting contains porosity attributed to solidification shrinkage. Porosity invariably occurs in the area of the casting that is last to solidify. The challenge faced by the technician is to use knowledge of the science of casting to plan the location of that porosity in an area of the spruing system away from the restoration(s).

Building on the earlier work of Ingersoll and Wandling[18] (1986), an expanded set of 17 separate recommendations for spruing, investing, wax elimination, and melting and casting procedures were created in 1992.[12] Collectively, these guidelines are referred to as the *laws of casting*. Included in these laws are the principles behind the buttonless casting technique. As with any set of regulations, there are penalties when these laws are not followed.

A three-unit fixed partial denture pattern is used to illustrate several key points related to the spruing, investing, and casting procedures.

Spruing

First law of casting

Attach the pattern sprue former to the thickest part of the wax pattern. As the molten alloy moves from the reservoir to the pattern margins, it should flow from areas of greater volume to areas of lesser volume (ie, the margins).

Begin by carefully evaluating the size, geometry, and configuration of the wax pattern(s) to be cast to identify any special requirements that may need to be considered (Fig 5-24). Select a prefabricated indirect sprue former of an appropriate gauge and length (Fig 5-25). Lute a wax pattern sprue former to the most practical portion of the occlusal/incisal surface of each wax pattern (Fig 5-26). Warm the prefabricated indirect sprue former and gently alter the shape to align with the curvature of the arch, as needed (Fig 5-27). If 18-gauge wax handles are to be applied, place them on the lingual surfaces of a metal-ceramic wax pattern *before* luting the patterns to the runner bar (Fig 5-28).

Except with thin anterior copings, do not place the pattern sprue former in a cutback area if an adjacent, fully contoured cusp is available. Molten metal flowing from a thin

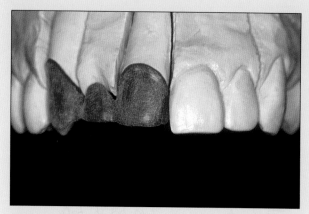

Fig 5-24 Three-unit fixed partial denture substructure (see chapter 4) after completion of the wax cutback.

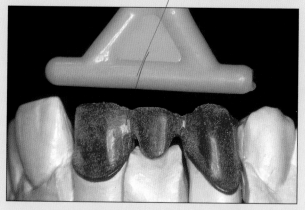

U-shape contact

Fig 5-25 This Ready Sprues has a runner bar with a diameter and length sized to support this fixed partial denture wax pattern.

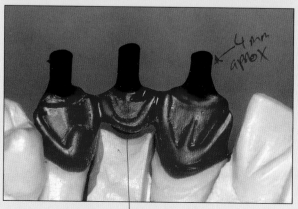

4 mm approx

Fig 5-26 Wax pattern sprue formers of an appropriate diameter (gauge) are selected and luted to each wax pattern.

porcelain space

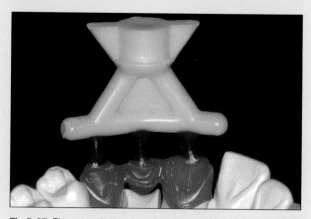

Fig 5-27 The runner bar portion of the indirect sprue former is luted to the three individual pattern sprue formers. Before being attached, the Ready Sprues can be warmed slightly and adjusted to mimic the actual curvature of the arch rather than allowed to remain straight.

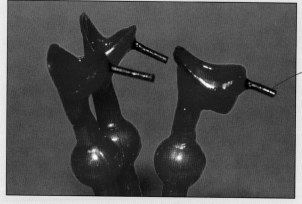

18 G lingual

Fig 5-28 Before securing the patterns to the runner bar, it is recommended that you add 18-gauge wax to the lingual surfaces. This step creates handles in the cast framework, thereby protecting the delicate cast metal margins.

region to a thicker region of the wax pattern may solidify before the mold is completely filled (cold shut). When using indirect spruing, be sure to select the appropriate-sized prefabricated sprue former (see Figs 5-25 and 5-27).

The penalties for not obeying this law are cold shuts, short margins, or incomplete castings.

Second law of casting

Orient wax patterns so that all of the restoration margins face the trailing edge when the ring is positioned in the casting machine. To identify that orientation, add a wax dot to the crucible former so you will know how to orient the

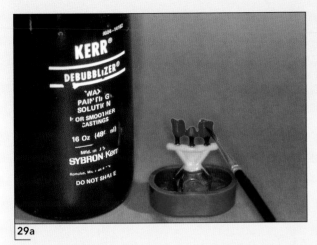
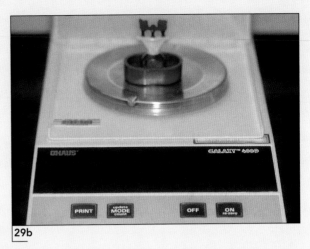

Figs 5-29a and 5-29b Apply a thin layer of debubblizer (wax pattern cleaner) to the wax patterns and indirect spruing system, and allow it to dry thoroughly before investing. Then weigh the assembly and calculate the amount of metal needed based on the density of the alloy (see appendix D).

ring in the casting cradle once those patterns have been invested (see Fig 5-6).

The penalties for not obeying this law are cold shuts, short margins, and incomplete castings.

Third law of casting

Position the wax patterns in a "cold zone" of the investment mold and the reservoir in the "heat center" of the casting ring. The coolest parts of the mold (cold zones) are located at the end of the ring and along the ring periphery. The hottest portion, or heat center, of the casting ring is located near the center of the ring as determined by the location of the largest mass of metal in the investment (see Fig 5-10). Limit the amount of investment covering the patterns to approximately 6.0 mm (¼ inch), and position the reservoir in the heat center[11,34] (see Figs 5-3 and 5-10). Adherence to this law increases the likelihood that casting porosity will occur in the reservoir rather than in the restoration.

The penalty for not obeying this law is porosity in the restorations.

Fourth law of casting

A reservoir must have sufficient molten alloy to accommodate the shrinkage that occurs within the restorations. Ideally, alloy that fills the pattern (restoration) areas will solidify first. As that molten metal solidifies, it shrinks and creates a vacuum. For complete casting to occur, the vacuum must be able to draw additional metal from an adjacent source—the reservoir. A runner bar can be an effective reservoir if its size is equal to or larger than the thickest cross-sectional area of the wax pattern (see Figs 5-5, 5-10b, and 5-25). Units sprued directly should include a round ball that potentially can serve as a reservoir in a properly designed spruing system (see Fig 5-16).

The penalties for not obeying this law are porosity in the restorations and/or suck-back porosity.

Fifth law of casting

Do not cast a button if a runner bar or other internal reservoir is used (see Fig 5-11). With indirect spruing, the largest mass of metal should be the reservoir (see Fig 5-10b). The presence of a button is counterproductive because it can draw available molten alloy from the bar, shift the heat center, and reduce the feed of metal to the restorations (see Fig 5-14). Likewise, the wax patterns should not be larger than the runner bar if the bar is to act as a true reservoir (see Figs 5-10b and 5-15). Weigh the sprued patterns and use the wax pattern–alloy conversion tables (appendix D) to calculate the amount of alloy needed (Fig 5-29).

The penalties for not obeying this law are porosity in the restorations, potential distortion during porcelain firing, and suck-back porosity.

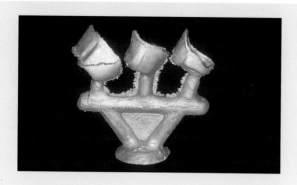

Fig 5-30 This casting has fins caused by excess wax pattern cleaner or improper heating of the mold.

too much heat or bublizer not dried out, or oven too hot.

Sixth law of casting

Turbulence must be minimized if not totally eliminated. Pathways for the flow of metal should be smooth, gradual, and without impediments. Eliminate sharp turns, restrictions, points, or impingements that might create turbulence and occlude air in the casting. Restrictions, or constrictions, can accelerate the metal's rate of flow and abrade the mold surface, possibly resulting in mold wash.[18]

The penalties for not obeying this law are voids in the casting and/or surface pitting. Voids can be created by the occlusion of air from turbulent metal flow. Mold wash can remove investment particles from the mold's inner surface and carry them ahead of the alloy. These entrapped particles can produce surface pits and incomplete margins.

Seventh law of casting

Select a casting ring of sufficient length and diameter to accommodate the patterns to be invested. The casting ring should be of sufficient size (length and diameter) to permit the patterns to be located 6.0 mm (¼ inch) apart and 6.0 mm (¼ inch) from the top of the investment. A minimum of 9.0 mm (⅜ inch) of investment should separate the patterns from the ring liner, if used (see Fig 5-3). If too little investment covers the wax patterns, the alloy is more likely to break through the mold. Conversely, filling the ring with too much investment may position the wax patterns too close to the heat center of the mold and impair the escape of gases. Insufficient investment between wax patterns and the casting ring (ringless technique) or casting ring liner can result in uneven investment expansion.

The penalties for not obeying this law are mold fracture, casting fins, and porosity in the restorations.

Investing and wax elimination

Eighth law of casting

Reduce the surface tension and increase the wettability of the wax patterns. Proper surface tension reduction is important because it enables the casting investment to cover the wax patterns completely and thus reduces the potential for air-bubble entrapment.[35] A wetting agent, such as a wax pattern cleaner, should be brushed or sprayed on the wax patterns and dried thoroughly before investing[11,12] (see Fig 5-29a). Apply the liquid sparingly. Too much wetting agent may create a surface film that can dilute and weaken the investment in that area and produce bubbles or fins on the casting (Fig 5-30). Too little surface tension reduction can be followed by increased air entrapment. When a wetting agent is applied correctly, the result is a clean wax surface, which improves the ability of the casting investment to wet the patterns more completely.

The penalty for not obeying this law is the formation of bubbles on the surface of the pattern as a result of the entrapment of air (too little wetting agent) or excess liquid (too much wetting agent).

Ninth law of casting

Weigh any bulk investment, and measure the investment liquid for a precise powder-to-liquid ratio. The correct proportions of powder to liquid and any required dilution of the special liquid with distilled water should be established for each type of alloy. Two key variables to consider relative to the powder-to-liquid ratio are (1) the total volume of liquid and (2) the concentration of the special liquid.

vibrator

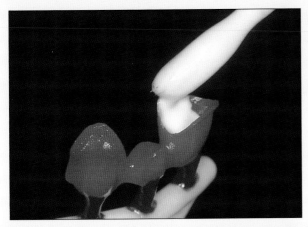

Fig 5-31 After vacuum mixing, carefully add a small portion of investment to the inside of the individual wax retainers to prevent the entrapment of air and to ensure complete wetting of the patterns.

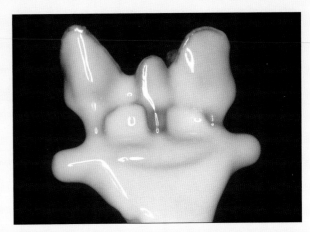

Fig 5-32 Once all of the wax surfaces have been covered by investment, place the casting ring in the crucible former, and fill the casting ring with enough investment to cover the wax patterns.

The total powder-to-liquid ratio to use is that recommended by the investment manufacturer.[11,12] If too little liquid is dispensed, the investment will be thick and may lack proper flow and workability. A thick mixture can also lead to too much investment expansion, which ultimately may result in loose-fitting castings. On the other hand, if too much investment liquid (100% colloidal silica or special liquid and water) is used in proportion to the weight of powder, a thinner mixture results. That thin investment mixture will have less expansion, and the resulting castings may be tighter fitting than desired.

The concentration of special liquid also directly affects expansion. For example, if 100% of this liquid is used, more expansion occurs as compared to a dilution using just 50% special liquid and 50% distilled water.

The penalty for not obeying this law is ill-fitting castings.

Tenth law of casting

Avoid the incorporation of air into the casting investment, and remove the ammonia gas by-product of phosphate-bonded investments by mixing under vacuum. Vacuum mixing removes more air and gaseous by-products than does hand spatulation (Figs 5-31 and 5-32). Areas of the mold that contain dense, bubble-free investment will expand more uniformly than sections with large voids (entrapped air). The mixing time depends on the type of investment used and the mixing speed (slow-speed versus high-speed mixing).

The penalties for not obeying this law are small nodules on the casting, a weak mold, or distortion of the casting.

Eleventh law of casting

Allow the casting investment to set completely before initiating the wax elimination procedure. If setting of the investment is not complete at the time a ring or mold (ringless technique) is placed in the oven, the mold may be weak and unable to withstand the pressure and expansion produced by the formation of steam in the early stage of heating. The investment could develop cracks and actually fracture. For best results, wax elimination should be initiated only after the investment has been allowed to remain undisturbed for the recommended setting time. If invested patterns are not to be cast immediately after setting, keep the investment hydrated by storing the work in a sealed container or plastic bag. If the casting investment is allowed to dry out, it is difficult to replace the free water in the interior of the investment and achieve total rehydration.

The penalties for not obeying this law are mold cracking/blowout or casting fins (see Fig 5-30).

Twelfth law of casting

Use a wax elimination technique that is appropriate for the type of patterns involved (wax versus plastic) and recommended for the type of casting alloy selected. Plastic sprue formers should be heated slowly to allow the plastic to soften, melt, and gradually flow out of the mold without exerting pressure on the investment walls. The safest way to achieve this is by using a two-stage wax elimination

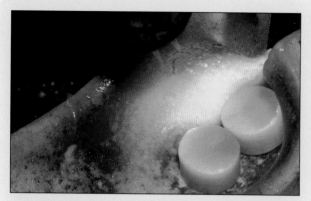

Fig 5-33a Most base metal alloys do not pool when heated, so you should use the fewest ingots possible and place them in contact with each other in the crucible.

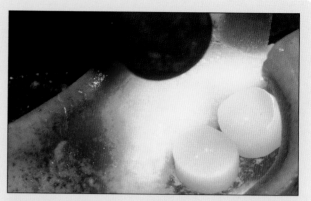

Fig 5-33b Through mutual contact, the ingots can heat uniformly.

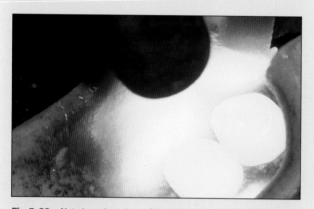

Fig 5-33c Note how the edges of the ingots have rounded and remain in contact, but the ingots have not pooled.

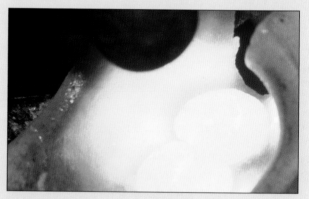

Fig 5-33d These ingots are now molten under an oxide surface skin and are ready to cast. Know how to recognize the appearance of the molten state for a base metal alloy, because it is different from that of high-noble and noble alloys.

technique.[23] Set the oven for a slow to moderate rate of rise to permit the heat to move through the investment and achieve uniform expansion. If wax elimination is incomplete, the channels of the spruing system may be partially blocked by wax or plastic residue (carbon). During casting, air may not be able to escape completely as the metal enters the mold.[23,24] Therefore, use at least a 30-minute heat soaking at 427°C (800°F) for the first wax elimination stage. After completion of this first stage, heat the ring to the recommended high temperature setting for the desired hold time.

The penalties for not obeying this law are cold shuts, short margins, mold cracks, and/or casting fins (see Fig 5-30).

Melting and casting

Thirteenth law of casting

Adequate heat must be available to properly melt and cast the alloy.[1] The selected heat source should be capable of melting a metal-ceramic alloy to the point of sufficient fluidity for casting. Prolonged heating, caused by an improperly adjusted torch, can prevent the alloy from attaining the fluidity needed for complete mold filling and compensation for heat loss.[1] Too much heat, or too high a temperature, also can burn off minor alloying elements through vaporization and/or oxidation (burned metal).[12] Ingots of high-noble and noble alloys will slump and flow together to form one molten mass, but most base metal alloys do not pool (Fig 5-33).

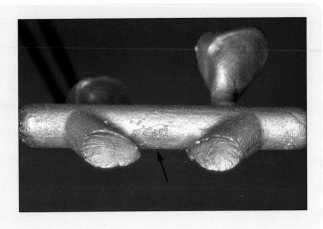

Fig 5-34 When no button is cast and the reservoir is the last portion of the casting to solidify, the porosity should appear on the underside of the bar *(arrow)*, away from the restorations (cast in nickel-chromium-beryllium alloy).

The penalties for not obeying this law are cold shuts, short margins, or rough castings, and/or investment breakdown (too much heat).

Fourteenth law of casting

When torch casting, use the reducing zone of the flame, not the oxidizing zone, to melt the alloy (see Fig 5-21). An improperly adjusted torch can add carbon or oxygen to an alloy while it is being heated. A melt achieved by the exclusive use of the reducing zone of the flame minimizes the likelihood of metal oxidation and gas absorption and helps to ensure a proper melt (see Fig 5-21).

The penalties for not obeying this law are porosity (from gas absorption) and/or a change in the alloy's coefficient of thermal expansion (due to alloy contamination).

Fifteenth law of casting

Provide enough force to cause the liquid alloy to flow into the heated mold. Adjust the casting machine to the requirements of each alloy. Low-density metals typically require more windings of a centrifugal casting arm as compared to high-density gold-based alloys. However, do not overwind the casting machine.[11,12,36]

The penalties for not obeying this law are cold shuts, short margins, incomplete castings, mold fractures, and/or fins (too much force).

Sixteenth law of casting

Cast toward the margins of the wax patterns. Place the heated ring in the casting cradle using the orientation dot as a guide so the pattern margins face the trailing edge (the second law). In a centrifugal casting machine, the metal will flow downward and to the right, taking advantage of the centrifugal, rotational, and gravitational forces on the molten alloy.[18,37]

The penalties for not obeying this law are cold shut, short margins, and otherwise incomplete castings.

Seventeenth law of casting

Do not quench the ring immediately after casting. Allow the alloy and the investment to cool to room temperature. Uneven cooling and shrinkage between alloy and investment can apply tensile forces to the casting.[38] After casting, the alloy may not possess sufficient strength to resist these forces, and the restoration could tear if quenched.

The penalty for not obeying this law is hot tears in the restoration.

Judging Success in Casting

Casting success typically is associated with a complete well-fitting restoration, coping, or substructure. However, the true challenge in the casting process is to direct the location of the casting porosity to a noncritical area. With indirect spruing, the most ideal location for porosity to reside is the undersurface of the runner bar opposite the restorations (Fig 5-34). When direct spruing includes a reservoir, the side of the ball opposite the restoration is an ideal location for casting porosity to occur (Fig 5-35).

Subjective castability testing using abstract mesh patterns has *not* been shown to correlate well with the actual casting parameters (high temperature for the mold and melting range for alloys)[24] (Fig 5-36). Replicas of metal-ceramic substructures (Fig 5-37) should be used in lieu of abstract patterns such as the Whitlock test.[24]

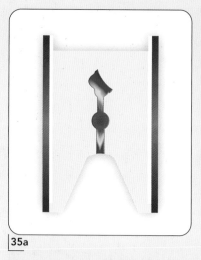
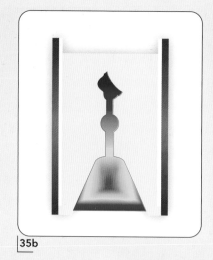
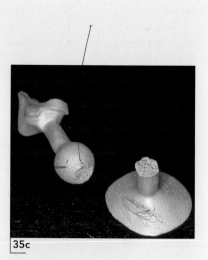

Fig 5-35a Illustration of how a button can shift the heat center and lead to an incomplete casting when using direct spruing.

Fig 5-35b When the wax pattern is weighed and cast with the proper volume of metal for direct spruing, the pattern area can solidify properly and cast a complete restoration.

Fig 5-35c With direct spruing, when alloy solidification occurs in the area of the reservoir ball, the porosity should appear on the side opposite the restoration. In this case the porosity resides on the underside of the reservoir ball. The large round base was thin and lacked sufficient mass, illustrating the principle depicted in Fig 5-35a.

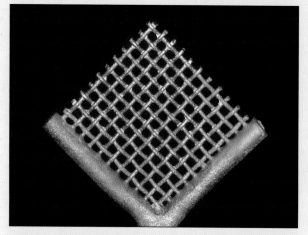

Fig 5-36a A nickel-chromium-beryllium alloy reproduced 100% of this abstract mesh pattern.

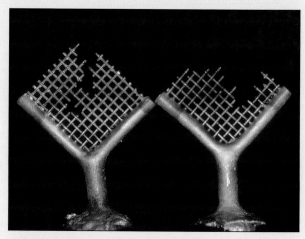

Fig 5-36b The best performance by this palladium-silver alloy using this abstract test was 85.5% reproduction of the mesh pattern *(left)*, and its worst performance was 53.6% *(right)*.

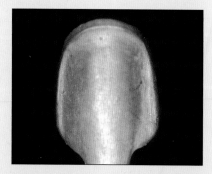

Fig 5-37 The same palladium-silver alloy shown in Fig 5-36b produced a smooth, complete replica casting based on a metal-ceramic substructure.

Fig 5-38 If the runner bar is too small and a button is present, the bar may be cast adequately, but there is a greater likelihood that the restorations will be incomplete (see also Fig 5-14). Note the dense surface and absence of porosity on the underside of the bar, an indication that the button supported the bar rather than the patterns.

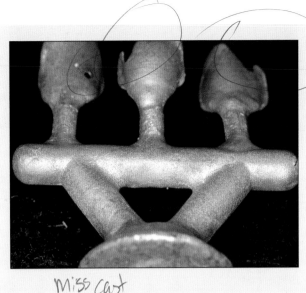

miss cast
runner bar not big enough

Analyzing Casting Failures

Despite concerted efforts to follow the recommended procedures outlined in this chapter, casting failures and mishaps are bound to occur in the dental laboratory (Fig 5-38). Errors in technique and, on occasion, material failures can unexpectedly result in unsatisfactory castings. By standardizing your technique and paying strict attention to each step involved in spruing, investing, and casting, it is often possible to minimize the number of actual miscasts and to control the location of solidification shrinkage (see Figs 5-33 to Fig 5-35). Proper storage and rotation of casting investment inventories also will help ensure consistent and accurate performance.

When casting failures do occur, troubleshoot each miscast to diagnose the cause or causes of the problem, so corrective measures can be taken before you make additional castings. Mackert[11] (1988) reported one of the most comprehensive methods to assess casting failures from preparation of a custom impression tray to waxing, spruing, investing, wax elimination, and, ultimately, melting of the alloy.

Summary

The very nature of the differences between metal-ceramic alloys and conventional gold-based crown-and-bridge metals necessitates certain adjustments to your waxing, spruing, and investing techniques. Whether it is in understanding the demands of low-density alloys, selecting an appropriate spruing technique (direct versus indirect), or determining how to properly cast a high-fusing alloy, knowledge of the theoretical aspects of waxing, spruing, and investing is required. This chapter brings together the fundamental principles of these technical procedures in the laws of casting with emphasis on the buttonless casting technique.

Before proceeding to the discussion of metal finishing (chapter 7), you must first understand how dental porcelain bonds to a metal-ceramic alloy (chapter 6). In this way, you will gain a better appreciation of the materials, procedures, and technique used to prepare the cast restoration to receive porcelain and maintain the porcelain-metal bond.

References

1. Myers RA. Study of the causes of discontinuity of metal in sprues during pressure casting. J Am Dent Assoc 1936;23:554–568. *Casting "discontinuity" is attributed to (1) insufficient pressure, (2) insufficient heating of the metal, and (3) insufficient volume of alloy.*

2. Anusavice KJ. Phillips' Science of Dental Materials, ed 11. Philadelphia: Saunders, 2003.

3. Dykema RW, Goodacre CJ, Phillips RW. Johnston's Modern Practice in Fixed Prosthodontics, ed 4. Philadelphia: Saunders, 1986: 161–163.

4. Naylor WP, Young JM. Non-Gold Base Dental Casting Alloys. Vol I: Alternatives to Type III gold [ADA156672]. Brooks AFB, Texas: USAF School of Aerospace Medicine, 1985:19–25.

5. Naylor WP. Non-Gold Base Dental Casting Alloys. Vol II: Porcelain-fused-to-metal alloys [ADA173766]. Brooks AFB, Texas: USAF School of Aerospace Medicine, 1986:75–99.

6. Nielsen JP, Ollermann R. Suck-back porosity. Quintessence Dent Technol 1976;1:61–65.
If no reservoir is provided, alloy is drawn from the sprue, so the pattern area becomes a source of molten alloy for the button. Flaring the sprue former at its attachment to the wax pattern reduces the potential for suck-back porosity.

7. Rousseau CH. The Rousseau casting system: A foundation for esthetic restorations. Trends Tech Contemp Dent Lab 1984;1(3): 26–29.

8. Dootz ER, Asgar K. Solidification patterns of single crowns and three-unit bridge castings. Quintessence Dent Technol 1986;10: 299–305.
Classic article documenting a Type III gold alloy entering and solidifying in a scattered pattern. A Pd-Ag metal-ceramic alloy fills the mold in one direction.

9. Young HM, Coffey JP, Caswell CW. Sprue design and its effect on the castability of ceramometal alloys. J Prosthet Dent 1987;57: 160–164.
Evaluates three spruing methods and concludes that indirect spruing is significantly better than direct spruing.

10. Young HM, Marguelles-Bonnet R, Mohammed H. The relationship of metal volume and sprue design to porosity in nonprecious castings. Quintessence Dent Technol 1987;11:399–404.
Authors evaluate five different spruing techniques and finds more porosity in the pontics.

11. Mackert JR Jr. An expert system for analysis of casting failures. Int J Prosthodont 1988;1:268–280.
Excellent reference for analyzing casting failures using flowchart, "Casting Failure Inference Network."

12. Naylor WP. Introduction to Metal Ceramic Technology, ed 1. Chicago: Quintessence, 1992:65–81.

13. McLean JW. The Science and Art of Dental Ceramics. Vol II: Bridge design and laboratory procedures in dental ceramics. Chicago: Quintessence, 1980:223–238.

14. Weber K. Casting mould design and spread in precious metal castings [in German]. Dent Labor (Munch)1977;25:363–367.
Weber describes locating patterns outside the heat center and into a cold zone of investment and narrowing the sprue former at the wax pattern (constricted spruing).

15. Tamura K. Essentials of Dental Technology. Fowler J (trans). Chicago: Quintessence, 1987:356, 378.

16. Yamamoto M. Metal-Ceramics: Principles and Methods of Makoto Yamamoto. Chicago: Quintessence, 1985:88-89.

17. Alleluia VV. The parameters of better casting, Part 1. Dent Lab Rev 1980;55(10):18–23.
This three-part series includes practical tips to improve casting results. Part 1 examines two-stage wax elimination and proper position of wax patterns in the mold.

18. Ingersoll CE, Wandling RA. Laws of casting. Harmony Notes, Jan 2–3. Amherst, NY: Williams Dental, 1986.

19. Civjan S, Huget EF, Godfrey GD, Lichtenberger H, Frank WA. Effects of heat treatment on mechanical properties of two nickel-chromium-based casting alloys. J Dent Res 1972;51:1537–1545.
Authors explain how the use of a smaller melt eliminated a button and enhanced solidification.

20. Wight TA, Grisius RJ, Gaugler RW. Evaluation of three variables affecting the casting of base metal alloys. J Prosthet Dent 1980; 43:415–418.
Casting with narrow-diameter sprue formers (1.0-mm width) had more defects than patterns cast with 2.0- and 3.0-mm wide ingate sprue formers. Also recommends 18-gauge wax vents.

21. Compagni R, Faucher RR, Youdelis RA. Effects of sprue design, casting machine, and heat source on casting porosity. J Prosthet Dent 1984;52:41–45.
Sprue design had more influence on casting results than did the type of casting machine or the method of alloy heating.

22. Verrett RG, Duke ES. The effect of sprue attachment design on castability and porosity. J Prosthet Dent 1989;61:418–424.
A straight, flared sprue former produced better casting with less porosity than did constricted spruing.

23. Tombasco T, Reilly RP. A comparison of burnout temperatures and their effects on elimination of plastic sprues. Trends Tech Contemp Dent Lab 1987;Dec:36–39.
Authors describe a two-stage wax elimination technique for plastic sprue formers.

24. Naylor WP, Moore BK, Phillips RW, Goodacre CJ, Munoz CA. Comparison of two tests to determine the castability of dental alloys. Int J Prosthodont 1990;3(5):413–424.
Whitlock test was not a good predictor of castability, and investment type had a greater effect on castability.

25. Barreto MT, Goldberg AJ, Nitkin DA, Mumford G. Effect of investment on casting high-fusing alloys. J Prosthet Dent 1980;44: 504–507.
Castability was affected by the pairing of alloy and investment.

26. Hinman RW, Tesk JA, Whitlock RP, Parry EE, Durkowski JS. A technique for characterizing casting behavior of dental alloys. J Dent Res 1985;64:134–138.
Authors recommend an abstract polyester sieve pattern to quantify alloy castability. (Author's note: Read Naylor et al.[24])

27. Teteruck WR, Mumford G. The fit of certain dental casting alloys using different investing materials and techniques. J Prosthet Dent 1966;16:910–927.
Alloy-investment interactions occur and should be considered to improve casting.

28. Davis DR. Potential health hazards of ceramic ring lining material. J Prosthet Dent 1987;57:362–369.
Size of ceramic ring liner fibers is a potential health concern.

29. Priest G, Horner JA. Fibrous ceramic aluminum silicate as an alternative to asbestos liners. J Prosthet Dent 1980;44:51–56.
Authors use scanning electron micrographs (SEMs) to point out potential health hazards of asbestos, and suggests using fibrous ceramic aluminum silicate. (Author's note: Read Naylor et al.[30])

30. Naylor WP, Moore BK, Phillips RW. A topographical assessment of casting ring liners using scanning electron microscopy (SEM). Quintessence Dent Technol 1987;11:413–420.
Authors found ceramic liner particles of a size recognized as potentially harmful for asbestos.

31. Dental Laboratory Technology, USAF Manual 162-6. Department of the Air Force. November, 1982:53–54.

32. Cascone P. Quartz or clay? . . . A never ending saga. Thermotrol Technician 1977;31:1, 4.
This newsletter, produced by former JF Jelenko & Co, outlines the rationale for using quartz rather than clay crucibles for casting metal-ceramic alloys.

33. Winings JR. Using aluminous oxide abrasives in porcelain-bonded-to-metal fabrication. J Prosthet Dent 1981;46(3):345–347.
Winings describes uses of nonrecycled 50- and 25-μm aluminous oxide abrasives.

34. Phillips RW. Studies on the density of castings as related to their position in the ring. J Am Dent Assoc 1947;35:329–342.

    Gold fills the mold in less than 1 second; solidification does not occur for several seconds. The distance from pattern to end of the ring (0.225 inch) has been rounded to ¼ inch (or 6.0 mm) by others.

35. Johnson A, Winstanley RB. Air-bubble entrapment as affected by investment technique, pattern angle, and use of a surface tension-reduction agent. Int J Prosthodont 1994;7:35–42.

    Authors describe techniques to reduce air entrapment on wax patterns/castings.

36. Goodsir L. Casting low density alloys. Thermotrol Technician 1973; 27(5):2, 4.

    Goodsir suggests a larger-diameter sprue former and increased acceleration when casting low-density alloys because more metal produces large buttons.

37. Ogura H, Raptis CN, Asgar K. Inner surface roughness of complete cast crowns made by centrifugal casting machines. J Prosthet Dent 1981;45:529–535.

    Variables affecting casting surface roughness are (1) alloy type, (2) mold temperature, (3) alloy casting temperature, (4) type of casting machine, (5) sandblasting (airborne-particle abrasion), and (6) location in the mold. The trailing edges of castings are rougher than the leading edges. Higher casting and mold temperatures produce rougher castings, especially with base metal alloys.

38. Cascone P. Fractures in ceramic alloy. Thermotrol Technician 1976; 30(4):1, 3.

    Hot tears occur as the metal tries to shrink on solidification but is restrained by the investment.

CHAPTER 6

How Does Dental Porcelain Bond to Metal?

Four types of bounding:
1) van der Walls forces etc

Mechanisms of Porcelain-Metal Attachment

No text on the metal-ceramic restoration would be complete without some discussion of how dental porcelain "bonds" or "adheres" to its underlying metal substructure. The exact mechanisms responsible for bonding are unknown; however, several theories are believed to provide acceptable explanations for the interrelationship at the porcelain-metal interface. Understanding these theoretical considerations of porcelain bonding is just as important as mastering the technical skills of porcelain application is to the overall success of the metal-ceramic restoration.

Use of the word *bond* might imply that the relationship between dental porcelain and metal is purely chemical.[1] Indeed, chemical bonds do play a primary role, but several nonchemical mechanisms are also believed to contribute to the bonding of dental porcelain to its underlying metal substructure.[2] Whether this attachment is chemical, mechanical, or physical in nature is not simply an academic point. Knowing how to establish and then maintain an optimum porcelain-to-metal bond is critical from a technical viewpoint as well.

At least four theories have been proposed to explain the processes involved in porcelain-to-metal bonding: (*1*) van der Waals forces, (*2*) mechanical retention, (*3*) compression bonding, and (*4*) direct chemical bonding.[2–6] While not everyone accepts all four of these proposed explanations, most experts generally agree that the chemical form of attachment is the predominant and most significant mechanism.[3]

van der Waals forces

The attraction between charged atoms of metal and porcelain that are in intimate contact yet do not actually exchange electrons is derived from *van der Waals forces*.[2,3] These are secondary forces generated more by this physical attraction between charged particles (Fig 6-1) than by an actual shar-

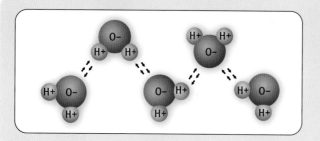

Fig 6-1 The attraction between the positively charged hydrogen (H+) of one water molecule and the negatively charged oxygen (O–) of an adjacent water molecule is one of the clearest examples of van der Waals forces.

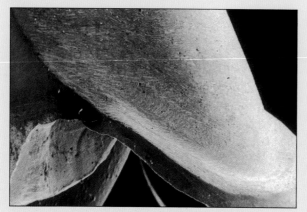

Fig 6-2 This scanning electron micrograph of a finished metal coping reveals numerous surface irregularities capable of providing mechanical retention for the fired porcelain.

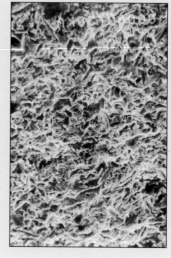

Fig 6-3 Airborne-particle abrasion of the porcelain-bearing surface with aluminum oxide removes surface contaminants and oxides while leaving a matte finish for improved porcelain bonding. The surface irregularities also enhance micromechanical retention.

mechanical retention
wonder wall

ing or exchange of electrons as is seen in primary (chemical) bonding. Because nearly all of the positive and negative charges present in the atoms are satisfied in a single molecule, van der Waals forces typically are weak[7] with minimal attraction between one molecule and another.

It is also believed that bonding entails true adhesion, but only to the extent to which the metal substructure is wetted by the softened dental porcelain.[3] The better the wetting of the metal surface by the opaque layer, the greater the van der Waals forces of attraction. Furthermore, porcelain's adhesion to metal can be diminished or enhanced by alterations in the surface character (texture) of the porcelain-bearing areas of the substructure. For example, a rough, contaminated metal surface will inhibit wetting and, hence, reduce the van der Waals bond strength. On the other hand, slight texturing of that same surface via finishing with uncontaminated aluminum oxide abrasive wheels/points, carbide burs, or diamond instruments followed by airborne-particle abrasion (blasting) with 50-μm aluminum oxide particles promotes wetting by the liquid porcelain. Improved wetting

is then accompanied by an increase in adhesion through van der Waals forces.

Even under optimum conditions, van der Waals forces undoubtedly are only minor contributors to the overall porcelain-metal attachment mechanism.

Mechanical retention

The porcelain-bearing area of a metal casting contains microscopic irregularities into which opaque porcelain may flow when heated (Fig 6-2). Airborne-particle abrasion of the metal with nonrecycled aluminum oxide, followed by steam cleaning, is believed to enhance mechanical retention further by eliminating microscopic surface metal projections and other irregularities, referred to as *stress concentrations* or stress raisers,[8] while increasing the overall surface area available for bonding (Fig 6-3). This cleansing step also removes contaminants from the porcelain-bearing surface in preparation for oxidation and subsequent opaque porcelain application.

porcelain needs to be compatible w/ metal

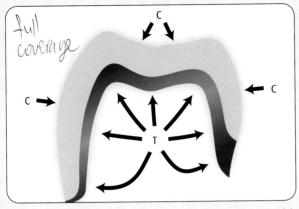

full coverage

Fig 6-4 In an ideal metal-ceramic restoration with complete porcelain coverage, the metal is believed to be under tension (T), which puts the veneer porcelain under compression (C).

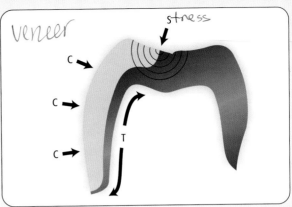

veneer *stress*

Fig 6-5 In a restoration with a partial porcelain veneer, stresses (S) may arise at the porcelain-metal junction, with limited compression (C) on the facial porcelain and tension (T) in the underlying metal substructure.

It is the opaque porcelain that fills the many surface irregularities on the metal, initiates bonding of the porcelain to metal, and serves as a foundation for color development. Nevertheless, the degree to which mechanical retention contributes to bonding may be relatively limited. Dental porcelain does not require a roughened area for bonding to occur. In fact, porcelain will fuse to a well-polished surface,[3] but some surface roughness is effective in increasing bonding forces.[9] Consequently, mechanical retention alone is not believed to be sufficient to entirely explain how dental porcelain adheres to a metal substructure.

> Dental porcelain is strongest under compression and weakest under tension; therefore, if the coefficient of thermal expansion of the metal substrate is greater than that of the porcelain placed over it, then the porcelain is placed under compression upon cooling.

3) Compression bonding

Dental porcelain is strongest under compression and weakest under tension; therefore, if the coefficient of thermal expansion (CTE) of the metal substrate is greater than that of the porcelain placed over it, then the porcelain is placed under compression upon cooling[4,10] (Fig 6-4). As a restoration cools, the metal substructure contracts at a faster rate than the ceramic veneer, but that contraction is resisted by the porcelain due to its lower CTE. This difference in contraction rates creates tensile forces on the metal and corresponding compressive forces on the ceramic veneer.[9] As noted in chapter 4, Yamamoto indicated that compressive forces are greater at the metal-porcelain interface for a dis-

tance of approximately 2.0 mm than they are at the external surface.[9] A "neutral zone" exists beyond this 2.0-mm distance, and areas of porcelain thicker than 2.0 mm likely are under tensile stresses.

One point not often made is that the theory of compression bonding assumes that the restoration in question is designed with complete and not partial veneer (ie, metal occlusal or lingual) porcelain coverage (Fig 6-5). Without the wrap-around effect created by complete porcelain coverage, there is less likelihood that "compression bonding" will develop fully. As a result, a partially veneered restoration may not encompass sufficient porcelain-bearing surfaces to exert significant compressive bonding forces.

Despite the stresses that are believed to arise at the porcelain-metal junction, the partial veneer (metal occlusal or lingual) substructure is still regarded as a very successful substructure design for anterior and posterior restorations.

4) Chemical bonding

It is generally recognized that the single most significant mechanism of porcelain-metal attachment is a chemical (molecular) bond between the oxides in dental porcelain and the oxides on the metal surface.[3,4,6] In fact, some believe that two mechanisms may occur within the chemical bonding process.[4]

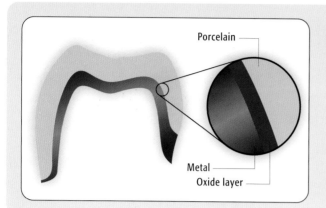

Fig 6-6 At a very basic level, a metal-ceramic restoration is made up of a metal substructure, a porcelain veneer, and (preferably) an intermediary monomolecular oxide layer.

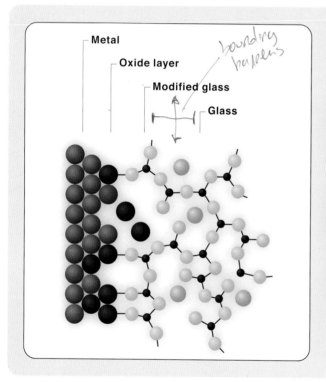

Fig 6-7 (left) The surface oxides produced by the metal substructure chemically bond with the oxides in the porcelain veneer and produce a zone of modified glass.

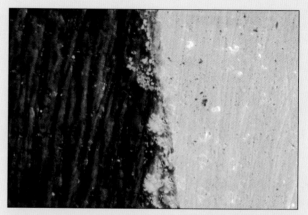

Fig 6-8 (above) The oxide layer of the metal (left) chemically bonds with the oxides in the opaque layer (right) (original magnification ×1,000). Note how porcelain has flowed into surface irregularities and areas of porosity, resulting in micromechanical retention.

"Sandwich" theory

According to one hypothesis, the oxide layer is permanently bonded to the metal substructure on one side with the dental porcelain on the other side (Fig 6-6). The oxide layer itself is sandwiched between the metal substructure and the opaque porcelain under this so-called sandwich theory, and the possible presence of a thick oxide layer would weaken the attachment of metal to porcelain.

Oxide dissolution theory

The second and more likely theory suggests that the metal surface oxides dissolve or are dissolved by the opaque layer. The porcelain is then brought into atomic contact with the metal surface for enhanced wetting and direct chemical bonding, permitting metal and porcelain to share electrons[4,9] (Fig 6-7). Both covalent and ionic bonds are thought to form, but only a monomolecular (single) layer of oxides is required for chemical bonding to occur.

There is still much to understand about what takes place at the metal surface–porcelain interface, as evidenced by the fact that these proposed methods of porcelain bonding are theories. Nonetheless, chemical bonding is generally recognized as the primary mechanism responsible for the porcelain-metal attachment (Fig 6-8).

Fig 6-9 These three oxidized copings were made with noble alloys, yet their color and character (eg, texture, thickness) appear to be markedly different. The Olympia casting (Jelenko) *(left)* is medium gray and has a moderate level of oxidation. The high-palladium–copper alloy Naturelle (Pentron) *(center)* has the darkest color (dark brown to black) and the highest level of oxidation. The Ivoclar Vivadent W-1 casting *(right)*, a palladium-silver alloy, exhibits a light-gray oxide layer. The differences in the appearance of the oxidized castings are most distinct when the high palladium–copper unit *(left)* is compared with the palladium-silver (tin only) alloy coping *(right)*. Note that this palladium-silver alloy produced a relatively thin layer of a light-gray oxide.

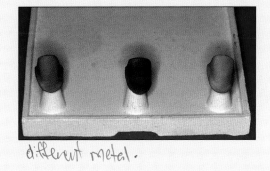

different metal.

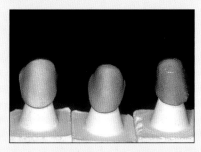

Fig 6-10 Three different base metal alloys: nickel-chromium-beryllium *(left)*; nickel-chromium (beryllium-free) *(center)*; and cobalt-chromium *(right)*. Each casting produces a distinct oxidation when properly oxidized according to the manufacturers' recommended instructions.

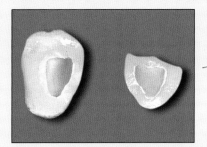

— degassing stage of oxydation

Fig 6-11 Porcelain-metal bond failures can occur through the oxide layer itself if that layer is too thick or poorly adherent. Note how the ideal straw-like color of the oxide layer remains bonded to the porcelain and cleanly separates from the metal surface.

porcelain breakage of metal means oxydation didn't bond correctly

Oxidation

Oxidation is one of the principal steps in the preparation of the metal substructure for porcelain bonding.[4,5] Once metal-ceramic castings have been properly finished, they are thoroughly cleaned, after which the castings are heat-treated (oxidized) in a porcelain furnace (in air or in a vacuum) to a designated temperature for a specified period of time (according to the manufacturer's instructions).[5]

There is no single standard oxidizing technique for all alloys on the market. On the contrary, the type of atmosphere (vacuum or air) and the high-temperature setting/duration differ among the numerous high noble, noble, and base metal-ceramic alloys.[5] Furthermore, the chemical makeup of the oxides differs among systems according to variations in the type and quantity of minor alloying elements.

Oxidizable trace elements, such as tin, indium, and iron, are commonly included in noble ceramic alloys to produce an adherent oxide layer (Fig 6-9). These metals are needed because gold, palladium, and other noble elements do not oxidize. That is why it is necessary to hold high noble and noble alloy substructures at a prescribed temperature for several minutes, so the nonnoble trace elements can form the required oxide layer.

By comparison, base metal alloys *do* oxidize, and oxidize quite readily. Still, trace elements are added to their formulations to facilitate the formation of a particular type of surface oxide layer required by each alloy to establish a stable bond (Fig 6-10). The oxidation procedure may even be carried out in a vacuum to minimize the amount of oxide formation. The hold time at the recommended high temperature setting may even be reduced, if not completely omitted. Allowing certain base metal alloys to oxidize in air or to remain too long at high temperature can lead to overoxidation and is likely to result in an excessively thick, nonadherent oxide layer, which is often responsible for porcelain bond failures (Fig 6-11).

Evaluating an oxidized casting

It is important to think of oxidation not just as a procedure but as a process. As such, the appearance of each oxidized casting should be visually assessed to ensure that the settings for temperature, time, and atmosphere (vacuum firing versus air firing) for the porcelain furnace are correct before firing. Only by visually analyzing the end result can one be assured that the recommended appearance of that oxide layer has been achieved. Otherwise, the by-product of this procedure may simply be a poorly oxidized substructure.

Properly oxidized castings often have a distinctive color and character (eg, texture, thickness) that vary among alloy systems and sometimes even among alloys within the same system (see Fig 6-10). Variations outside the expected results should be reassessed and perhaps discussed with the alloy manufacturer.

It is also important to point out that some manufacturers recommend omitting the oxidation step and minimizing the number of firings to which castings are subjected. In the late 1970s, it was noted that oxidation heat softened certain types of alloys through molecular rearrangement, resulting in marginal distortion and a decrease in porcelain bond strength.[11] These potential limitations aside, most modern-day alloy manufacturers regard the oxidation process as an essential step in the fabrication of the metal-ceramic restoration.

To avoid possible laboratory errors, follow the manufacturer's recommendations and do not apply broad, generic processing instructions to every alloy. But remember, the recommended firing temperatures are only general guidelines that should be adjusted to accommodate the unique demands of each type (horizontal muffle versus vertical muffle) and brand of porcelain furnace. Again, a successful outcome is determined by visually inspecting restorations after the oxidation step to ensure that the appearance recommended by the alloy manufacturer has been achieved.

Postoxidation Treatment

As might be expected, recommendations for the postoxidation treatment also vary according to the type and brand of alloy used. With some products, including several of the noble and base metals,[5] the first oxides formed may be the most desirable for porcelain bonding. For these alloys, it is best not to remove the oxide layer but to proceed directly to the application of opaque porcelain. For other types of alloys, manufacturers recommend either removing or at least modifying the oxide layer.

Removing/modifying the oxide layer

Should the manufacturer recommend removal or reduction of the oxide film on porcelain-bearing areas following oxidation, two principal methods can be used: acid treatment* (chemical method) or nonacid treatment (mechanical method).

Acid treatment

Several different acids can be used to reduce or eliminate surface oxides, including hydrofluoric acid, hydrochloric acid, or dilute sulfuric acid.[1,9] The potential hazards posed by these chemicals require that they be both stored and used in clearly marked, resealable plastic bottles.[12] For added safety, acid-containing containers should be maintained in a hooded area in the laboratory. It is also advisable to wear protective rubber gloves and eye protection and to use rubber-tipped instruments for all procedures requiring acid use. Expect the type of acid, and even the recommendation to use acids, to vary with the different alloy systems and manufacturers.

To reduce the risk of injury associated with the potential mishandling of acids, consider using a hydrofluoric acid substitute such as NoSan (Triodent).

Nonacid treatment

Not everyone is eager to handle acids on a routine basis, especially when a mechanical method of oxide removal or reduction is readily available. Castings can be airborne-particle abraded with 50-μm aluminum oxide particles. Only nonrecycled aluminum oxide (white) should be used to avoid possible contamination of the porcelain-bearing surface of the metal substructure[13] (see Fig 5-23). Traditionally, sand was used for "blasting" complete gold crowns to remove investment residue. The term "sandblasting" has carried over into the vocabulary of metal-ceramic terminology, but it is more appropriate to refer to this procedure as *airborne-particle abrasion*.[14] Steam clean or ultrasonically clean the casting in distilled water for 10 to 15 minutes before applying the opaque porcelain.

The cost of an airborne-particle abrasion unit and the need to maintain an adequate supply of aluminum oxide powders are well worth the initial investment and the ongoing expense. Direct skin contact with either hydrofluoric or sulfuric acid can cause very serious injury and requires immediate medical attention,*[12] making nonacid treatment the preferred method.

---

*Note: For safety reasons, the use of caustic chemical agents such as hydrofluoric acid (HF) or sulfuric acid (H_2SO_4) is discouraged when airborne-particle abrasion with 50-μm aluminum oxide particles can achieve a similar outcome.

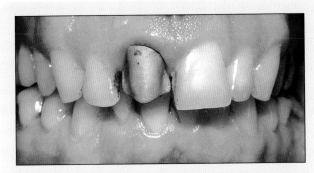

Fig 6-12a This type of bond failure is often referred to as a *loss of attachment* or a *delamination* of the porcelain from the metal substructure.

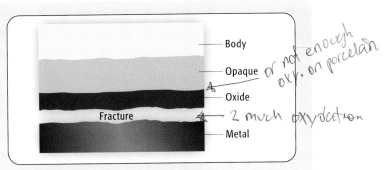

[handwritten annotation: or not enough oxi. on porcelain]

[handwritten annotation: 2 much oxydation]

Fig 6-12b Complete detachment from the metal by the dental porcelain may be caused by excessive oxide formation or a poorly adherent oxide layer.

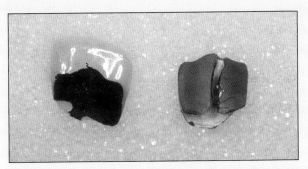

Fig 6-13a Note how the heavy greenish oxides are bonded to the porcelain *(left)*, yet a substantial amount of oxidation remains on the metal substructure *(right)* of this cobalt-chromium casting.

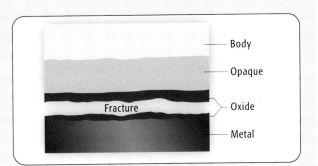

Fig 6-13b The bond failure shown in Fig 6-13a likely occurred through the thick oxide layer, leaving oxides on both porcelain and metal.

Porcelain-Metal Bond Failures

Metal-ceramic alloys, whether high-noble, noble, or base metals, oxidize differently because of variations in their composition. If the oxidation process is not performed properly, the subsequent porcelain-metal bond may be weak and fail. The consequences of bond failures, whether immediate or delayed, obviously are costly.

Porcelain delamination

With base metal alloys, separation of the porcelain veneer from the metal substrate is primarily the result of a loss of the "attachment" of an oxide layer that either is too thick or is poorly adherent to the metal substructure.[15] The porcelain and oxide film retain their bond yet become detached or delaminated at the porcelain-metal junction (Fig 6-12). Overoxidation has been a particular problem with the heavily oxidizing base metal alloys and has been linked to increased bond failures. In other instances, bond failures are not the result of a loss of the chemical bond between the ceramic and the oxide layer. Rather, the porcelain may actually remain visibly attached to the metal surface oxides, but the bond fails within the oxide layer itself (Fig 6-13). This problem can be attributed to the formation of a thick and poorly adherent oxide layer.

Likewise, excessive absorption of oxides by the ceramic layer can lower the porcelain's CTE, alter the final shade

[handwritten: noble metal is better, less chances have it turn gray]

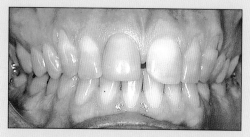

Fig 6-14 The metal-ceramic restoration on the maxillary right central incisor was fabricated with a high palladium–copper alloy, but the opaque porcelain could mask the metal and control the dark oxidation layer. Note the very distinct graying of the porcelain. This restoration must be remade because such a color shift cannot be corrected with surface stains.

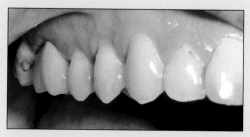

Fig 6-15 The placement of another brand of dental porcelain on a different high-palladium alloy did not result in any discoloration of the porcelain on the metal-ceramic crown on the maxillary right first molar. Perhaps the greater thickness of porcelain, fewer body bakes, or improved masking ability of a different opaque porcelain prevented discoloration.

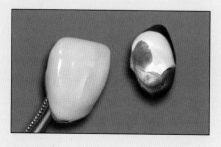

[handwritten: porce. not adhering to metal correctly]

Fig 6-16 The cracking of the porcelain on the base metal alloy unit *(left)* is an indication of a possible porcelain-metal incompatibility that could lead to an immediate or a delayed bond failure *(right)*. Improper substructure design (eg, too much free-standing porcelain) also should be ruled out as a possible cause of a structural failure in the porcelain veneer.

(causing a graying or bluing), or do both[5,16] (Fig 6-14). Changes in the shade of the porcelain may not be noticeable in posterior restorations, particularly if a greater thickness of porcelain masks any dark oxides (Fig 6-15). Such shade shifts can occur even with noble metal alloys.[5,16] Moreover, the oxide-masking ability of opaques is not the same for all brands of dental porcelains.[10] Some opaque porcelains are able to mask certain oxides better than others.

Incompatible materials

Bond failures are not always attributable to improper oxidation, but may actually be caused by a physical incompatibility between the dental porcelain and the metal-ceramic alloy being used. Differences in the CTE between the veneering porcelain and the metal may be at the maximum limit of the acceptable thermal compatibility range yet be sufficiently large to cause cracking of the ceramic veneer (Fig 6-16, *left*) or so far outside the desirable range as to result in porcelain debonding[9] (see Fig 6-16, *right*) (see chapters 2 and 3).

Bear in mind that cracking also can occur with a thermally compatible alloy and porcelain pairing because the thickness of unsupported porcelain is beyond the desired 2.0-mm maximum dimension.[9]

Overoxidation/underoxidation

As stated previously, the oxidation process varies for alloys of different compositions, and it should not be taken for granted. Bear in mind that no single technique can be used for every type of metal-ceramic alloy. Careful processing followed by a visual assessment of the postoxidation appearance of each casting will ensure that the procedure was carried out correctly. Castings that are either overoxidized or underoxidized should be reprocessed until a uniform oxide of the desired color and thickness, as recommended by the alloy manufacturer, has formed. Overoxidation, if undetected, may eventually lead to bond failure with "cleavage" of the bond through an excessively thick oxide layer (see Figs 6-13a and 6-13b).

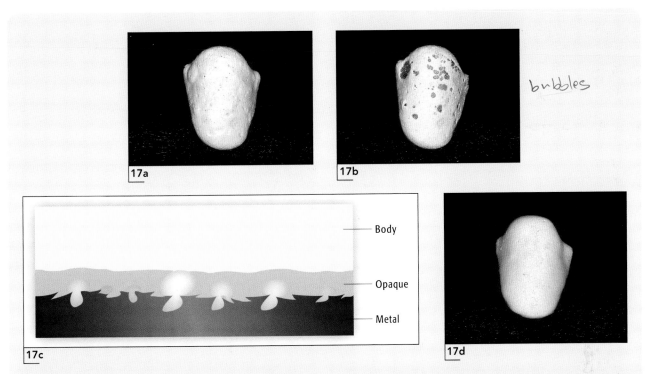

bubbles

Fig 6-17a Although the manufacturer's directions were followed, bubbling of the opaque porcelain occurred on this high-palladium–copper alloy.

Fig 6-17b Removal of the opaque bubbles revealed areas where the porcelain either did not bond or debonded during the opaque firing cycle.

Fig 6-17c Surface or subsurface contaminants may be reponsible for the bubble formation during porcelain firing.

Fig 6-17d Merely refinishing this casting removed the surface and subsurface contamination and resulted in an appropriate porcelain-metal bond.

Contamination

Very often, castings that demonstrate some evidence of contamination may not have to be remade. Should surface debonding occur, refinishing the substructure's porcelain-bearing surface may be all that is necessary in some instances (Fig 6-17). But before taking this course of action, make certain that the level of contamination is not extensive. To minimize potential problems it is best to use only clean, uncontaminated finishing instruments. For added safety and to prevent cross-contamination, dedicate a set of finishing abrasives for each type of alloy used.

Summary

The porcelain-metal bond is established through a variety of complex processes, and our understanding of the bonding mechanisms involved continues to grow. This chapter explains the theories behind the bonding process, how to optimize the porcelain-metal bond, and how to identify different types of bond failures. In chapter 7 you will learn how to prepare the metal substructure for the application of dental porcelain through proper adjusting, finishing, and oxidation techniques.

References

1. Sarkar NK, Verret M, Eyer CS, Jeansonne EE. Role of gallium in alloy-porcelain bonding. J Prosthet Dent 1985;53:190–194.

2. Bagby M, Marshall SJ, Marshall GW Jr. Metal ceramic compatibility: A review of the literature. J Prosthet Dent 1990;63:21–25.
   Authors attribute porcelain bonding to three mechanisms: van der Waals forces, mechanical interlocking, and chemical bonding, and then discusses thermomechanical compatibility.

3. Lacy AM. The chemical nature of dental porcelain. Dent Clin North Am 1977;21:661–667.
   Lacy reviews van der Waals forces, mechanical bonding, and chemical bonding of porcelain. (Author's note: No mention of mismatch of coefficients of thermal expansion.)

4. McLean JW. The Science and Art of Dental Ceramics. Vol II: Bridge design and laboratory procedures in dental ceramics. Chicago: Quintessence, 1980:31–36.
Reviews three theories for porcelain bonding (excluding van der Waals forces).

5. Naylor WP. Non-Gold Base Dental Casting Alloys. Vol II: Porcelain-fused-to-metal alloys [ADA173766]. Brooks AFB, Texas: USAF School of Aerospace Medicine, 1986:100–108.

6. Murakami I, Schulman A. Aspects of metal-ceramic bonding. Dent Clin North Am 1987;31:333–346.
Authors review four theories of dental porcelain bonding in metal-ceramic restorations.

7. Anusavice KJ. Phillips' Science of Dental Materials, ed 11. Philadelphia: Saunders, 2003:22,26.
Explaination of van der Waals forces.

8. Riley EJ. Ceramo-metal restoration. State of the science. Dent Clin North Am 1977;21:669–682.
Riley presents engineering principles for fixed-partial denture design, metal preparation, and the porcelain bond.

9. Yamamoto M. Metal-Ceramics: Principles and Methods of Makoto Yamamoto. Chicago: Quintessence, 1985:189–190.
Author believes compressive forces are greater at the metal-porcelain interface within the first 2.0 mm (approximately) than they are at the external surface. Tensile forces exist in porcelain thicker than 2.0 mm.

10. Coffey JP, Anusavice KJ, DeHoff PH, Lee RB, Hojjatie B. Influence of contraction mismatch and cooling rate on flexural failure of PFM systems. J Dent Res 1988;67:61–65.
Laboratory study supports theory that in porcelain-fused-to-metal restorations the metal should have a higher CTE than the porcelain (a positive expansion coefficient mismatch).

11. Stein RS, Kuwata M. A dentist and a dental technologist analyze current ceramo-metal procedures. Dent Clin North Am 1977;21:729–749.

12. Wilson GA, Sanger RG, Boswick JA. Accidental hydrofluoric acid burns of the hand. J Am Dent Assoc 1979;99:57–58.
Authors provide a protocol for the management of a hydrofluoric acid chemical burn.

13. Winings JR. Using aluminous oxide abrasives in porcelain-bonded-to-metal fabrication. J Prosthet Dent 1981;46:345–347.
Winings uses a hand-held unit (Paasche Air Eraser) and a larger, self-contained Micro Blaster unit with two hoses and two diameter tips to air-particle abrade castings.

14. Glossary of prosthodontic terms. J Prosthet Dent 2005;94:10–92.

15. Mackert JR, Ringle RD, Fairhurst C. Oxide wrinkling and porcelain adherence on nonprecious alloys [abstract #377]. J Dent Res 1981;60A(special issue):405.
Poorly adherent and wrinkled appearance of oxides on base-metal alloys linked to poor porcelain bond.

16. Stavridakis MM, Papazoglou E, Seghi RR, Johnston WM, Brantley WA. Effect of different high-palladium metal-ceramic alloys on the color of opaque and dentin porcelain. J Prosthet Dent 2004;92:170–178.

CHAPTER 7

Preparation of the Metal Substructure for Porcelain

If you were meticulous when waxing, preparation of the cast substructure should proceed quickly. However, if the substructure was poorly designed or hastily constructed, you may need to start over or allocate additional time for the adjusting and finishing procedures. Familiarity with the principles of substructure design (see chapter 4) will help you to identify any such flaws in your work. It is critical that errors be caught by this stage, for metal preparation is the last opportunity you will have to correct them.

Thinking Ahead

A number of different procedures must be completed to transform a casting into a metal substructure ready for the application of opaque porcelain. To maximize the potential for success on a consistent basis, think ahead to identify what needs to be accomplished for each successive step.

Casting appraisal

Evaluate the quality of the casting using a microscope, magnification loupes, or another form of magnification. Closely inspect the work for any defects produced as a result of the casting process (Fig 7-1).[1] Make certain the casting is dense and no porosity is located in the restoration itself (Fig 7-2a). Check the margins. Are they complete and sharp? If so, inspect the intaglio (interior) surface of the restoration for the presence of nodules or excessive surface roughness (Fig 7-2b).

In the event that defects are detected, make note of them, and determine how they might be prevented in subsequent cases. If the casting is judged to be inadequate for any reason (eg, incomplete margins, porosity, an unacceptable fit, excessive roughness), do not even begin finishing the metal substructure for porcelain. Also, avoid the temptation to seat the casting on its master die because you may irreparably damage the gypsum and waste a great deal of time in the process. Instead, reject the casting and rewax the case.

Important

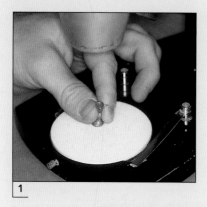
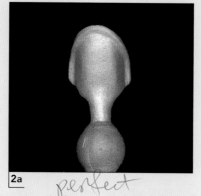
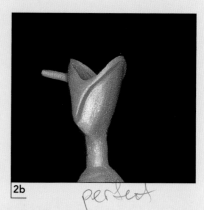

perfect *perfect*

Fig 7-1 Inspection of the intaglio surface of castings requires the aid of some form of magnification.

Fig 7-2a The completed casting should be dense and free of defects. Note the smooth transition from the sprue to the restoration, which is a direct result of the care taken during spruing.

Fig 7-2b The margins of the casting should be complete and sharp.

suck-back / a hole could be on incisal

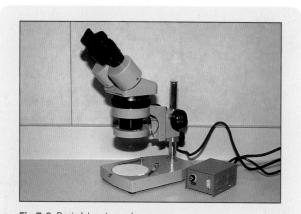

Fig 7-3 Basic laboratory microscope.

Armamentarium

You might think you have to surround yourself with a large assortment of equipment and materials to perform even some very simple tasks. Actually, once you understand what is involved in metal preparation and master a technique, you will find that very few items are required for these procedures (see appendix E).

The armamentarium for adjusting and finishing the metal substructure can best be divided into three categories: *(1)* equipment, *(2)* instruments, and *(3)* materials.

Equipment

A variety of equipment is needed in the dental laboratory. This equipment can be divided into the general categories of magnification, laboratory handpieces, and alloy-recovery devices.

Magnification

A laboratory microscope and magnification loupes are valuable tools that can be used for a multitude of procedures, from waxing margins to adjusting metal substructures right through to finishing the final restoration (Fig 7-3).[1] The growing popularity of using some form of magnification in dental technology has led to the development of different types and styles of microscopes (see appendix E). For most laboratory procedures, a magnification level between 7× and 20× is adequate. Should you need to purchase a microscope, choose one that features a good external light source and adequate working distance under the tube head. A design that permits mounting above the laboratory bench top leaves the immediate work area free of clutter. Such a configuration not only makes it easier for you to perform tasks but also helps to reduce exposure of this equipment to the debris

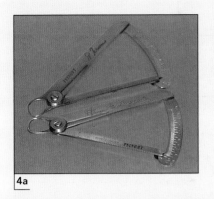 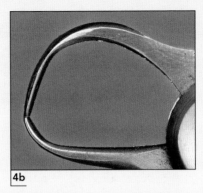 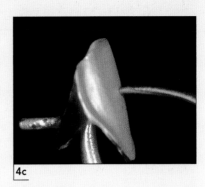

Fig 7-4a The measuring caliper for metal (Pfingst) *(top)* looks similar to the measuring caliper for wax (Pfingst) *(bottom)*.

Fig 7-4b The tips of the metal-measuring caliper have flat ends and are smaller in diameter than those of the wax-measuring caliper.

Fig 7-4c Use the metal-measuring caliper to take multiple measurements of different sections of the porcelain-bearing area.

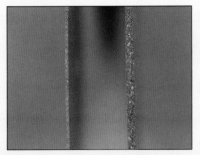 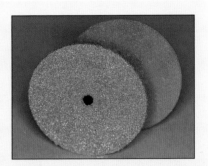

Fig 7-5a Select either a thin *(left)* or thick *(right)* carborundum disk for despruing.

Fig 7-5b Coarse *(foreground)* and fine *(background)* carborundum disks.

generated during grinding and polishing procedures. But select a microscope based on the overall quality of the unit, not merely on how it can be mounted in a dental laboratory.

Laboratory handpieces

Metal finishing and polishing can be accomplished with a laboratory handpiece, but some procedures can be performed using a bench-top lathe. A variable speed laboratory handpiece is preferred for most tasks and accepts commonly used abrasives (eg, stones, diamond instruments, carbide burs, mandrels for disks). Having the ability to adjust the rotary speed gives the operator control and reduces the risk of possibly damaging the cast restoration.

Alloy recovery device

A portable dust-collection device is valuable because it allows the recovery of precious elements lost during sprue

removal, metal finishing, and metal polishing. Small, commercially available hand-held units are recommended. The collected dust can be sent to a metal refining company for processing in exchange for money or ingots of dental alloy. A device to consider is the 1.5 horsepower Hippo Portable Hand-Held Vac (RE Williams).

Instruments

One instrument that is essential for the metal-finishing procedures is a metal caliper (Fig 7-4). You will use this gauge throughout the adjusting and finishing stages to measure the thickness of metal in both the porcelain-bearing and the nonporcelain areas. Likewise, finishing instruments are available for performing a variety of tasks such as sprue removal (Fig 7-5), metal recontouring, finishing the porcelain-bearing surfaces, and smoothing and polishing the nonporcelain sections of a casting.

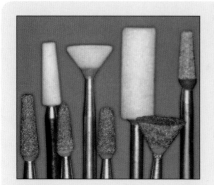

Fig 7-6 Assorted ceramic stones for metal finishing.

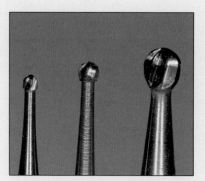

Fig 7-7 Three commonly used round carbide burs for fitting and adjusting: No. ½ *(left)*, No. 2 *(center)*, and No. 8 *(right)*.

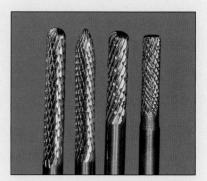

Fig 7-8 Carbide burs for adjusting and finishing the porcelain-bearing areas of a metal substructure. Note the varied shapes and geometries.

crown little bits

Rough cuts

Exercise caution when selecting finishing instruments because the composition of certain types of abrasives can actually contaminate the metal and jeopardize the porcelain-metal bond. Debris left behind on the porcelain-bearing areas by some silicone and carborundum abrasives (or from the abrasive binder) can release gases when the restoration is later heated. These gaseous by-products are capable of expanding to 80 times their original volume, producing bubbling of the opaque porcelain, and otherwise interfering with the formation of an adherent porcelain-metal bond.[2]

To prevent potential problems associated with surface contamination, use a ceramic abrasive (Fig 7-6), carbide fissure bur, or carbide finishing bur (Figs 7-7 and 7-8) for metal preparation whenever possible,[2] or use these instruments in the final stages of surface preparation.

Materials

Among the materials you will want to include in your armamentarium are disclosing agents, articulating film, and abrasives such as nonrecycled 50-μm aluminum oxide and glass beads.

Metal-Finishing Procedures

Before beginning any metal finishing, make sure all residual investment has been removed from the casting. Quite frequently, debris will remain in the intaglio surface or cling to the occlusal or lingual surfaces. Care should be taken when airborne-particle abrading because it has been shown that both aluminum oxide and glass beads can damage a restoration's delicate margins.[3]

Likewise, remember to thoroughly clean the sectioned sprues before storing the spent alloy. If the metal is to be recast, any investment attached to it may end up in the next casting and cause pitting or a miscast margin.

As with most laboratory procedures, metal finishing should proceed in an orderly fashion. The basic goal of preparing a substructure is to take the metal through a sequence of finishing steps, beginning with coarse abrasives and ending with a fine abrasive instrument.

Removing the sprue

After you have inspected the casting and judged it to be satisfactory, the next step is to remove the sprue(s). Some technicians prefer to use a bench-top lathe for despruing because it can be quicker, easier, and safer than using a

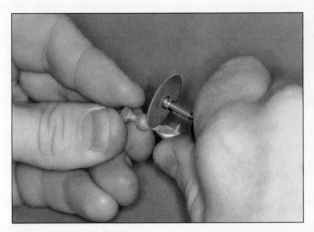

Fig 7-9a Holding the handpiece with a strong thumb grip, make a cut in the sprue on the facial surface as close to the restoration as possible. Rotate the casting 180 degrees, and make a second cut on the lingual surface of the sprue.

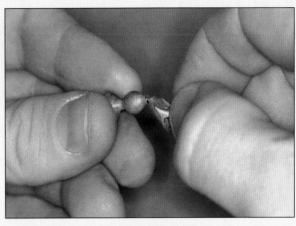

Fig 7-9b With two cuts on opposite sides, the restoration is alternately moved facially and lingually (rocked) until the coping separates from the sprue.

don't put it on the die right away, make sure everything is done properly on casting & remove anything in future

handpiece. Others like the convenience and added control offered by a slow-speed handpiece. Aside from selecting your choice of equipment (handpiece versus lathe), you must decide whether to use a thin fine-grit or a thick coarse-grit carborundum disk mounted on a mandrel (see Fig 7-5). The thicker disks have several disadvantages: they generate more heat, produce more metal debris (dust), and remove excessive amounts of alloy. However, they are stronger and less likely to break during sprue removal.

With the restoration held securely in one hand, carefully section the sprue, cutting as close as possible to the restoration without contacting the work itself (Fig 7-9a). If you are uncertain how close to make the cut, err on the safe side and leave some additional sprue length on the restoration; the sprue-restoration attachment area can always be recontoured later. Be advised that a significant amount of frictional heat can be generated during this process. To avoid injury to your fingers, make the cuts using light, intermittent pressure.

When despruing, be extremely careful not to damage any adjacent restorations. Avoid distractions during this critical task, especially when using a high-speed lathe. As an added safety measure, switch on the lathe's evacuation system, adjust the plastic shield to protect yourself from flying debris, and wear safety glasses with side shields. It is not necessary to cut completely through the diameter of a sprue. Instead, make a partial cut on one side, rotate the

> The basic goal of preparing a substructure is to take the metal through a sequence of finishing steps, beginning with coarse abrasives and ending with fine abrasive instruments.

casting, and make a similar cut on the opposite side. At this point you should be able to move the restoration back and forth (Fig 7-9b) until it detaches from the sprue.

Fitting the cast restoration

After despruing, the next step is to fit the restoration to its die. Assess the fit of the casting first before removing remnants of the sprues, initiating any surface finishing procedures, or reducing the porcelain-bearing areas; these procedures will result in unnecessary metal loss should the casting fit be unsatisfactory and require a laboratory remake.

In this way you will ensure, at the earliest possible time, that the fit and quality of the casting are satisfactory before proceeding with any additional work. Likewise, if the intaglio surface of the restoration requires extensive adjustment, determine if metal finishing can be completed satisfactorily without a risk of perforating the metal substructure in the porcelain-bearing areas.

In most cases, the master cast is your only reference for the prepared tooth or teeth; therefore, care should be taken not to damage it. One small chip of the gypsum margin during metal finishing may necessitate extensive chairside adjustment by the dentist or result in a clinically unacceptable restoration. Whenever possible, repour the final impression to obtain a second die on which to seat the work if a

Using this tech ⊗→ ⊗ don't rush it

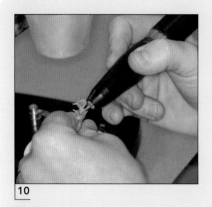

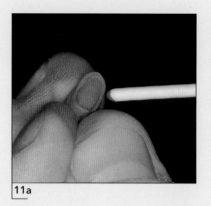

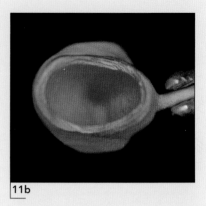

Fig 7-10 A No. ½ round carbide bur is ideal for removing small nodules and making minor adjustments to the intaglio surface. Note the use of a weaker pencil grip.

Fig 7-11a Occlude (Pascal) disclosing agent can be sprayed into the inside of a casting.

Fig 7-11b After being sprayed with Occlude, the casting has a thin, uniform layer of the disclosing medium.

second die is not already available. This relatively inexpensive and simple procedure can save a great deal of time and help ensure an accurate and well-fitting final restoration.

From your initial inspection of the inside of the casting, you may have already identified obvious irregularities. Attempt to remove any weakly attached nodules with a metal instrument such as a discoid carver. If that proves unsuccessful, grind away the irregularities with the aid of magnification (Fig 7-10) using a small (No. ½) round carbide bur (see Fig 7-7).[1]

Next, apply a disclosing medium to the intaglio surface of the casting, and fit it to the die. There are a number of commercial products on the market designed for this type of application, including aerosol spray indicators such as Occlude (Pascal) (Fig 7-11a) and paint-on liquids such as Crown Fit Indicator (KerrLab) and AccuFilm IV (Parkell). These products can be used to disclose either the die or the restoration. Both techniques work well; however, when a marking medium is brushed onto or sprayed into the interior surface of a casting (Fig 7-11b), it can build up internally with repeated applications. Depending on the extent of the adjustment needed and the amount of material applied, periodic steam cleaning of the restoration may be necessary to prevent such buildup.

It is easier, neater, and probably less time-consuming to coat a second die with a very thin layer of disclosing material (Fig 7-12a) and gently seat the restoration on it (Fig 7-12b). Remove the restoration from the die, and inspect the internal surface of the casting for any indication of a

transfer of the marking medium (Fig 7-12c). Also, examine the die itself for evidence of contact that may not have transferred to the casting (Fig 7-12d). Make necessary adjustments using a small round carbide bur (Fig 7-13). Repeat this process until the restoration is completely seated (Fig 7-14). If the fit of the restoration is less than perfect (eg, if it is over- or underexpanded), make note of this outcome, so you can change your investing technique for future cases and determine if the casting must be remade. If all of the preceding procedures were performed correctly, the restoration should seat completely. Assuming the fit is satisfactory, return the casting to the master die for final confirmation of the fit.

Recontouring the sprue area

With the fit assured, remove the casting from the die and carefully reduce the areas where remnants of sprues remain using a coarse ceramic abrasive such as a heatless stone (Fig 7-15). This sprue attachment area must be recontoured so that the casting can be returned to the mounted master cast and properly articulated. Also, if the casting has suckback porosity at the junction of the sprue and restoration, it may not become apparent until this area of the metal is finished. It is better to know before proceeding if such porosity is present, because the casting may not be usable. It is not advisable to grind the casting while it is on the master die.

can make a duplicate die

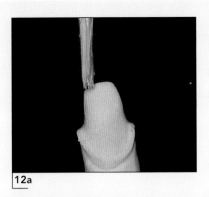
12a

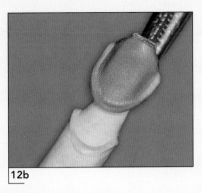
12b

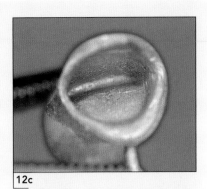
12c

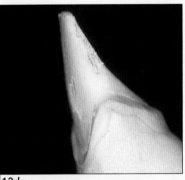
12d

Fig 7-12a Gypsum die painted with AccuFilm IV (Parkell).

Fig 7-12b The casting is gently and slowly seated on the stone die covered with the disclosing medium.

Fig 7-12c If resistance is met, the casting is removed; if not, it is seated completely. Areas of binding will transfer the disclosing medium from die to casting. Repeat this step, and adjust the casting if the mark appears in the same location a second time (ie, mark twice, cut once).

Fig 7-12d In some instances, the disclosing agent on the die itself may be slightly abraded, indicating that an adjustment is needed.

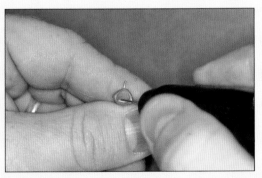

Fig 7-13 Grind the marked area on the inside of the casting using a small carbide bur in an electric handpiece and light, intermittent pressure.

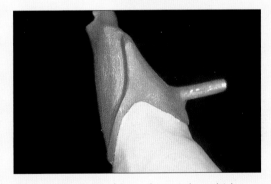

Fig 7-14 Lateral view of the casting seated completely.

Fig 7-15 With the fit confirmed, the remaining sprue can be removed and that area grossly finished with a heatless stone (Mizzy) or similar instrument.

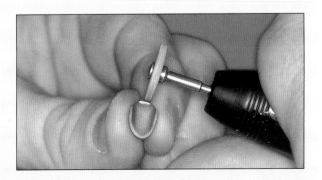

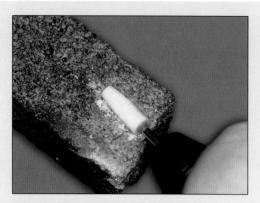

Fig 7-16 Use a sharpening stone to adjust a large ceramic stone to your preferred shape and size.

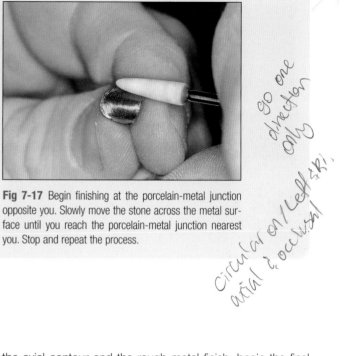

Fig 7-17 Begin finishing at the porcelain-metal junction opposite you. Slowly move the stone across the metal surface until you reach the porcelain-metal junction nearest you. Stop and repeat the process.

Finishing the porcelain-bearing surface

Assuming no suck-back porosity is present, you are now ready to begin the rough finishing of the restoration. Start by using the metal caliper to measure the thickness of metal across the entire porcelain-bearing surface (see Fig 7-4). If any areas require reduction, adjust them first. If the wax was cut back appropriately, some sections may be thicker than others in order for the porcelain to be uniform. Should you find an excessively thick area, reduce it to the appropriate dimension for the clinical case and the type of alloy used.

During these adjusting and finishing procedures, continue to check the thickness of the casting periodically to be sure the metal is not inadvertently overreduced. Failure to take frequent measurements of the metal thickness can unexpectedly lead to perforation of the substructure. Very small perforations can be repaired by presoldering, but only in extenuating circumstances. It is better to remake the restoration if the perforation is extensive or a large area has been thinned excessively and weakened the substructure. You do not want to leave behind sharp angles or concavities, but you do want to create a sharp, well-defined butt joint (interface) at the porcelain-metal junction.

Again using a heatless stone, perform any gross reduction of axial surfaces, and measure the thickness of the area where the sprue was attached. Once you are satisfied with

> Failure to take frequent measurements of the metal thickness can unexpectedly lead to perforation of the substructure.

the axial contour and the rough metal finish, begin the final preparation of the porcelain-bearing surface of the restoration.

The steps taken in this final finishing stage are intended to:

- Smooth the porcelain surface, making it free of sharp angles and potential stress raisers.
- Create microscopic undercuts (as described in chapter 6) to gain mechanical retention.
- Increase the surface contact area for the opaque dental porcelain veneer.
- Reduce the contact angle of the porcelain as it is being applied.

Although the finished surface is slightly rough for mechanical retention, it will still allow the dental porcelain to readily wet the metal.

Selection of an abrasive is critical.[2] Use a clean, ceramic-bound abrasive that has never come in contact with any other type of metal. Avoid any possibility of metal cross-contamination by keeping your abrasives separated by alloy type. Stock abrasives can be reshaped with a sharpening stone if desired (Fig 7-16). Do not use an abrasive finer than a fine ceramic stone (Fig 7-17), and especially do not use a rubber wheel to smooth porcelain-bearing areas. Residue from the rubber wheel will contaminate the surface, reduce the mechanical undercuts on the surface, and increase the contact angle of the porcelain mixture, which can adversely affect the wettability of the ceramic during sintering.[2]

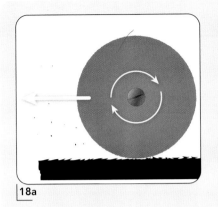

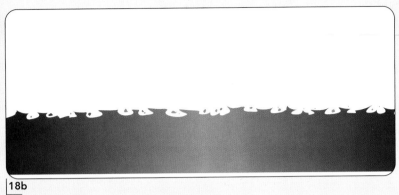

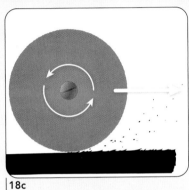

Fig 7-18a Avoid finishing in many directions because this creates irregularities on the metal surface.

Fig 7-18b Some of the irregularities may retain debris that can later contaminate the porcelain.

Fig 7-18c Finish the metal in one direction. Unidirectional finishing should leave the metal surface smooth and minimize surface debris and irregularities.

Avoid haphazard finishing in many directions because you can actually trap debris in the small surface irregularities (Figs 7-18a and 7-18b). By finishing the porcelain-bearing surfaces in one direction only and by rotating the abrasive toward you, the metal is pulled in your direction, thereby reducing surface imperfections and minimizing debris entrapment (Fig 7-18c). A properly finished porcelain-bearing area should have a smooth, satin finish.

If a thin facial metal collar is included in the substructure design, expect to devote extra attention to this area during finishing. Technically, a 0.5-mm beveled tooth preparation requires more than a 0.5-mm metal collar.[4] The actual width of the collar should include the height of the bevel externally plus the thickness of the metal substructure. If you wish to reduce the collar width, now is the time to do so. A straight shank No. 8 round carbide bur is recommended for this procedure (Fig 7-19). To lessen the risks of damaging the restoration, select a sharp bur, and make certain to rotate it toward you. This particular procedure lends itself to being performed under magnification. If the metal collar is adjusted below the 0.5-mm dimension, the facial porcelain placed in that area will lack proper bulk and will be subject to stresses should the thinned metal flex. Of course, if there is no facial bevel and a rounded shoulder or chamfer preparation has been used, the facial metal can be thinned to the recommended minimum thickness for the type of alloy used. Remember to recheck the thickness of the porcelain-bearing areas periodically.

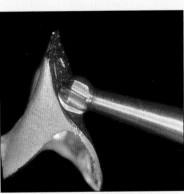

#8 gives roundness

Fig 7-19 The sharp external line angle of the porcelain-metal junction can be restored or refined with a No. 8 round carbide bur, especially across the facial metal collar (if present).

Finishing the nonporcelain surfaces

The next step in preparing the metal substructure for porcelain is to finish the nonporcelain surfaces (Fig 7-20a). There are several schools of thought on how to handle this phase of metal preparation. One approach is to do minimal finishing of all nonporcelain areas until after the porcelain has been built up, contoured, and glazed. The belief is that anything more than a light finishing of the nonporcelain areas will

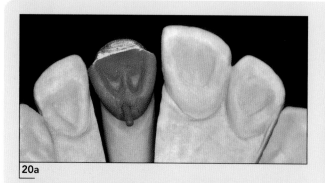
20a

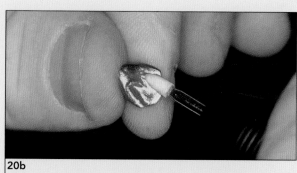
20b

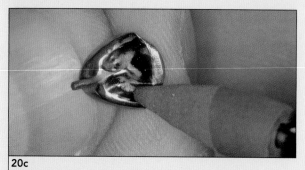
20c

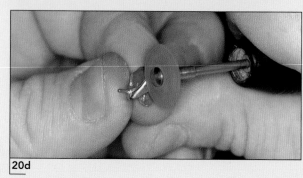
20d

Fig 7-20a The nonporcelain area can either be airborne-particle abraded and cleaned or rubber polished to remove scratches and irregularities before the porcelain is applied. Identify the location of any occlusal contacts before beginning the polishing procedure.

Fig 7-20b If the lingual surface is rough or contains irregularities, use a brown stone. Generally, a smooth casting requires only gentle finishing with a fine white ceramic stone.

Fig 7-20c Follow the fine ceramic stone with a green polishing point.

Fig 7-20d Use a rubber polishing wheel to smooth axial surfaces.

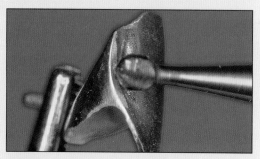

Fig 7-21 Polishing may have rounded the porcelain-metal junction, so refine this junction with a No. 8 round carbide bur.

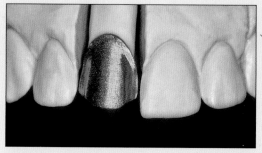

Fig 7-22 Facial view of the porcelain-bearing area of the finished substructure.

promote surface oxidation and increase the risk of contaminating those surfaces that are to receive porcelain.

A second approach entails preliminary finishing of all nonporcelain areas through the rubber wheel stage.[5] The belief here is that there are three important benefits to rubber wheeling these surfaces at this stage. First, rough areas and scratches can be eliminated *before* the porcelain has been applied; this reduces the risk that the ceramic veneer will become contaminated during the final polishing. Second, preliminary polishing of the nonporcelain areas may prevent

some problems from occurring during a subsequent procedure. For example, opaque porcelain is very coarse and cannot be glazed, so it must be covered completely with a layer of dentin or enamel porcelain. Once the porcelain buildup is complete, any excessive finishing of the nonporcelain surfaces could expose opaque at the porcelain-metal junction. And third, extensive adjusting and polishing of the metal after the porcelain has been glazed could generate and transfer unwanted and potentially damaging heat to the porcelain.

[handwritten: everything rounded, all surface sa blasted]

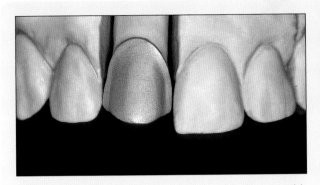

Fig 7-23 Facial view of the same substructure after airborne-particle abrasion with nonrecycled aluminum oxide particles.

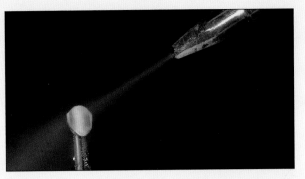

Fig 7-24 Steam clean the substructure after airborne-particle abrasion with aluminum oxide. As a matter of safety and to avoid potential injuries, wear safety glasses with side shields, and perform all steam-cleaning procedures over a sink and out of the way of other personnel.

[handwritten: 1. steam clean it, never touch surface 2. ultrasonic water + use hemostat to handle]

Be sure to place the restoration on the cast to check the occlusion, then adjust any occluding surfaces according to the predetermined occlusal scheme (see Fig 7-20a). Use a ceramic abrasive to rough finish the metal lingual and axial surfaces. After this step, switch to a finer ceramic stone (Fig 7-20b). At this point you may simply airborne-particle abrade and steam clean the restoration in preparation for oxidation or continue finishing the nonporcelain area with a rubber instrument. As mentioned previously, one concern is that rubber finishing at this point could possibly contaminate the metal surface. However, if the restoration has been airborne-particle abraded and steam cleaned or cleaned ultrasonically prior to oxidation, contamination should not be a problem. If you choose to smooth the nonporcelain surfaces now, use a rubber point to refine the lingual anatomy (Fig 7-20c) and a rubber wheel to go over the axial surfaces (Fig 7-20d).

Refine the porcelain-metal junction again if you need to restore the 90-degree butt joint (Fig 7-21). The porcelain-bearing surface should now take on a satin finish, and the nonporcelain-bearing areas should be smoothed just short of a final polish (Fig 7-22). Do not use any polishing agents (eg, buffing bar compound, tripoli, or rouge).

Metal loss during processing

Key steps such as casting, cutting of a sprue, seating a casting, and metal finishing of porcelain-bearing areas require the removal of alloy. When high-noble and noble metals are used, these losses are significant enough to warrant that steps be undertaken to capture spent metal and the dust generated during finishing. In one study involving 6 dental laboratory technicians, the mean overall weight loss of a gold-palladium alloy during procedures to a total of 323 anterior, premolar, and molar copings was 0.413 g (29%).[6] The smallest amount of alloy was lost during casting (8.92%), followed by sprue removal (17.59%) and seating of the restoration (34.03%). As might be expected, the largest amount (39.46%) was lost during the finishing of the porcelain-bearing areas.

Cleaning Procedures

After the substructure has been adjusted and finished, it should be cleaned thoroughly. First, airborne-particle abrade the porcelain-bearing surfaces (Fig 7-23) with 50-μm nonrecycled, pure aluminum oxide particles (see Fig 5-23). It is important to recognize that airborne-particle abrasion can have potentially damaging effects on a restoration irrespective of the type of abrasive being used. Suggestions for minimizing damage include using low pressure, short blast duration, and small-particle abrasives.[7] It has been shown that glass beads can be more damaging because of their large particle mass than aluminum oxide.[8] Therefore, great care should be taken with any procedure involving the use of air abrasives.

Second, steam clean the entire work again (Fig 7-24) or clean it ultrasonically in distilled water for 10 to 15 minutes.

margin above gum line or below?

Clinical crown prep under gum

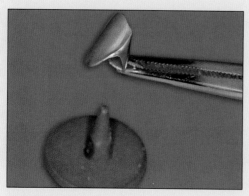

Fig 7-25a Using the cast 18-gauge handle, carefully place the cleaned casting on an individual sagger tray (Vident). The casting is ready to be oxidized.

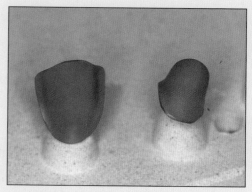

Fig 7-25b Multiple units can be placed on a larger sagger tray and oxidized together. These castings made with Protocol (Ivoclar Vivadent) were oxidized at 1,010°C for 5 minutes under vacuum.

tooth profile starts at CEJ

always lay it on special trays

Oxidizing the Anterior Single-Unit Restoration

The finished and cleaned substructure should be of the appropriate thickness for the type of casting alloy used and the clinical case requirements. Assuming that no additional changes are necessary, the substructure is ready to be oxidized. Take special care not to touch the porcelain-bearing areas with your fingers to avoid contaminating these surfaces with oils and debris transferred from your skin.

Place the cleaned castings on a sagger tray (Fig 7-25a), and oxidize the metal substructure according to the manufacturer's directions for high temperature, hold time (if any), and atmosphere (air or vacuum) (Fig 7-25b).

Finishing Other Types of Single-Unit Restorations

The technique for fitting, adjusting/finishing, and oxidizing the prepared metal substructure also applies to the other types of restorations described in chapter 4 (ie, anterior substructures with a porcelain lingual surface, posterior substructures with a metal occlusal surface, and posterior substructures with a porcelain occlusal surface). These substructures should be finished to a smooth surface, airborne-particle abraded with nonrecycled 50-μm aluminum oxide particles, and oxidized according to the same technique used for the single-unit anterior restoration.

Finishing a Fixed Partial Denture

The technique for finishing a fixed partial denture is very similar to that used for a single-unit restoration. Carefully cut the sprues and remove the cast framework from the spruing system (Fig 7-26; see also Fig 7-9b). Inspect the intaglio surface of each retainer under a microscope or with magnification loupes, and remove any nodules or other obvious defects that might prevent complete seating of the casting. Do not attempt to seat the framework on the master cast without this visual inspection.

The next step in finishing a fixed partial denture is to fit the retainers individually; each one should be adjusted in the same manner as that used for a single-unit crown (Fig 7-27). After you have separately fit the retainer castings, carefully attempt to seat the one-piece framework on an uncut master cast or a master cast with very stable dies (Fig 7-28a). Do not use pressure to seat the work; if the casting does not fit, the gypsum dies can be easily abraded and irreparably damaged.

Once the fixed partial denture is in place, gently press each retainer separately to determine if the restoration fits securely (Figs 7-28b and 7-28c). If the prosthesis is ill-fitting, it will probably "rock" on the cast when the retainers are alternately depressed (Figs 7-28d and 7-28e). If the fit is not completely satisfactory, use an ultra-fine cut-off disk to section through one of the connector areas (Fig 7-29), and plan to presolder the prosthesis. Before sectioning the framework, select the least favorable joint. Now is your chance to improve a connector area that has identifiable flaws. If the fit is acceptable, continue the metal-finishing procedure following the steps outlined above (see Figs 7-15 to 7-24).

Fig 7-26 Additional care must be taken when despruing a fixed partial denture because it is easy to break carborundum disks. After making cuts on both the facial and lingual aspects, rock the prosthesis backward and forward to separate it from the runner bar.

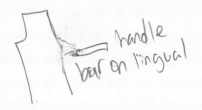

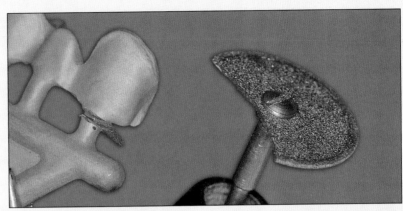

Fig 7-27a Carefully seat each fixed partial denture retainer on its individual die.

Fig 7-27b Examine the intaglio surface of each retainer for areas where the disclosing medium (AccuFilm IV) has been transferred from die to casting. Mark again and repeat this step. Adjust only those areas with repeat marking, and use a small round carbide bur.

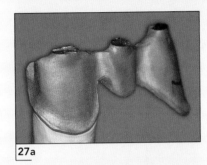

27a

27b

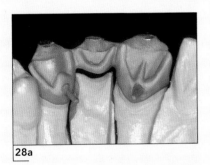

28a

28b

28c

Fig 7-28a Once adjusted, verify the fit of the fixed partial denture on the master cast. Use a solid cast if one is available.

Fig 7-28b To make certain the one-piece framework does not rock, lightly depress the anterior retainer and observe the distal retainer.

Fig 7-28c Next, lightly depress the distal retainer and observe the anterior retainer for evidence of rocking.

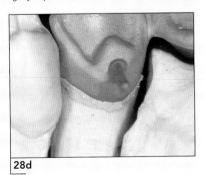

28d

28e

29

Fig 7-28d If the one-piece framework fits the cast well, no movement should be detected in the canine retainer when the opposite incisor retainer is depressed.

Fig 7-28e On the other hand, if the prosthesis is ill-fitting, the canine retainer will lift from its die when the incisor retainer is depressed. If this occurs, the framework should be sectioned and presoldered.

Fig 7-29 Section the connector that has the least desirable dimensions of occlusogingival height and buccolingual thickness width, and use the presoldering procedure to correct discrepancies in the selected joint.

Soldering a fixed partial denture

Several circumstances encountered in fabricating fixed partial dentures require a soldering procedure to complete the case. The three situations you are most likely to encounter are:

1. A fixed partial denture framework cast entirely in a ceramic alloy that may not fit on the master cast as well as you would like.
2. A prosthesis that is so large or so complex that you would rather not attempt to cast it in one piece.
3. A case that calls for joining dissimilar metals. With posterior restorations, this might involve soldering a Type III or Type IV gold retainer to a metal-ceramic component.

Soldering versus brazing

When a filler metal (solder) is heated to a liquidus temperature *not exceeding* 450°C (842°F), the process is defined as *soldering*. The term *brazing* refers to heating a filler metal to a liquidus temperature above 450°C (842°F).[9] Practically speaking, most metal-ceramic solders have a flow point well above the 450°C threshold, so technically, these metals are used to join components by brazing rather than soldering. However, the term soldering is deeply engrained in the vocabulary of dental laboratory technology and unlikely to change. (Note: Some textbooks use a temperature of 425°C (797°F) to differentiate between soldering and brazing procedures, but 450°C is generally more accepted.[10])

Types of soldering

In dentistry, two basic soldering techniques are used: *presoldering* and *postsoldering*. They are distinguished by *(a)* the stage at which they are performed in the fabrication process of a metal-ceramic restoration and *(b)* the composition of the solders that must be used. Solders are not pure metals but alloys designed to flow at specific temperatures.

Presoldering

When a soldering procedure involves uniting components of the same alloy before the porcelain is fired to the substructure, that process is referred to as *presoldering* (or preceramic soldering). The solder used for presoldering is a high-fusing alloy similar in composition to the parent metal of the components to be joined. With presoldering, you must use a high-temperature, phosphate-bonded soldering investment.

Postsoldering

If the components to be joined are made of different alloys (eg, Type III or Type IV gold and a ceramic alloy) or the porcelain application has been completed (glazed) and the metal polished, you must use a low-fusing gold solder and join the components by postsoldering (or postceramic soldering).[11] The term *postsoldering* is used because the soldering process occurs after the ceramic veneer has been glazed and the work is essentially complete (the metal has been polished).[12] With postsoldering, a low-temperature, gypsum-bonded soldering investment must used to avoid damaging the glazed porcelain surface.

Because most situations requiring the soldering of a metal-ceramic fixed partial denture occur prior to the application of porcelain, only the presoldering procedure is presented.

Presoldering a fixed partial denture

The most common situation that warrants soldering is when a fixed partial denture framework does not fit the uncut master cast but the retainers do fit their individual dies. As a general rule, you have two choices: either rewax and recast the work, or section and presolder the substructure. However, if a fixed partial denture has been cast in one piece and does not fit, it should be presoldered immediately after the connector has been cut. Do not continue finishing the restoration until after the soldering has been performed and a proper fit of the restoration has been confirmed. The added bulk of the prefinished metal will strengthen the prosthesis and help it resist exposure to the high soldering temperatures. Regardless of whether it was planned or not, presoldering is a relatively simple procedure with most metal-ceramic alloys.

Materials

Select the appropriate solder and soldering investment for the components to be joined. High-fusing metal-ceramic alloys require a phosphate-bonded soldering investment. This type of refractory material resists slumping when mixed properly, undergoes minimal expansion, and remains stable at the high temperatures required to join high-fusing metal-ceramic alloy components.

The presolder you choose must be matched to the parent alloy. For best results, use the presolder recommended by each alloy manufacturer (see Table 3-4). Presolders are carefully formulated to melt several hundred degrees *below* the parent alloy and several hundred degrees *above* the fusion temperature of the dental porcelain veneer.

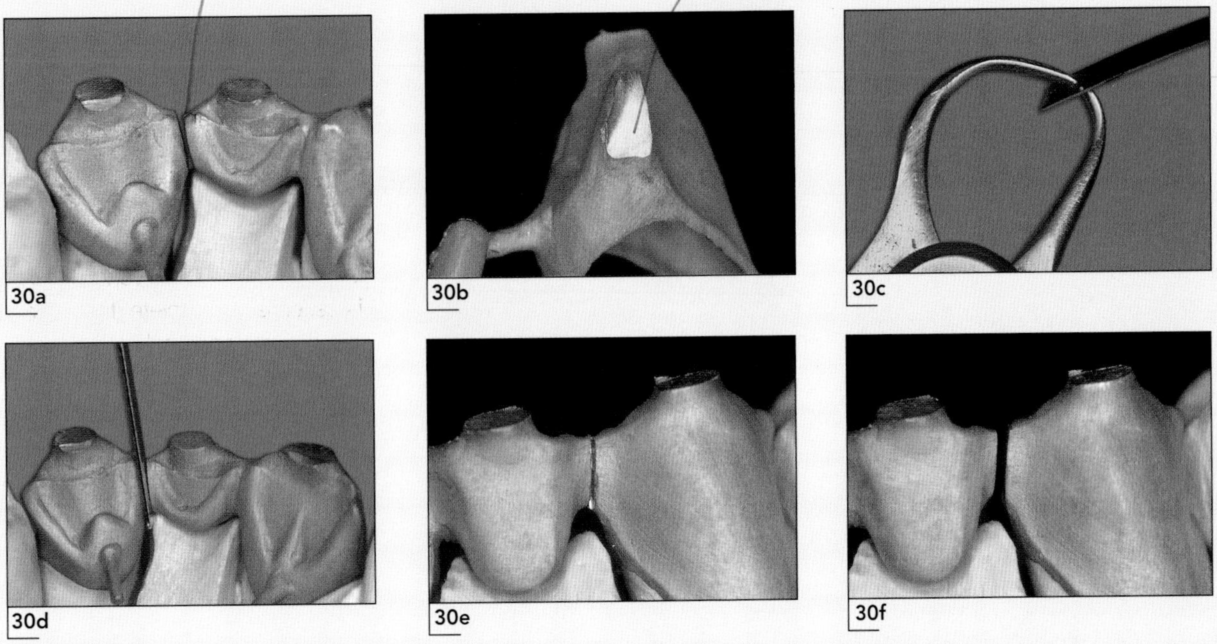

↑ abat 1.0 mm

pear shaped joint

30a

30b

30c

30d

30e

30f

Fig 7-30a The two components of the fixed partial denture are repositioned on the master cast.

Fig 7-30b Properly finished surface of a connector area. Note the triangular form of the joint, which provides sufficient height and breadth for anterior restorations.

Fig 7-30c Use metal calipers to measure the thickness of the solder strip. This strip of presolder measures 0.3 mm.

Fig 7-30d Use the 0.3-mm-thick solder strip to size the solder gap. If the strip cannot be inserted into the solder gap, the area should be enlarged slightly. If a solder gap of less than 0.3 mm is desired, adjust the thickness of the solder by lightly grinding the sides of the strip.

Fig 7-30e This gap is too small to allow for a sufficient amount of solder. It should be opened to approximately 0.3 mm for this high-palladium–silver-gold alloy.

Fig 7-30f This solder gap is larger than the desired 0.3-mm gap distance.

Adjusting the solder gap

Section the fixed partial denture at the connector area that has the least desirable height, facial-lingual width, and shape. After all, if you must solder a new connector, you may as well replace a cast joint that was less than ideal in design. Next, using a stable master cast, verify that the individual retainers seat completely on their respective dies (Fig 7-30a). Overlooked discrepancies in seating or orientation obviously will result in an ill-fitting soldered restoration.

Check the internal surfaces of the solder gap. They should be smooth and lightly finished (Fig 7-30b) with a rubber wheel[13] or fine sandpaper disks.[14] To provide adequate room for the solder, the gap should be opened to a dimension of approximately 0.3 mm (Figs 7-30c and 7-30d). If the solder gap is too small, the setting and thermal expansion that occur during the soldering procedure could close the opening to the point that the investment cracks (Fig 7-30e). On the other hand, if the gap is too large, an excessive amount of solder will be needed to fill the space, and the joint will be weak (Fig 7-30f). Recommended gap distances vary for different casting alloys, so consult the manufacturer of your alloy for specific guidelines.

Preparing the solder

There are at least three methods that can be used to estimate the amount of solder needed for a particular connector area.

1. *Perform freehand soldering.*

   This is the least complicated technique and involves little preparation. Simply place one end of a long solder strip into the connector area and allow the soldering torch to heat the solder freely (Fig 7-31). This technique is quick and easy, but it is not well controlled. It carries the risk of applying too much solder to the joint area, which can dramatically increase the amount of time required for metal finishing.

2. *Cut and fit a length of solder.*

   A second and more predictable method is to cut a length of solder and fit it to the gap to be soldered. Seat the sec-

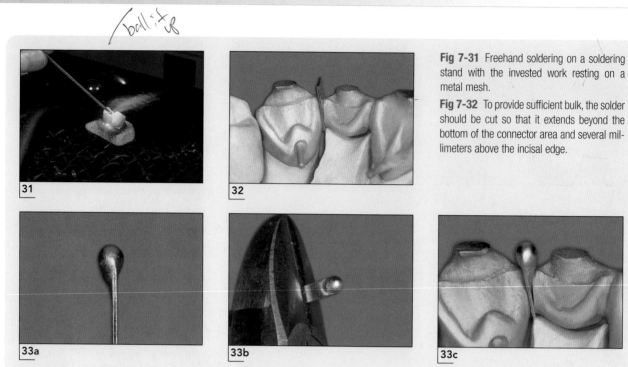

Fig 7-31 Freehand soldering on a soldering stand with the invested work resting on a metal mesh.

Fig 7-32 To provide sufficient bulk, the solder should be cut so that it extends beyond the bottom of the connector area and several millimeters above the incisal edge.

Fig 7-33a Insert one end of the solder strip into a properly adjusted torch until that end rounds, forming a so-called tadpole, as shown here.

Fig 7-33b Using wire cutters, trim the tadpole end of the solder strip to the desired length.

Fig 7-33c Position the solder in the prepared joint space so that the tadpole head sits above the incisal edge. The cut end should extend just beyond the full length of the connector area to provide sufficient bulk of solder for the gap.

tioned fixed partial denture securely on the master cast and place the piece of solder in the top of the prepared joint. Use a metal finishing stone to adjust the solder gap until it can accept and retain the solder strip, or if a gap of less than 0.3 mm is required, taper the solder strip. Cut the end of the solder strip so it extends several millimeters above the top of the connector area (Fig 7-32). The cut and adjusted piece of solder should contact the two components to be joined and remain in position after placement.

3. *Create a "tadpole" solder strip.*

The third and recommended approach is to create a "tadpole" piece of solder by placing one end of a solder strip directly in the soldering torch flame until the tip rounds (Fig 7-33a). Cut this tadpole end from the strip and adjust the opposite straight end until the head of the tadpole extends *above* the connector area and the cut end extends *below* the planned joint (Figs 7-33b and 7-33c)

Luting the restoration

For a proper solder relationship, the master cast must be an accurate replica of the patient's mouth. Seat the casting on the master cast; if necessary, trim the tissue area away from the prepared tooth. In the laboratory, you can use a solid cast without removable dies poured directly from the impression or a master cast with very stable removable dies. If you are unable to pour an additional, accurate cast from the impression, and if either the cast has been damaged or the removable dies have been damaged or are not stable, you will need to obtain a solder index directly from the patient.

With the units seated on the cast, make a stone index directly from the working cast. Alternatively, use a material with minimal setting expansion, such as some acrylic resins or a cyanoacrylate cement, to lute the two components together.[15-17] Do not use any form of sticky wax or modeling plastic (compound) because these materials will not provide the desired level of dimensional stability.

In laboratory comparisons, the dimensional accuracy of Pattern Resin (GC) and DuraLay (Reliance Dental) in indexing fixed partial dentures was found to be comparable.[17] However, a difference in the mean setting times was noteworthy: DuraLay required approximately 7 minutes compared to just 3 minutes for the Pattern Resin. In contrast, the manufacturers report setting times of "approximately" 5 minutes for DuraLay and 4 minutes for Pattern Resin.

This laboratory study compared the dimensional accuracy of assembled implant frameworks using these two

Resn material
to bond it together - (-In lab is bar across -)

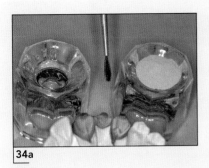

34a

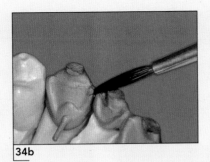

34b

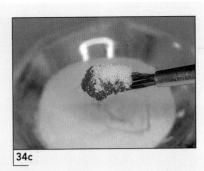

34c

Fig 7-34a To join the metal components together, use an acrylic resin with low polymerization shrinkage, such as Pattern Resin LS (GC). Dispense a small quantity of powder and liquid in separate dampen dishes, and select a small, clean brush.

Fig 7-34b Using the small brush, carefully wet the connector area with monomer.

Fig 7-34c Use the tip of the moistened brush to pick up a small amount of powder. Do not plunge the wetted brush into the acrylic resin powder because that will overload your brush, as shown. If the resin is too dry, it will bead up and not flow into the gap. Either rewet the mix or start again with a wetter brush and a smaller portion of material.

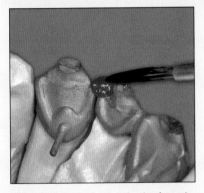

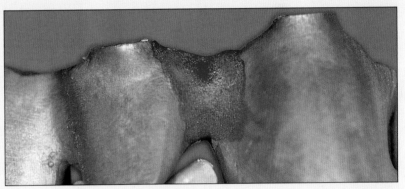

Fig 7-34d Lightly dab just the tip of a moistened brush into the powder to create a small, moist ball of resin on the brush tip. Place the small ball of resin at the incisal edges of the connector areas and let it flow down into the gap.

Fig 7-34e A properly luted joint should be neat and free of excess material, and it should provide sufficient bulk for strength—no more, no less.

acrylic resins after 15 minutes of polymerization.[17] Frameworks were visually assessed for fit at 15 minutes, 2 hours, and 24 hours postpolymerization. The quality of fit was 100% acceptable only at 15 minutes.[17] Since that study was reported, the Pattern Resin product has been replaced with Pattern Resin LS (low shrinkage) that, according to the manufacturer, also has a 4-minute setting time. Given that time is critical when making any type of index, a product with dimensional accuracy and a short setting time is preferred. Consequently, solder assemblies should be invested as soon as possible after completion of polymerization.[17]

Technique

Place a small quantity of resin powder and liquid monomer in separate dampen dishes (Fig 7-34a). Wet the connector area with the monomer (Fig 7-34b) and then use the tip of the moistened brush to pick up a small quantity of powder. Remove the brush quickly from the powder to avoid the formation of a large clump of resin (Fig 7-34c), but make certain the mix is not so dry as to inhibit its flow. Place the wetted mixture at the top of the connector area (Fig 7-34d) and gently move it down into the joint (connector) space (Fig 7-34e).

After the units have been properly luted together and the acrylic resin has completely polymerized, invest the fixed partial denture assembly immediately, preferably within 15 minutes or less to minimize potential distortion.[17]

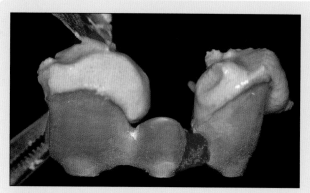

Fig 7-35a For small fixed partial dentures, fill the individual retainers with presoldering investment, and protect the margins of the retainers.

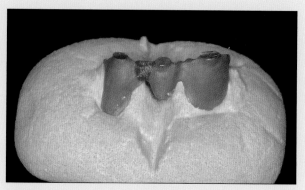

Fig 7-35b The invested fixed partial denture before trimming. Note that a V-shaped groove has been created under the connector area. This enables the torch frame to heat the metal components more easily, yet investment still supports the pontic.

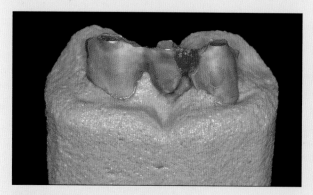

Fig 7-35c Facial view of the trimmed investment patty. Note that all sharp line angles have been removed.

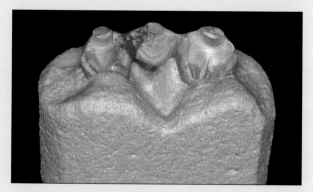

Fig 7-35d Lingual view of trimmed investment patty. The cast 18-gauge handles on the lingual surface have been covered with investment to secure the two components.

Investing

The goal of presoldering is to heat the parent alloy until it reaches a temperature high enough to allow the solder to flow into the prepared joint space, wet the parent metal, and join the components.

To invest, mix the soldering investment according to the manufacturer's instructions. Carefully pour the investment into the boxed index, or if the units are small and no index was used, fill each abutment with investment (Fig 7-35a). Place a small patty of investment (approximately 9.0 mm thick) on a glass slab, and gently seat the restoration on the patty (Fig 7-35b). Make certain that only the restoration margins are covered with the soldering investment. To prevent the casting from settling into the mix, place the glass slab in a vibration-free area. Allow the investment to bench set for

the amount of time specified by the investment manufacturer. For optimum heat transfer, every effort must be made to fully expose the casting's facial, incisal/occlusal, and lingual surfaces. If these areas are covered, the investment—rather than the metal components—will absorb the heat, which will hinder the solder's flow.

To minimize the amount of heat required for soldering, trim the set material around the entire periphery to within 6.0 mm of the casting. Reduce the investment base to a maximum thickness of 9.0 mm, if it is greater than this dimension (Fig 7-35c). Smooth any sharp line angles, and remove the investment under the solder gap to make certain the area is clean and open for air flow (Fig 7-35d). Keeping this area clean also ensures that any residual investment does not end up in the solder joint where it can cause pitting and porosity.

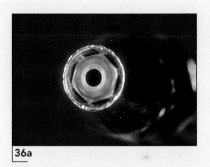

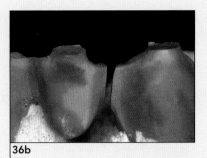

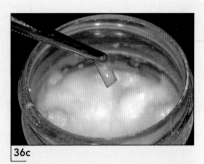

Fig 7-36a Single-orifice soldering tip on a Magic Wand torch (Ivoclar Vivadent).

Fig 7-36b Facial view of the airborne-particle abraded connector area.

Fig 7-36c A fluoride-containing flux for presoldering (High Fusing Bondal Flux, Ivoclar Vivadent). A properly mixed flux should be moist and have a smooth, creamy consistency. Dip the cut solder strip into the presolder flux, and wipe off any excess so that only a light coating remains.

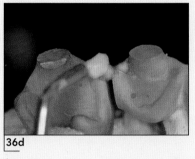

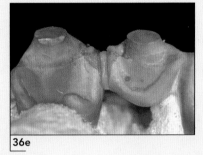

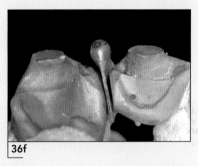

Fig 7-36d Place a small quantity of flux in the joint itself.

Fig 7-36e The presoldering flux should readily wet the joint.

Fig 7-36f Place the fluxed tadpole high-fusing solder into the connector area. Slowly move the soldering torch from left to right across the exposed framework on the lingual side until the metal is heated uniformly. Be certain to use the reducing tip of the flame (see Fig 5-21a).

Soldering

To obtain the proper expansion and to burn off the acrylic resin luting agent, insert the invested work in a burnout oven set at room temperature. Slowly raise the temperature to 649°C (1,200°F) over a 30-minute period, and hold the work at this temperature for at least 10 minutes.

While the investment is being heated and the acrylic resin is burning off, assemble the soldering torch, solder, and related equipment. Use a propane/oxygen (or natural gas/oxygen if propane is not available) mixture as your heat source, and select a single-orifice soldering torch tip (Fig 7-36a; see also Fig 5-21a). A single-orifice tip will form a concentrated flame enabling you to control the flow of the solder. As when casting, do not use acetylene or air and natural gas as a heat source. After eliminating the acrylic resin, remove the work from the furnace. The connector area should be free of debris with no signs of residual luting agent and soldering investment. If debris is evident in the connector area or the alloy is heavily oxidized, allow the substructure to cool, and gently airborne-particle abrade the joint with aluminum oxide (Fig 7-36b).

Some but not all ceramic alloys require or benefit from the use of a fluoride-containing flux for presoldering. Gener-

ally, alloys with a high gold content do not readily oxidize, so a soldering flux is not necessary. It has also been argued that flux can contaminate the alloy and discolor the porcelain; however, this is not a factor provided the metal is properly finished and cleaned following the soldering procedure. If a flux is used, make certain the mix is smooth by adding water and stirring it well. Then dip the solder in the flux and remove any excess material (Fig 7-36c).

Transfer the work to a tripod heated by a Bunsen burner and covered with metal mesh. The Bunsen burner will prevent the investment from rapid loss of heat during the soldering procedure. Apply only a small amount of flux to the connector area itself (Figs 7-36d and 7-36e), and carefully insert the prepared tadpole high-fusing solder (Fig 7-36f).

Solder always flows toward heat (ie, the flame). To work this to your advantage when using the freehand technique, place the solder on the side opposite that of the flame. If the work has metal lingual/occlusal surfaces, apply the heat from the lingual aspect, so the thinner facial regions are protected while the thicker portions of the casting are being heated.

With the two other techniques, position the cut solder strip or tadpole in the joint awaiting the application of heat. Begin the soldering process by warming the entire restoration with the reducing portion of the flame and focusing on

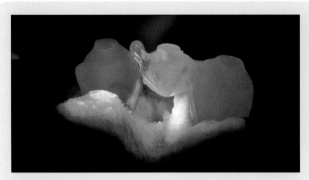

Fig 7-36g As heating continues, focus on the connector area, and watch as the head of the tadpole disappears as the solder slumps and flows into the prepared connector area.

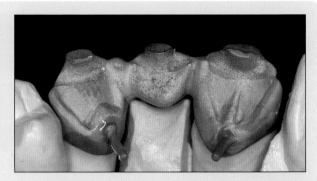

Fig 7-36h Lingual view of airborne-particle abraded fixed partial denture after presoldering. Confirm the proper fit of the prosthesis. Note that some solder has extended onto the lingual surface of the pontic. This overflow can be removed during metal finishing.

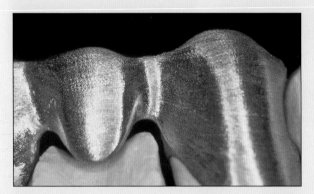

Fig 7-37a Facial view of the soldered connector area of the finished framework. Note that the joint is dense, complete, and virtually indistinguishable from the adjacent parent alloy components.

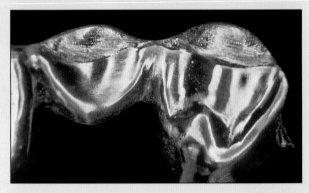

Fig 7-37b The nonporcelain areas can be finished through the rubber wheel/point stage to remove scratches and rough areas prior to oxidation and the application of porcelain.

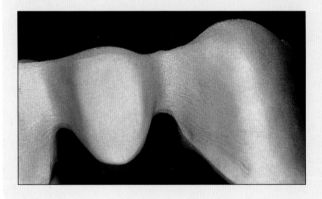

Fig 7-38 Facial view of airborne-particle abraded and cleaned soldered connector area. The soldered joint is barely discernable by its light yellow hue.

the exposed metal components and solder. It is not necessary to heat the investment. The goal is to heat the parent alloy. Move the soldering torch left to right and visually monitor the metal as the units take on heat to ensure both sides of the solder gap are the same color. This is your best visual indicator of a uniform temperature. Continue heating the parent alloy and positioning the flame to allow the solder to slump and be pulled or drawn through the solder gap (Fig 7-36g). Once the solder has melted and flowed completely, withdraw the flame and allow the work to cool to room tem-

perature. Retrieve the fixed partial denture from the investment, airborne particle abrade the metal with nonrecycled 50-µm aluminum oxide particles, and steam clean or ultrasonically clean the prosthesis framework (Fig 7-36h). Check the fit of the substructure on the master cast as described previously only after the intaglio surfaces have been inspected to ensure there is no debris.

Once you have confirmed the fit, adjust and finish the porcelain-bearing and nonporcelain-bearing areas of the prosthesis as described previously (Figs 7-37a and 7-37b).

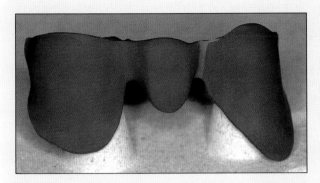

Fig 7-39 Labial view of the framework after oxidation. The oxide layer of Protocol alloy is uniform in color and appearance.

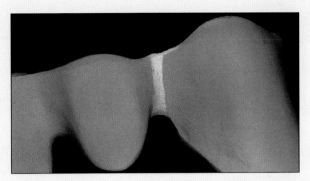

Fig 7-40 Close-up view of the solder joint after oxidation. The yellow hue of the presolder is now readily apparent, and the solder joint is dense and free of contamination and porosity.

When the metal finishing is complete, again airborne-particle abrade the restoration with aluminum oxide (Fig 7-38), and again steam clean or ultrasonically clean the work in distilled water. You are now ready to oxidize the metal in preparation for the application of opaque porcelain.

Oxidizing the substructure

Even though the prosthesis was presoldered, the oxidation procedure is the same as that used for a single-unit restoration (see Fig 7-25). Select an appropriate sagger tray to support both retainers and carefully place the entire assembly on the muffle stand. Take care to avoid touching the prepared metal substructure to prevent possible contamination of the porcelain-bearing surfaces. If you planned ahead when preparing the substructure, you should have handles on each retainer to facilitate handling (see Fig 7-30b)

Oxidize the framework under the conditions of time, temperature, and atmosphere recommended by the alloy manufacturer. Following completion of the oxidation firing cycle, inspect the metal surface to ensure a uniform oxide was produced that is free of contamination (Fig 7-39). The presoldered connector area will likely have a distinctive color that is different from the parent alloys (Fig 7-40), which is normal.

Summary

Adjusting and finishing a metal-ceramic substructure are relatively simple procedures, but they must be performed correctly if they are to enhance rather than jeopardize the porcelain-metal bond. With fixed partial dentures, presolder-

ing should not be considered an obstacle to obtaining a well-fitting prosthesis. And metal-ceramic substructures should be properly oxidized to prepare the metal surface to form a stable and enduring porcelain-metal bond.

Now that you know how to adjust/finish and oxidize a single-unit substructure and presolder a fixed partial denture, you are ready to proceed to chapter 8 to learn the techniques for applying porcelain to these substructures.

References

1. West AJ, Goodacre CJ, Moore BK, Dykema RW. A comparison of four techniques for fabricating collarless metal-ceramic crowns. J Prosthet Dent 1985;54:636–642.
   Intaglio surface of castings is adjusted under a microscope using a No. ½ round carbide bur.

2. Yamamoto M. Metal-Ceramics: Principles and Methods of Makoto Yamamoto. Chicago: Quintessence, 1985:106–157.
   Author reviews metal preparation for porcelain bonding.

3. Felton DA, Bayne SC, Kanoy BE, White JT. Effect of air abrasives on marginal configurations of porcelain-fused-to-metal alloys: An SEM analysis. J Prosthet Dent 1991;65:38–43.
   A comparison of abrasion with 25-μm Al_2O_3 and 25-μm glass beads under 80 psi indicates that all margins were shorted for all alloys by both abrasives.

4. McLean JW. The Science and Art of Dental Ceramics. Vol I: The nature of dental ceramics and their clinical use. Chicago: Quintessence, 1979:273–285.

5. Rosenstiel SF, Land MF, Fujimoto J. Contemporary Fixed Prosthodontics. St Louis: Mosby, 1988:499.

6. Soh G. Loss of alloy in the fabrication of metal ceramic crowns. Int J Prosthodont 1991;4:361–363.
   Soh reports mean alloy loss of 0.413 g (29%) and greater losses for maxillary anterior copings during finishing of the porcelain-bearing areas.

7. Peutzfeldt A, Asmussen E. Distortion of alloy by sandblasting. Am J Dent 1996;9(2):65–66.
Negative effects are greater with an increase in pressure, a decrease in metal thickness, and larger particle sizes.

8. Mansueto MA, Verrett RG, Phoenix RD. Microabrasion of cast metal margins—A warning. J Prosthodont 2007;16:136–140.
Minimize negative effects by increasing the distance from handpiece to casting, decreasing exposure time, or using particles with less mass.

9. Anusavice KJ. Phillips' Science of Dental Materials, ed 11. Philadelphia: Saunders, 2003,608–620.

10. Powers JM, Sakaguchi RL. Craig's Restorative Dental Materials, ed 12. St Louis: Mosby, 2006:375.
Authors state that brazing *is performed above 425°C, and* soldering *is performed below 425°C.*

11. O'Brien WJ. Dental Materials and Their Selection, ed 4. Chicago: Quintessence, 2008:256–257.
O'Brien describes brazing metal-ceramic fixed partial dentures.

12. Ianzano JA, Johansen R, Shiu A. Postceramic soldering in fixed prosthodontics. Quintessence Dent Technol 1989;13:69–74.
Authors present clinical and laboratory steps for successful soldering.

13. Eissmann HF, Rudd KD, Morrow RM (eds). Dental Laboratory Procedures. Fixed Partial Dentures, vol II. St Louis: Mosby, 1980: 313–326.
Authors review soldering materials and techniques.

14. Shillingburg HT, Hobo S, Whitsett LD, Jacobi R, Brackett SE. Fundamentals of Fixed Prosthodontics, ed 3. Chicago: Quintessence, 1997:526.

15. Cho GC, Chee WW. Efficient soldering index materials for fixed partial dentures and implant substructures. J Prosthet Dent 1995; 73:424–427.

16. McLean JW. The Science and Art of Dental Ceramics. Vol II: Bridge design and laboratory procedures in dental ceramics. Chicago: Quintessence, 1980:357–362.

17. McDonnell T, Houston F, Byrne D, Gorman C, Claffey N. The effect of time lapse on the accuracy of two acrylic resins used to assemble an implant framework for soldering. J Prosthet Dent 2004;91: 538–540.
Implant frameworks indexed with DuraLay and GC Pattern Resin had a passive fit at 15 minutes but unacceptable fit at 2 hours and 24 hours.

CHAPTER 8

Applying Porcelain to the Metal Substructure

The application of dental porcelain to the metal substructure is perhaps the single most demanding procedure in the fabrication of a metal-ceramic restoration. As a rule, the technical skills needed for this process require considerable effort to develop and perfect. Moreover, the instruments and techniques used for porcelain buildups are so numerous and varied, it would be impossible to include a comprehensive review of all of them. Therefore, the buildup techniques presented in this chapter depict a basic approach to porcelain application that can serve as a springboard for the developing ceramist. Once the technical fundamentals are mastered, the potential for improvement and incorporating more advanced techniques is limitless.[1] Initially, however, it is essential to acquire basic skills founded on sound principles for success in the fabrication of a functional and esthetically pleasing restoration.

> Once the technical fundamentals are mastered, the potential for improvement and incorporating more advanced techniques is limitless.

Instruments and Equipment

The armamentarium for applying porcelain as described in this chapter is quite simple (Fig 8-1) and at the very least should include some of the following items (see also appendix E).

Brushes

Ceramist brushes are essential to any porcelain kit, especially high-quality sable porcelain brushes. These instruments are available in sizes ranging from the smallest No. 000 to the largest No. 10 and are used for building (or stacking) dental porcelain. Try a number of different brands and sizes for opaque application, body buildup, and internal layer application, as well as characterization (staining and glazing), to determine what works best in your hands. Avoid less expensive substitutes, if at all possible.

Sable brushes are the standard because they permit easy manipulation of the porcelain. Their added cost is more than recouped through improved working efficiency and durability. A simple test can be used to identify a high-quality brush. Moisten the bristles thoroughly and then remove the moisture either by shaking the brush or pulling the bristles across a tissue or sponge. If the brush is high quality, the bristles will readily form a sharp tip or *point*. This point enables the ceramist to pick up porcelain from the glass slab or tray and improves control during placement of porcelain on the crown buildup. Worn or inferior-quality brushes will not point as described. A technique for pointing a brush is presented later.

A basic instrument kit should include a number of frequently used brushes (Fig 8-2). A large No. 10 brush, often referred to as a *whipping brush*, has a large surface area,

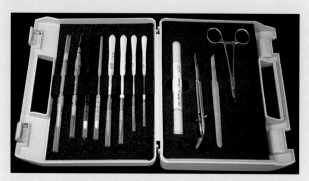

Fig 8-1a Porcelain kit (Renfert) containing the essential instruments for buildup procedures as well as for characterization (staining and glazing).

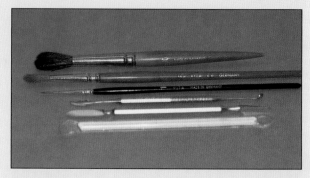

Fig 8-1b *(top to bottom)* Instruments from a Vita porcelain kit (Vident) include a large No. 10 whipping brush, No. 6 and No. 1 brushes for porcelain application, metal carving instruments, and a glass mixing rod.

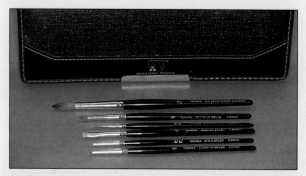

Fig 8-2a Assortment of brushes from a porcelain kit. The large brush is used in porcelain buildup, and the smaller brushes are designed for staining and glazing or for removing porcelain from exposed metal.

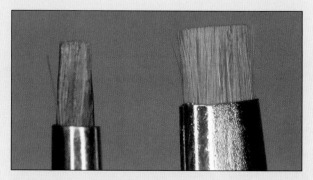

Fig 8-2b Small and large stiff-bristle brushes are used to remove dry porcelain from nonporcelain areas such as metal margins, porcelain-metal junctions, and the intaglio (inside) surface of the metal substructure.

soft bristles, and a delicate action that make it ideal for smoothing the porcelain buildup or contouring, condensing, and even removing excess porcelain. Flat brushes with relatively stiff bristles are also important. These large- and small-sized brushes should be kept dry because they are used exclusively to remove porcelain particles from non-porcelain areas and from the intaglio surface of a coping or fixed partial denture retainer prior to firing. Finally, very small No. 0 to No. 000 sable brushes are required for the placement of stains or very small increments of porcelain. These brushes are useful anywhere maximum control is necessary.

Carving instruments

Porcelain carving instruments, designed for shaping and sculpturing porcelain buildups, are offered in diverse shapes and sizes. Many are rigid and some have at least one serrated edge. As a group, carving instruments serve two

principal functions: *(1)* those with a serrated handle can be used to condense wet porcelain; *(2)* instruments with blades (Fig 8-3) or small discoid carvers can be used to build porcelain, shape the buildup, and carve the porcelain as will be demonstrated in the technique sections that follow.

Spatulas

Some ceramists prefer to include a small, flexible, metal spatula in their armamentarium to dispense and mix porcelain. If you choose to mix porcelain with a metal instrument, exercise caution. As with all ceramic materials, dental porcelain can easily abrade metallic surfaces, particularly if appreciable pressure is applied during mixing. Small metal fragments generated during mixing may then be introduced into the wet porcelain as contaminants that can dramatically discolor the mix as well as the fired porcelain restoration. With careful use, the metal mixing spatula

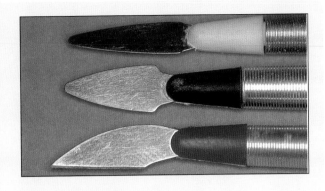

Fig 8-3 Belle de St Claire carving instruments (KerrLab) for stacking and shaping the porcelain buildup. Note the straight cutting edge on the flexible blade of the knife *(bottom)*.

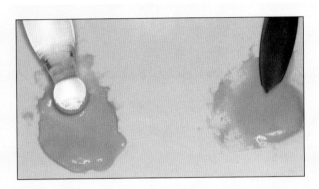

Fig 8-4 A glass rod *(left)* is better suited for mixing porcelain than is a metal instrument *(right)*. Porcelain can abrade the metal instrument, contaminate the opaque mix, and discolor the fired porcelain. The mixes are of the same shade of opaque porcelain, but the mixture on the right has a lower value due to metal contamination from aggressive mixing with a metal instrument.

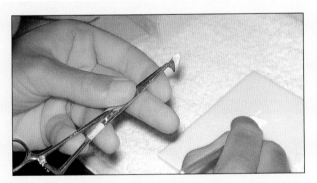

Fig 8-5a A hemostat (straight or curved) attached to the cast 18-gauge handle on the metal substructure improves access to all areas of the restoration during porcelain application.

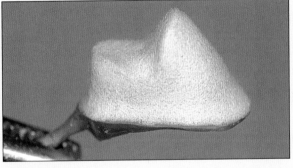

Fig 8-5b A cast metal handle is particularly useful for copings with minimal exposed metal because it helps to avoid possible damage to delicate metal margins.

need not be abraded. However, substituting a glass mixing rod for the metal spatula can revent this problem altogether (Fig 8-4).

Razor knives

Another necessity is some type of razor knife equipped with a thin, flexible blade for carving the porcelain buildup (see Fig 8-3). Thicker knives or scalpel blades are less desirable substitutes because of their greater bulk and lack of flexibility.

Hemostats

A small, straight or curved hemostat is needed to hold the work during the opaquing process and at certain times during porcelain additions and condensation (Fig 8-5a). Hemostats can be modified to hold the cast substructure securely without damaging the metal margins. If an 18-gauge handle has been added to the lingual collar, it can provide a convenient, safe, and secure grip for removing a restoration from the working cast and holding it during condensation, especially for restorations with minimal exposed metal (Fig 8-5b). The handle can always be shortened after the restoration has

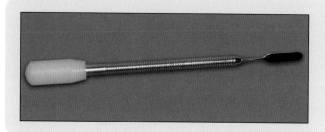

Fig 8-6 A mallet can be used to lightly tap the working cast and condense the porcelain buildup in a very controlled manner.

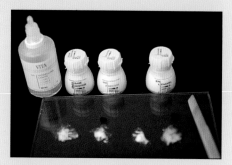

Fig 8-7a A large ceramic or glass slab is recommended for the buildup procedure. The larger working area accommodates the mixing and storing of dentin, enamel, and translucent porcelains, as well as various modifiers.

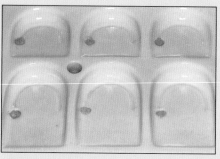

Fig 8-7b Ceramic tray (Tanaka Dental) with an airtight lid and individual recessed areas keeps porcelains moist by using wicks that draw liquid from a reservoir below the tray.

been fully fabricated and left intact only during the try-in procedure to facilitate removal of the work from the patient's mouth. This modification is especially convenient during intraoral, custom characterization with surface stains. Obviously, the handle is removed, and the metal is polished after glazing and before final cementation.

Condensing mallets

A condensing mallet is a useful porcelain instrument (Fig 8-6). Lightly tapping the working cast while the restoration is still on it is yet another way to condense the porcelain buildup. The value of such a procedure is discussed in greater depth later in the presentation of different porcelain buildup techniques.

Glass or ceramic mixing slabs

Finally, a glass slab, ceramic tile, or ceramic tray can serve as a useful palate for mixing and storing porcelains during the buildup procedure (Fig 8-7a). Initially a small mixing slab will suffice. As modifiers are added and more complex buildups are attempted, a larger working surface will be required to accommodate the different porcelain mixtures. Porcelain that is mixed on a glass slab or ceramic tile and left unused will eventually dry out and have to be discarded.

To avoid waste of material, some manufacturers offer special ceramic trays designed to keep the porcelain powders moist even when not in use. Liquid is stored in a reservoir, and a wick draws moisture to each individual well containing a separate porcelain mixture (Fig 8-7b). These trays typically have airtight lids to prevent evaporation

Porcelain Furnaces

A porcelain furnace, or oven, is one of the more expensive equipment items required for the production of metal-ceramic restorations. Although at least three types of porcelain ovens are available—manual, automatic, and programmable—programmable units are the industry standard (Figs 8-8 to Fig 8-10).

Common to all porcelain furnaces is an adjustable rate of rise from the low entry temperature to the high firing temperature and the capability to create a reduced atmospheric pressure (at 700 to 740 mm of mercury). The rates of rise and cooling also can be programmed for different processing steps. Manufacturers generally provide a recommended rate of rise for their particular porcelain system (see appendix A). However, this rate of heating and cooling may vary with different brands of porcelain and types of casting alloys.

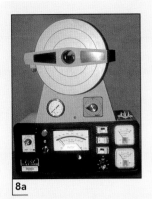
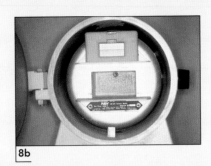
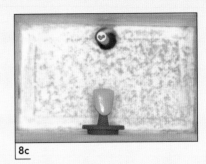

Fig 8-8a Manual porcelain furnace (Ney Mark III, JM Ney).

Fig 8-8b Interior of the front-loading porcelain furnace with a horizontal muffle. The operator works the vacuum manually as well as opens and closes the muffle door.

Fig 8-8c The restoration is positioned manually under the thermocouple to ensure consistent and uniform heating in this front-loading porcelain furnace.

Fig 8-9a Automated, programmable porcelain furnace with a vertical muffle (Multimat 99, Dentsply).

Fig 8-9b Early design of a vertical-loading porcelain furnace. The work was placed on the center of the ceramic platform and raised automatically into the muffle.

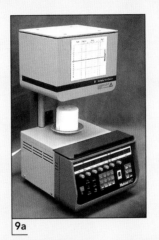
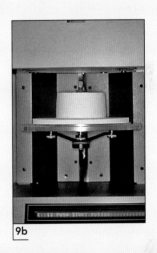

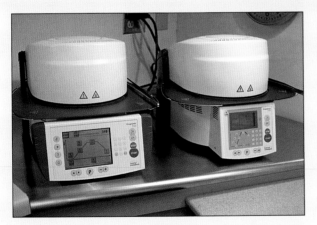
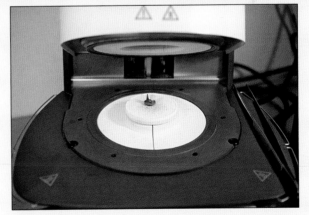

Fig 8-10a Programat P500 *(left)* and Programat P300 *(right)* (Ivoclar Vivadent) are examples of contemporary porcelain furnaces.

Fig 8-10b The muffle of the Programat P500 furnace closes over the ceramic platform. The "clam shell" design of the vertical muffle ensures that the work does not move.

Most furnaces can be set to hold the work at a specified temperature for a certain length of time as needed for the firing schedule. The ability to hold work at a high temperature for a prescribed time interval is essential during oxidation of the metal substructure and glazing of the finished restoration.

Evolving technology and designs

Historically, porcelain furnaces were not only categorized as manual, automatic, or programmable, but they also were divided into three basic types depending on the manner of entry into the muffle.

If the work was inserted from the front of the muffle to the back (horizontally), the unit was referred to as a *front-loading furnace* (see Figs 8-8b and 8-8c). Ovens with a front-loading muffle tended to be hotter in the back of the muffle and cooler near the door. As a result, differences could be observed between the appearance of porcelain fired in the back of the firing chamber and work fired in the front. The variation in the appearance of the fired porcelain may have been particularly noticeable during the metal oxidation cycle. Those substructures oxidized in the rear-most portion of the muffle could come out with different oxide formation than those heated in the front near the door due to variations in the internal temperature.

In vertical-loading furnaces, the second category, the restoration is placed in the center of the platform and is raised up into the furnace muffle (see Fig 8-9b). The vertical-loading design reportedly provides a more uniform temperature distribution throughout the muffle and allows the work to be completely surrounded by the heating elements.

The final category includes ovens with a vertical muffle and a "clam shell" design in which the work remains stable on the stand. Instead of the platform moving vertically toward the muffle, the opposite occurs: The muffle rotates downward and closes over the work, thus the reference to a clam shell (see Fig 8-10b). This design is an improvement over older furnaces where restorations had to remain stable while traveling in and out of the muffle. The clam shell design makes loading and unloading restorations much easier.

Porcelain Condensation

The process of condensing dental porcelain actually refers to any action that results in tighter packing of the unfired porcelain. As porcelain particles move closer together, air and moisture previously occupying the space between these particles move towards the outer surface of the buildup. This process is essential, because liquid or air that remains trapped in the unfired porcelain creates voids (porosities) in the fired ceramic. In fact, the powder-liquid ratio can affect porcelain density and total porosity.[2] One

study found that the best density and porosity levels were achieved with a low powder-liquid ratio (2.56 to 2.85 g/mL) for some dental porcelains and with a medium powder-liquid ratio (2.64 to 3.07 g/mL) for other porcelain brands.[2]

The presence of voids in fired porcelain not only weakens the restoration but also diminishes its esthetic qualities, both its color and translucency. From a structural perspective, it is easy to appreciate how the presence of voids throughout porcelain can weaken the material; they occupy space that could otherwise be filled by porcelain. But how does porosity adversely affect the optical qualities of a ceramic? As light passes through a translucent material—such as dental porcelain—and strikes an air bubble, the light is scattered in all directions rather than passing completely through the area. The visual impact of many small voids scattering light in all directions is that the restoration takes on a cloudy, opaque appearance rather than with reduced translucency. More voids and greater opacification translate into a loss of color due to a poor condensation technique.

Another advantage of well-condensed porcelain is a reduction in firing shrinkage. All porcelains shrink when sintered because of the loss of moisture and the increase in density. If overbuilt by at least 10% (and no more than 15%), this increased size is an approximation of the estimated shrinkage that occurs during the firing cycle. This physical change occurs as porcelain particles become molten, fuse together (vitrify), and form a smaller mass. It stands to reason that condensation also increases the density of the unfired ceramic by physically forcing the particles to move closer to one another before they fuse together. Increased density in an unfired buildup translates to less shrinkage during firing.

Finally, the porcelain-to-metal bond is maximized when the porcelain-bearing areas of the substructure are covered by a layer of opaque porcelain that wets the metal thoroughly, is well condensed, and has a minimum of voids (ie, air and water entrapment).

At least five different methods of porcelain condensation are recognized: *(1)* capillary action, *(2)* vibration, *(3)* spatulation, *(4)* whipping, and *(5)* dry powder addition.[3]

> At least five different methods of porcelain condensation are recognized: capillary action, vibration, spatulation, whipping, and dry powder addition.

Capillary action

The technique of blotting wet porcelain with facial tissue, gauze, or blotting paper relies on surface tension (capillary action) to withdraw liquid from the buildup. The mechanics are simple. Surface tension is the force that causes all liquids to contract to their smallest possible surface area.[4] This property accounts for the transformation of water droplets into a spheric mass. In a wet bulk of porcelain, it is surface tension that helps to pack the particles more tightly during vibration and blotting. When blotting alone is used, only available moisture near the surface is drawn off, so some additional action is needed to bring liquid from the interior to the surface. Free water molecules that exist in the buildup are forced to the surface when an absorbent material comes in contact with the wet exterior porcelain. The porcelain particles are then able to move into the space formerly occupied by the free water molecules. As the buildup becomes more condensed, it also becomes firmer (more dense) and slightly smaller in size. For this cycle of capillary action to occur, continuous blotting is needed to remove surface moisture.

However, capillary action with blotting does not remove all the available liquid from the interior of the mass. For maximum efficiency, capillary action with blotting should be accompanied by some other condensation technique, typically vibration. For example, the cyclic action of vibration or whipping brings additional moisture to the porcelain surface where it can be removed via capillary action with blotting. This cycle of vibration and blotting is repeated until free liquid can no longer be forced to the surface of the porcelain.

Vibration

The easiest and simplest form of vibration is created by passing a serrated instrument over the neck of a hemostat in which the restoration is held,[5] or by merely tapping the hemostat neck very lightly. Alternatively, if the restoration is left on the cast, the entire cast can be tapped or vibrated. Whether the restoration is condensed on a hemostat or a cast, any vibratory action forces free water to the porcelain surface. At that point, blotting material can be placed on the wet buildup to initiate capillary action as well.

Several devices also have been designed to provide mechanical vibration, such as vibrating brushes, spatulas, and ultrasonic condensers. For the beginner, ultrasonic equipment should be limited to the final stages of condensation, reserving preliminary condensation for some other method (eg, gentle tapping). Usually, a delicate touch is all that is required to initiate the vibratory mechanism. Without this gentle initial condensation, the fragile wet buildup could readily slump or shift, or the layers of porcelain could simply run together. Should such movement occur and go undetected, the appearance of the resulting fired porcelain is likely to be adversely affected.

Spatulation

With this form of condensation, a spatula or porcelain carver is used to apply, then rub (or pat) the porcelain buildup to force liquid to the surface.[4,5] This technique brings with it a greater likelihood of porcelain dislodgement, particularly if too much pressure is applied and especially with the initial buildup. An undetected dislodgement or separation between layers or between opaqued porcelain and metal could result in porcelain cracks.[5] The spatulation technique is a less favored condensation method and is not recommended for beginners who have yet to master vibration and capillary action.

Whipping

Whipping is actually nothing more than a variation of the vibration technique. As the porcelain is built up, a No. 10 sable brush is rapidly moved over the porcelain surface with a "whipping" motion, thus the name. The whipping action drives fluid to the outer surface where it can be blotted.

Dry powder addition

This approach to porcelain condensation may be the least widely known and used of all the methods described. The technique, also referred to as the *brush application method*, requires dry porcelain powder to be sprinkled on an area of wet porcelain using existing liquid in the buildup to wet the powder additions.[6] As you might imagine, estimating the correct volume of powder to add and then placing that powder in an appropriate position on the restoration is not without its problems. For the beginner, the technique can be more time-consuming and less predictable than other methods.

Where appropriate, several of these methods of porcelain condensation will be illustrated in the technique sections that follow. There may not be total agreement as to which condensation method or methods are most effective. Nonetheless, it is universally recognized that voids must be eliminated from fired porcelain or minimized as much as possible. The first and possibly most critical step in creating a dense, void-free buildup is proper mixing and subsequent handling of the wet porcelain.

> Surface tension is the force that causes all liquids to contract to their smallest possible surface area.

147

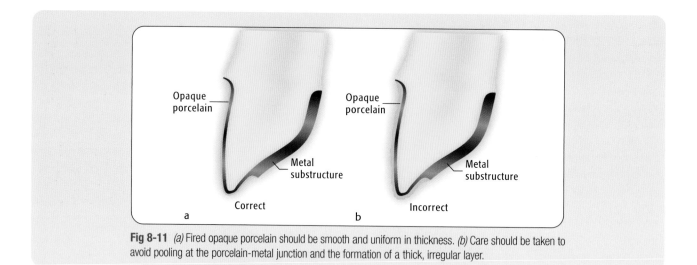

Fig 8-11 *(a)* Fired opaque porcelain should be smooth and uniform in thickness. *(b)* Care should be taken to avoid pooling at the porcelain-metal junction and the formation of a thick, irregular layer.

Opaquing the Metal Substructure

At this point, it is assumed that the metal has been properly finished, cleaned, and oxidized, and that any postoxidation treatment recommended by the alloy manufacturer has been followed. If this is the case, the areas of the substructure that will be veneered with porcelain must not be touched and should be protected from dust, oils from the skin, and any other form of contamination. When the ceramist is satisfied that proper procedures have been followed and the substructure is ready for veneering, the first material to be applied is the opaque porcelain.

Functions of the opaque porcelain

As mentioned in chapter 2, opaque porcelain serves three functions critical to the success of the completed restoration: *(1)* it establishes the porcelain-to-metal bond; *(2)* it masks the color of the metal substructure; and *(3)* it initiates the development of the selected shade of dental porcelain.

The thickness of opaque porcelain required to adequately mask the surface oxide layer varies from one brand of porcelain to another and certainly differs from one metal-ceramic alloy to the next. The range of thicknesses generally believed to be appropriate for opaque porcelain is 0.2 to 0.3 mm,[3,7–9] although some authors recommend a dimension as little as 0.1 to 0.15 mm.[10] In one study of older porcelain systems (Ceramco [Dentsply] and Vita VMK-68 [Vident]) using a uniform 0.3-mm opaque layer, the recommended body porcelain thickness ranged from 0.5 to 1.0 mm depending on both the shade and the brand of porcelain selected.[7]

Obviously, because the formation of the porcelain-to-metal bond rests with the opaque porcelain, proper applica-

tion and firing of this initial ceramic layer are essential. Yet opaque porcelains can be sintered up to 60°C above and 40°C below their recommended firing temperature without an adverse effect on the final color.[11] In terms of actual application, opaque porcelain is usually applied with one of three methods: *(1)* glass rod, *(2)* brush, or *(3)* spray.

Once the delivery method has been selected, the substructure can be opaqued using one of two techniques. Some ceramists attempt to completely mask the metal with a single application and firing, relying on a second opaque application only if some areas were not well masked. Other ceramists plan two separate firings, with the first application being a thin "wash" fired to the temperature recommended for the particular brand of porcelain. This initial layer wets the metal surface and establishes the porcelain-metal bond only to be covered by a second, much thicker layer of opaque that is intended to mask the metal completely. Some opaque porcelains have a greater tendency to crack on firing if applied too thickly. While these cracks are of little concern and can be easily corrected with another opaque application, they eliminate any advantage in completing the opaquing process in a single application and firing.

Despite the differences in these two approaches to opaquing the metal substructure, the goal should be to wind up with no pooling of the opaque porcelain in areas such as the porcelain-metal junction and occlusal grooves. A correctly placed and fired opaque layer should be smooth and uniform in thickness (Fig 8-11a). If too much opaque is applied, it can pool or build up, forming a thick and highly irregular layer after firing (Fig 8-11b). Dental porcelain manufacturers provide guidelines for visual indicators for each porcelain firing step, including the opaque layer (see appendix A). When ceramists use a sound technique and follow recommended guidelines, they optimize the potential for a good outcome.

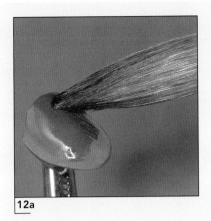
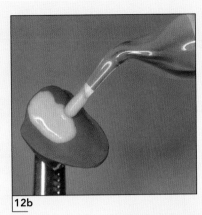
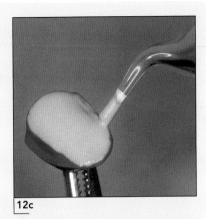

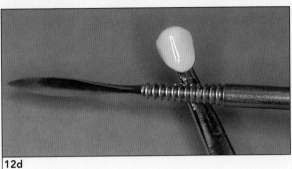

Fig 8-12a Areas to be opaqued on this oxidized restoration are lightly wetted with opaque liquid. The casting can be vibrated to thoroughly wet these surfaces.

Fig 8-12b Use the pointed tip of a glass rod (Tanaka Dental) to place opaque porcelain on the most convex surface of the restoration.

Fig 8-12c Again use the tip of the glass rod to move the opaque porcelain toward the porcelain-metal junction until the entire porcelain-bearing surface is covered.

Fig 8-12d Lightly tap the hemostat with a metal instrument to condense the opaque porcelain. Excess opaquing liquid will rise to the surface.

Anterior Single Crown with Metal Lingual Surface: Standard Buildup Technique

Mixing opaque porcelain

Generally, porcelain manufacturers provide a special liquid medium, rather than distilled water, to mix with their opaque powders. Select the recommended opaque shade for the body porcelain. Dispense an appropriate amount of opaque powders for the number of restorations to be fabricated, and place those powders on a glass or ceramic mixing slab. Do not place liquid directly on top of the porcelain because this may result in air entrapment within the material, which can lead to porosity in the mixed porcelain. As pointed out previously, it is ill advised to use a metal spatula for mixing dental porcelains. When course opaque porcelain particles are sandwiched between a glass or ceramic slab and a metal instrument, they can abrade the metal and lead to metal particles actually contaminating the mix (see Fig 8-4). Specially designed glass rods with a rounded tip on one end for mixing and a pointed tip on the other end for applying opaque porcelain can be used instead. Alternatively, opaque porcelain can be applied with a high-quality sable brush, but take care because brushes can entrap air bubbles and transfer them to the applied opaque.

Regardless of the application technique, if the porcelain powder soaks up the available liquid and appears dry, rehydrate it, but avoid incorporating too much liquid and creating a thin mixture.

Application of opaque porcelain

Glass rod technique

Using distilled water, lightly moisten the oxidized metal substructure to be veneered and gently vibrate the casting (Fig 8-12a). A wet substructure makes porcelain application easier and reduces the possibility of trapping air between the porcelain and the metal. The thin film of water also helps to draw the opaque particles onto the metal surface.

Use the pointed tip of the glass rod to apply the opaque porcelain. Begin by covering the most convex portion of the coping (Fig 8-12b). Move the opaque toward the porcelain-metal junction from one interproximal area (Fig 8-12c) to the other, and then cover the incisal edge. Lead the opaque over the incisal edge to cover the porcelain-bearing area on the lingual surface. After all the porcelain-bearing areas have been completely covered, lightly tap the hemostat, and the porcelain will settle into any concavities (Fig 8-12d). If the application starts in or near these concavities, the material tends to pool immediately, resulting in a thick opaque layer. Because concavities are often adjacent to porcelain-metal

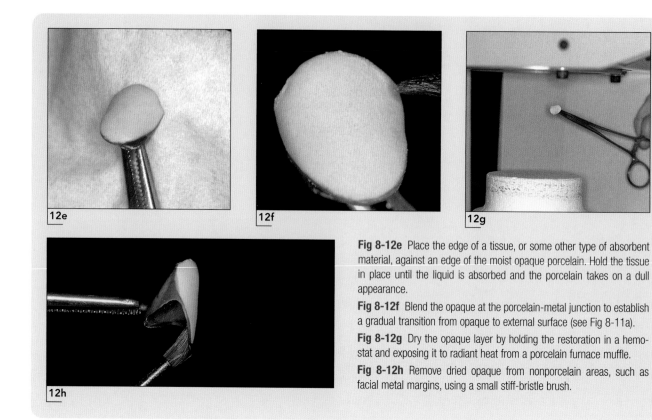

Fig 8-12e Place the edge of a tissue, or some other type of absorbent material, against an edge of the moist opaque porcelain. Hold the tissue in place until the liquid is absorbed and the porcelain takes on a dull appearance.

Fig 8-12f Blend the opaque at the porcelain-metal junction to establish a gradual transition from opaque to external surface (see Fig 8-11a).

Fig 8-12g Dry the opaque layer by holding the restoration in a hemostat and exposing it to radiant heat from a porcelain furnace muffle.

Fig 8-12h Remove dried opaque from nonporcelain areas, such as facial metal margins, using a small stiff-bristle brush.

junctions, any unnecessary thickness of opaque porcelain will result in a thin veneer of body porcelain or possible exposure of the opaque layer. Either situation will give the crown a very dull appearance because it causes the highly reflective opaque porcelain to be at or near the surface rather than completely covered by dentin porcelain. Such an outcome can present a significant esthetic and technical problem.

Furthermore, areas of exposed opaque porcelain are rough and must be covered by dentin or enamel body porcelain. If this roughness is near the gingival third, it has the potential to harbor bacteria and irritate the soft tissue. On the other hand, if the opaque porcelain is exposed on an area of occlusal contact, it will present a highly abrasive surface capable of wearing opposing restorations and natural tooth structure. Unfortunately, exposed opaque porcelain cannot be glazed or polished.

Generally, opaque porcelain is not blotted in the same way as body porcelain. However, it is sometimes helpful to remove excess liquid, particularly when attempting to mask the metal substructure with the initial application. Simply place a tissue or other absorbent blotter-type material gently against an edge of the moist opaque layer (Fig 8-12e). Although blotting the surface draws the liquid out by capil-

lary action and condenses the particles more tightly together, avoid blotting an entire surface. This action could lift the opaque layer off the metal substructure or otherwise disrupt the smooth surface.

If areas of the applied opaque porcelain appear rough and irregular, lightly tap the hemostat handle or move the serrations on a carver across the hemostat in a sawing motion. The vibrations created by either of these movements will condense and smooth the wet porcelain into a more uniform layer. If the opaque mix is too wet on the glass slab, blot it with a tissue and then continue. It is best to remove excess moisture before the opaque is applied to the metal.

Make any additions and gently blend the opaque at the porcelain-metal junction (Fig 8-12f). Lightly tap the hemostat again and dry the opaque by placing it in front of an open porcelain furnace muffle (Fig 8-12g). Carefully make a visual check to make certain that none of the opaque porcelain has extended past the porcelain-metal junction or onto nonveneered areas on the metal lingual surface. Remove any porcelain overextension with a stiff brush.

Dry the restoration in front of the muffle once more, and visually check again for any dried opaque porcelain on nonporcelain surfaces. Use the smaller stiff brush to remove this excess from the metal margin (Fig 8-12h). Be sure to inspect

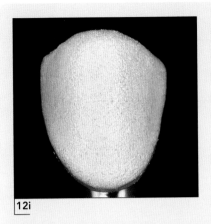 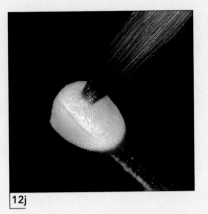 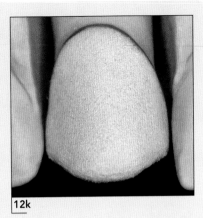

Fig 8-12i The visual indicator for a properly fired opaque layer is a sheen or an eggshell glisten.

Fig 8-12j If a second opaque application and firing is needed, wet the first layer with opaque medium and apply the second opaque layer.

Fig 8-12k The completed opaque layer masks the oxidized metal substructure. Inspect and clean the inside of the casting, and return it to its die and the master cast.

the intaglio surface of the coping. Remnants of porcelain left inside a substructure will be difficult to remove once the porcelain has been sintered. It is always easier to remove dried porcelain where it is not wanted at this stage; otherwise, fired porcelain must be ground off.

Put the restoration on a sagger tray and place the work in the middle of the muffle stand. Fire the work according to the manufacturer's instructions adjusted to the firing parameters of your particular porcelain furnace. A properly fired opaque layer will have a sheen or eggshell glisten (Fig 8-12i) or other visual indicators established by each porcelain manufacturer.

If a second application of opaque porcelain is required, as will generally be the case, lightly wet the surface with opaque liquid (Fig 8-12j). Apply the second opaque layer in the same manner as the first layer. Again, make every effort to keep this second layer as thin and uniform as possible. The second application should completely mask the metal oxide color. Remember to carefully clean porcelain from areas not intended for veneering, both inside and out. Examine the fired restoration to confirm complete, uniform masking of the metal and clean, well-defined porcelain-metal junctions. If metal coverage is incomplete, do not hesitate to apply additional opaque porcelain where necessary.

Carefully return the opaqued coping to the master die to confirm complete seating (Fig 8-12k). If the coping binds or fails to seat on the die, do not force it into place. Remove the restoration and reexamine the intaglio surface under magnification. Incomplete seating on the die often is an indication that some particle of opaque porcelain or other debris is inside the crown. It is imperative that the problem be identified and eliminated before proceeding. Always resist the temptation to force the restoration on the die. If a crown is forced into place, invariably the die will be abraded slightly or chipped. The result will be a restoration that seats on the die but not on the prepared tooth.

Brush technique

If you do not have a glass rod in your porcelain kit, you can apply the opaque with a ceramic brush. Select the appropriate shade, and mix the opaque porcelain as described previously. Lightly wet the metal with distilled water or opaque liquid, and then use the tip of your porcelain brush to lift a portion of the mixed opaque (Fig 8-13a).

Apply the porcelain on the most convex part of the wetted oxidized coping. Repeat the process several times until the porcelain-bearing area is completely covered with porcelain. Apply moderate-sized portions of opaque to min-

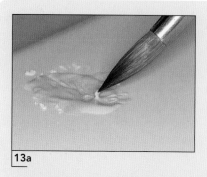
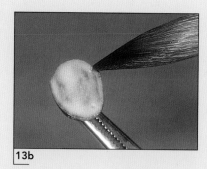
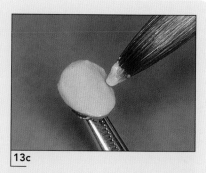

Fig 8-13a Opaque porcelain also can be applied with a brush. Load the tip of a large brush and carry the porcelain to the metal substructure.

Fig 8-13b Some ceramists apply and fire a thin initial layer of opaque to thoroughly wet the porcelain-bearing surface.

Fig 8-13c Others mask the oxidized surface completely with the first layer of opaque.

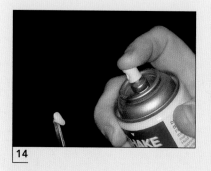
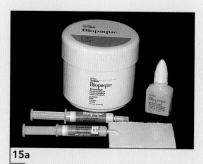
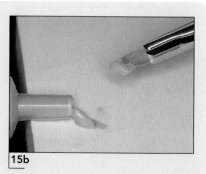

Fig 8-14 Spray opaques are available in a variety of shades.
Fig 8-15a Premixed opaques of various shades are available in individual syringes.

Fig 8-15b Mixed opaque can be dispensed from the syringe as needed and applied with a brush.

imize the number of additions and to decrease the potential for trapping air and introducing voids into the opaque layer.

You may fire this thin layer (Fig 8-13b), or alternatively, apply a thicker first layer (Fig 8-13c) and then fire the restoration. Apply a second layer of opaque as necessary to complete the masking of the substructure. After drying and firing the restoration, you should have a uniform layer of opaque.

Alternative methods

Conventional opaque porcelains are available in powdered form, but some companies offer spray opaques (Fig 8-14) and premixed opaques that can be applied with a brush (Fig 8-15). Large commercial laboratories often find it fast and economic to spray opaque applications on large numbers of castings at one time.

Application of dentin and enamel porcelain

The next step in the porcelain buildup procedure is to choose and properly mix the body porcelains that will be used to fabricate the porcelain veneer (see Fig 2-1 in chapter 2). All porcelain systems list a specific dentin and an enamel porcelain designed to reproduce a particular shade guide (Fig 8-16).

Tumble the individual porcelain jars to mix any fine particles that may have settled during storage (Fig 8-17a). Also be sure to wipe off any instrument used in dispensing or mixing any porcelain before inserting that instrument into a different bottle of powder. Dispense an adequate volume of dentin and enamel porcelain onto the mixing slab. Because dentin porcelain powders of different shades look the same

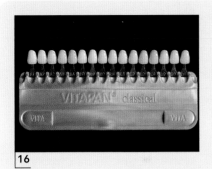

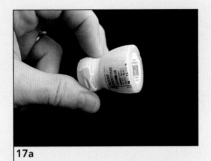

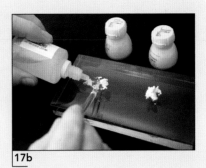

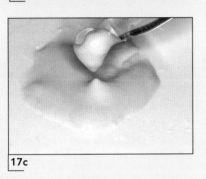

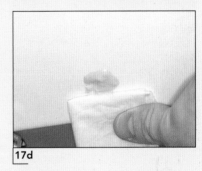

Fig 8-16 Vita Lumin Classical shade guide (Vident).

Fig 8-17a Tumble each porcelain jar before dispensing to thoroughly distribute fine particles that may have settled during storage.

Fig 8-17b Mix the body powders (dentin and enamel) with the recommended liquid. A commercial red color tag or food die can be added to the body porcelain to intensify the color and improve the level of contrast between layers.

Fig 8-17c When properly mixed, dentin porcelain should have a smooth, creamy consistency.

Fig 8-17d If too much liquid is added to the mix, use a tissue or blotting paper to remove excess liquid until the proper consistency is achieved.

once mixed, color tags (see chapter 2) can be added to vary the color intensity of each porcelain (Fig 8-17b). Be careful not to unintentionally mix the different powders (dentin, enamel, or opaque) with one another. Also, remember to discard the distilled water in which the brush used for opaquing was cleaned. This water contains particles that have intense pigmentation and are obviously very opaque. Even small amounts of opaque porcelain may alter the final shade and impair translucency should they contaminate the body powders.

> As the special liquids evaporate, only the water is lost, and the additives they contain remain in the porcelain.

Mixing dentin porcelains

The technique for mixing body porcelains is virtually the same as the one used to mix opaque porcelains. A glass rod is preferred to a metal spatula, and the liquid should be carefully added to the powder to prevent the entrapment of air.

Combine the liquid medium recommended by the porcelain manufacturer with each of the porcelains. Some brands are mixed with distilled water, while other manufacturers supply a special body porcelain liquid, referred to as *modeling liquid*, for this purpose. The advantages of these special liquids are that they usually evaporate more slowly than

water, and some are said to make the unfired porcelain mass more moldable and carvable. Tests found that modeling liquids increased dentin porcelain density by 2%, flexural strength by 5%, and microhardness (Vickers hardness) by 5%, but these changes were not statistically significant.[12]

A proper mix of body porcelain will have a thick creamy consistency (Fig 8-17c). If the porcelain on the glass slab begins to dry out during the buildup procedure, it should be rewetted with distilled water rather than with the special liquid. As the special liquids evaporate, only the water is lost, and the additives they contain remain in the porcelain. Adding only distilled water is generally adequate, although distilled water should not be mixed with some liquids, so always read the manufacturer's directions for specific recommendations.

Controlling moisture content in the mix

When all the porcelain particles are incorporated and a homogeneous mix is achieved, any excess moisture on the mixing slab should simply be blotted away with a tissue (Fig 8-17d). A mix that is too wet makes it challenging to build up the restoration or maintain the restoration's shape.

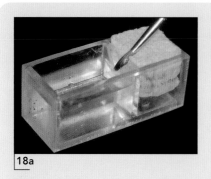
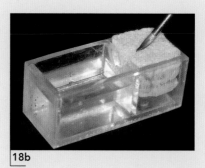
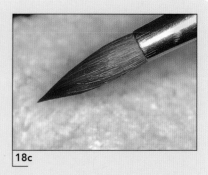

Fig 8-18a Wet the bristles in a distilled water bath, and drag the bristles through a V-shaped notch cut in an adjacent sponge while slowly rotating the brush.

Fig 8-18b Continue rotating the brush as it is dragged out of the distilled water and across the surface of the sponge.

Fig 8-18c The brush should have a distinct sharp point. It is not recommended to wet brushes by placing them in the mouth and simply twisting; the risk of infection alone discourages such a practice.

Conversely, if the porcelain is too dry, it is more difficult to apply to an existing layer, and air pockets can form between applications.

During the mixing procedure, avoid anything that might cause air entrapment. For example, do not fold the material onto itself, and avoid excessive stirring. To remove air bubbles in a buildup, a mixing instrument can be vibrated by pulling a serrated instrument across the handle. On occasion, air bubbles can be seen rising to the surface of the mix while vibrating.

As mentioned previously, another practice that should be avoided is rewetting porcelain that has completely dried out. When the liquid (water or modeling liquid) evaporates, air-filled voids are left behind in the mix. It is both impossible and impractical to try to eliminate these air pockets by reapplying liquid to moisten the porcelain. In fact, the voids are often so large and so numerous that you may be able to see the air bubbles in the mix. Vigorous condensation procedures cannot eliminate such large porosities. The porcelain, both on the mixing slab and in the buildup, should be monitored for its moisture level and rewetted with distilled water as necessary. In this way, porcelain is not allowed to dry out completely during the buildup procedure.

> Blotting relies on capillary action to draw the liquid toward the absorbent medium, and in the process, porcelain condenses in that same direction.

Applying dentin porcelain

The goal of the dentin porcelain buildup procedure is to apply and condense enough porcelain to create a restoration that is sufficiently overbuilt to accommodate the enamel veneer to be placed over the dentin layer and help to compensate for porcelain shrinkage.

Although some ceramists prefer to use spatulas,[13] most use a high-quality sable brush to create the porcelain buildup. The success of this buildup technique relies on a brush that is pointed (ie, transformed from a large blunt tip to a fine tapered point), which facilitates the pickup and placement of porcelain addition. Thus, the first step in the body buildup procedure requires a method to rapidly point ceramic brushes (Fig 8-18).

Some ceramists prefer to begin the buildup by applying dentin porcelain along the porcelain-metal junction and by thoroughly condensing the porcelain via alternating vibration and blotting. Such a practice is thought to reduce the tendency of body porcelain to pull away from these areas during firing because porcelain shrinks toward bulk. In general, the bulkiest area of a buildup on an anterior restoration is the midfacial region. Consequently, during the first body firing, porcelain pulls away from the porcelain-metal junction toward the center of the facial surface as it shrinks toward bulk. The method of first condensing at the porcelain-metal junction will be demonstrated with the application of opacious dentin.

However, the more common approach for a basic buildup is to simply build up the restoration to full contour and rely on sound condensation techniques to control shrinkage at the porcelain-metal junction. This technique will be illustrated for the standard buildup of a single-unit crown (Fig 8-19).

Because the lingual surface of this restoration has been restored in metal, the porcelain is condensed principally by blotting from the lingual aspect, as illustrated in Fig 8-19f. If the lingual surface were to be restored in porcelain, then

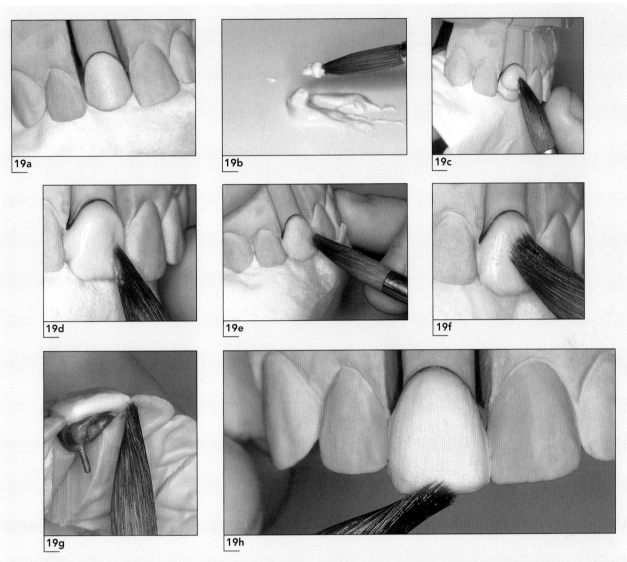

Fig 8-19a Carefully return the cleaned, opaqued coping to the master cast. Place folded tissue or blotting paper on the lingual side of the restoration.

Fig 8-19b To minimize the potential for entrapping air in the porcelain, move the tip of the pointed brush through the mixed dentin porcelain. Remove the brush with the dentin porcelain captured on the brush tip.

Fig 8-19c Apply the porcelain to the most convex surface (midfacial area) on the restoration.

Fig 8-19d Gently coax the porcelain toward the interproximal and incisal areas. Add more porcelain to the facial surface, and use a light tapping motion to move the porcelain along the porcelain-metal junction.

Fig 8-19e Move the porcelain down to the incisal edge, and lightly blot the buildup to condense the porcelain on the substructure. Place additional dentin porcelain in the incisal region, and move it from one interproximal area (mesial) to the other (distal).

Fig 8-19f To create the mesial-facial line angle, wipe the brush to dry it slightly and reduce the pointing, then lightly move it from the mesial-gingival area to the mesial-incisal area. Control the flow of the material and condense the buildup by periodically blotting the wet porcelain with the tissue. Dry the brush a little more to further flatten the tip, and returning to the mesial aspect, use light strokes from the gingival margin to the incisal margin over the entire facial surface to create the desired facial contour.

Fig 8-19g Point the brush and add additional dentin porcelain to the lingual aspect of the incisal edge. Smooth and condense the incisal edge from the lingual and facial aspects.

Fig 8-19h Add additional porcelain to complete the mesial and distal corners. The restoration should now possess the approximate shape of a central incisor. At this point, the dentin buildup should be slightly oversized (by 10% to 15%) but retain the outline of a central incisor.

blotting would have been done on both the facial and the lingual surfaces. Blotting relies on capillary action to draw the liquid toward the absorbent medium, and in the process, porcelain condenses in that same direction. Therefore, it is advisable to blot from as many orientations as possible (ie, facial, lingual, mesial, distal, incisal, and occlusal).

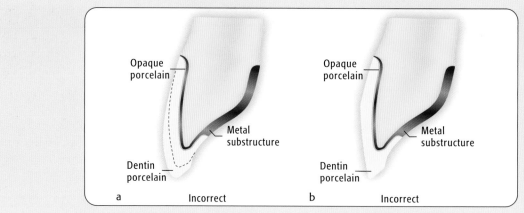

Fig 8-20 If dentin porcelain is overbuilt too much *(a)*, the amount of dentin remaining after the cutback may also be incorrect *(b)*.

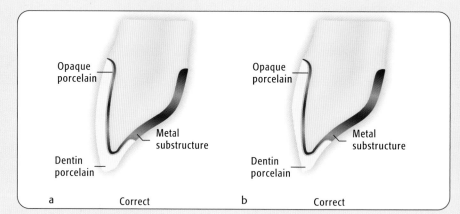

Fig 8-21 When the restoration has correct anatomic contours and slight overbuilding by 10% to 15% *(a)*, the dentin cutback will also be correct *(b)*.

Cutting back the dentin buildup

With the buildup complete, you are now ready to remove dentin porcelain from those areas of the crown where you would like to have enamel porcelain. The procedure of removing dentin porcelain to allow placement of a layer of enamel is referred to as the *dentin cutback*.

If too much dentin is overbuilt by mistake, the fired crown will be overcontoured even if the cutback is performed correctly (Fig 8-20). Therefore, it is imperative that the restoration be shaped to proper contour initially (Fig 8-21a) and that an appropriate amount of dentin porcelain is left to cover the opaque layer in the incisal and middle thirds of the crown (Fig 8-21b).

The illustrated technique should be considered a general approach to cutting back the dentin porcelain (Fig 8-22). The determination of how much dentin porcelain is removed and from which areas is governed by the esthetic demands of each particular case. In other words, no single standard cutback can be used for all patients. The amount of enamel and translucent porcelain that should be used to reproduce an individual crown will vary markedly with each patient. Therefore, look to the laboratory authorization (work order), clinician's sketch, or digital photograph (if provided) to determine the extent and depth of the dentin cutback (see Figs 8-22d and 8-22e).

Alternatively, you could use a knife to make these same facial cuts. At this point the restoration is ready for the application of enamel porcelain.

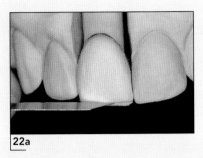

22a

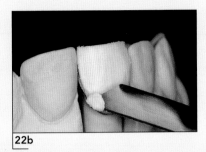

22b

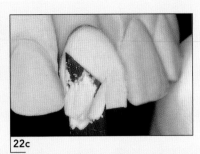

22c

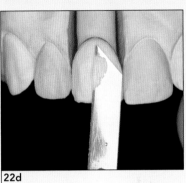

22d

Fig 8-22a Porcelain cutback procedure generally requires a razor knife and porcelain buildup brush. Use the razor knife to cut back the incisal edge between 1.0 and 1.5 mm.

Fig 8-22b Remove dentin porcelain at the mesial interproximal line angle. Extend the cut to the junction of the middle and gingival third for younger patients.

Fig 8-22c Cut across the middle third. Stop the cutback at the distal interproximal area.

Fig 8-22d At the distal interproximal line angle, make a cut from the incisal edge toward the gingival third as far as required for the esthetics of the case. Reduce the middle third of the facial surface as necessary.

Fig 8-22e The point where the incisal porcelain terminates in the cutback is determined by the enamel transition on a patient's tooth. Also, the depth of the cutback can be (A) a gradual transition replicated with a feather edge dentin cutback, (B) a noticeable delineation reproduced by a chamfer-like cut back, or (C) a distinct line recreated by a shoulder dentin cutback.

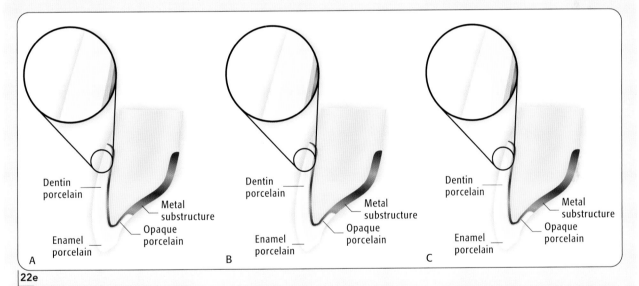

22e

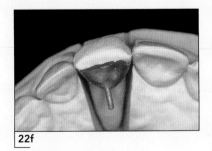

22f

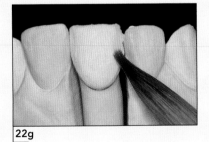

22g

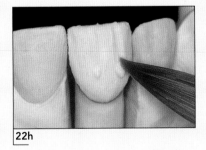

22h

Fig 8-22f Examine the restoration from an incisal view for symmetry and adequacy of the cutback.

Fig 8-22g Smooth the cutback areas with the porcelain brush so the transitions from dentin to enamel porcelain are gradual rather than abrupt. Assess the depth and incisal-gingival length of the cutback.

Fig 8-22h Mamelons may need to be developed in restorations for younger patients. With a pointed brush, create two depressions on the facial surface using vertical strokes from the incisal edge to the gingival margin. You can accentuate the incisal notches or fill them in for a more subtle appearance.

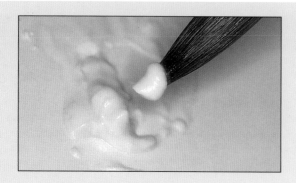

Fig 8-23 Use a mixing instrument to add buildup liquid (or distilled water) to the powder and stir gently. Generally, the enamel mix is slightly wetter than the dentin mix to facilitate its addition to a previously applied and condensed dentin layer. Ideally, mixed enamel porcelain should have a consistency that permits ready pick up by a pointed porcelain brush.

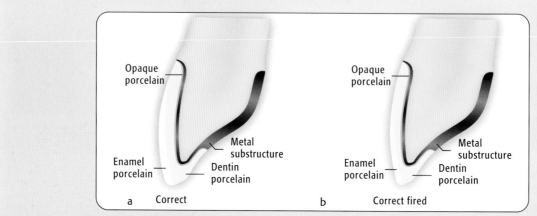

Fig 8-24 The goal is to create a crown with an enamel porcelain veneer placed over a correct thickness of dentin porcelain (a), so the fired restoration has the proper final contour and enamel coverage (b). Translucent porcelain can be applied over this buildup.

Mixing the enamel porcelain

The same recommendations for mixing opaque and dentin porcelain apply for the mixing of enamel porcelain. Use a mixing instrument to add buildup liquid (or distilled water) to the powder and stir gently (Fig 8-23).

Applying enamel porcelain

When applying the enamel porcelain layer (Figs 8-24 and 8-25), be careful in the placement of each increment to avoid trapping air between additions. Also, avoid "working" the new layer of porcelain into the initial dentin buildup; maintain the delineation between the two materials. By layering the enamel, you have a better opportunity of creating a well-defined junction between dentin and enamel porcelain. The combined dentin and enamel layers should be overbuilt by at least 10% (and no more than 15%) to approximate the estimated shrinkage that occurs during the firing cycle.

The esthetics of each case will vary such that in some instances the enamel porcelain is backed by dentin porce-

lain; or, you may have to extend enamel porcelain over the incisal edge and slightly onto the lingual surface. With a clean brush, remove any porcelain beyond the porcelain-metal junction with the brush tip. The restoration should be neat, clean, and slightly overbuilt to accommodate the firing shrinkage of the porcelain.

You can condense the porcelain buildup via the vibration method followed by capillary action with blotting (eg, a small mallet for tapping the cast) or the whipping technique followed by capillary action with blotting. However, when using the latter technique, avoid excess whipping because there is a tendency to pull particles of enamel porcelain down over the dentin layer and vice versa with each brush stroke. Such action can dilute the dentin color, diminish translucency, or lower of the value of the overall restoration as enamel particles are incorporated into the dentin layer. Whether for purposes of condensation or not, lightly moving the whipping brush over the buildup helps to smooth the surface and blend the enamel porcelain into the dentin layer (see Fig 8-25e).

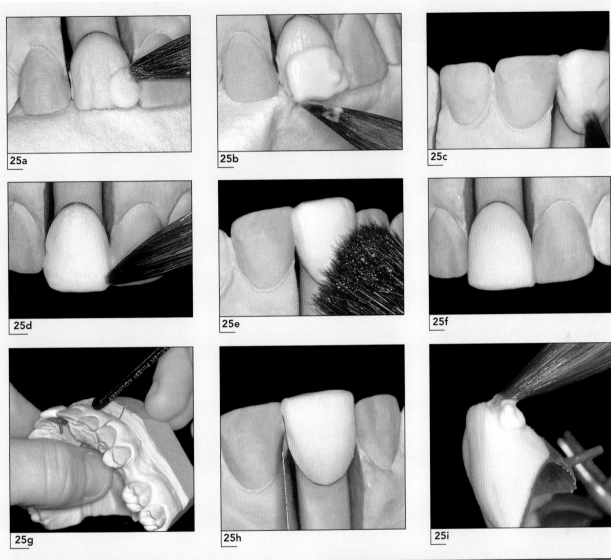

Fig 8-25a With a pointed brush, apply enamel porcelain to one corner of the cutback (mesial aspect shown).

Fig 8-25b Add more enamel porcelain and move it across the facial surface in the incisal third. Push the wet mix toward the middle third of the crown, and work it into the opposite (distal) interproximal line angle.

Fig 8-25c Blend the enamel porcelain at the junction of the middle and gingival thirds, and begin to establish the incisal edge. Condense the porcelain by blotting periodically.

Fig 8-25d With additional enamel porcelain, complete the incisal edge and the mesial-incisal line angle. Work your way along the incisal edge to create more of a distal-incisal line angle.

Fig 8-25e Blend the enamel porcelain into the gingival third on the facial surface. Re-create the interproximal contours and line angles.

Fig 8-25f Shape the mesial-incisal corner as required for each case. Examine the buildup from an incisal view and evaluate the overall shape. Make certain the restoration is slightly overbuilt.

Fig 8-25g Tap the cast lightly to condense the buildup and bring fluid to the surface for blotting.

Fig 8-25h Use a thin razor knife to cut and shape the mesial and distal interproximal areas. This procedure also removes any unwanted porcelain below the interproximal contact areas.

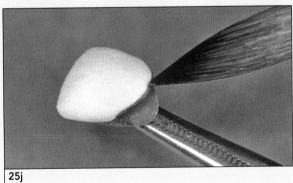

Fig 8-25i Carefully remove the crown from the master cast. Add enamel porcelain to the small dimples in each interproximal contact area. Using either enamel or translucent porcelain, overbuild these areas by about 0.5 mm to compensate for the porcelain shrinkage.

Fig 8-25j Remove excess porcelain beyond the porcelain-metal junction, and clean the facial metal collar (if present) of any porcelain with a small brush or a pointed porcelain buildup brush. Smooth the entire buildup with the whipping brush. Finally, inspect and clean the inside of the casting before firing the porcelain.

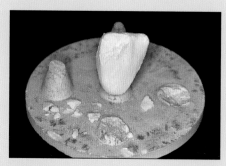

Fig 8-26 This wet porcelain buildup was not dried long enough or was suddenly exposed to high heat that produced steam and caused portions of the buildup to pop off the metal substructure.

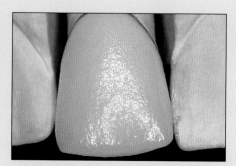

Fig 8-27 A properly fired porcelain body bake should have a pebbly or "orange peel" appearance. Examine the restoration for deficiencies in the outline and contour, such as an inadequate mesio-incisal corner. These discrepancies can be corrected with a second body bake.

Firing procedure

The large bulk of the buildup requires more time to dry and preheat than the opaque porcelain did. It is advisable to strictly adhere to the manufacturer's recommended drying times.

Put the restoration on a sagger tray and place it on the muffle stand of the porcelain furnace. Failure to thoroughly dry the buildup may cause the internal moisture to vaporize and actually pop parts of the unfired porcelain off the metal substructure (Fig 8-26).

Properly matured porcelain varies in appearance according to the different manufacturers' recommendations. However, most porcelains have a slightly rough, pebbly, or "orange peel" appearance when fired correctly (Fig 8-27).

Underfired porcelain

You want to avoid underfiring a restoration. Porcelain that has not matured properly can be identified by a lack of shine to the surface and a cloudy appearance, internally. The resulting porcelain also will be weak and brittle, and additional firings may not correct the problem. Restorations that are underfired often necessitate that the porcelain is stripped completely from the metal and rebuilt.

> To prevent or at least minimize the potential for under- or overfiring a restoration, learn to recognize the levels of porcelain maturation and the visual indicators manufacturers recommend for the various firing cycles.

Overfired porcelain

In contrast, overfired porcelain has a glazed appearance, and the surface has little, if any, of the desired pebbly appearance mentioned previously. Other problems that may be present with overfired porcelain are excessive translucency, slumping or rounding, and the general loss of anatomic contours.

To prevent or at least minimize the potential for under- or overfiring a restoration, learn to recognize the levels of porcelain maturation and the visual indicators manufacturers recommend for the various firing cycles.

Bisque stages of porcelain maturation

Porcelain systems have recommended firing parameters for each phase of the fabrication process: opaque, first body bake, second body bake, and glaze firing. The physical appearance of a restoration varies with the level of maturity resulting from the time and temperature settings used. Both color and translucency depend on the porcelain's level of maturity. This postfiring appearance of the predried vacuum-fired body porcelain buildup produces a restoration in a *bisque* stage. Three bisque stages are recognized: *low bisque, medium bisque,* and *high bisque.*[3,5,6]

Low bisque

This is the least mature stage of development for the ceramic veneer, characterized by a structure in which the grains of porcelain have just begun to soften and fuse at their contact angles.[4,6] The porcelain is both porous and weak. A porous surface is a concern because the ceramic is susceptible to contamination until maturation is complete and the outermost surface is sealed.

Medium bisque

In this next level of maturation, the porcelain grains have fused together more substantially. Less porosity is present, and it is evident that some shrinkage has occurred. The surface may still appear slightly porous but not to the level of a low-bisque firing. Any air that was retained internally and unable to escape will remain in the porcelain as voids.[6]

Externally, a sheen is apparent, but the ceramic lacks good color development and translucency.[5]

High bisque

A high-bisque bake is the desired stage of porcelain maturation. The grains have fused together, and the maximum amount of air has been eliminated for the level of condensation performed and the amount of vacuum used.[6] The exterior surface appearance may range from an "orange peel" to a smooth sheen; a smooth surface indicates the outer surface has been completely sealed. With shrinkage complete and voids eliminated as much as possible, the exterior surface retains texture, but most features appear rounded rather than sharp. At this high-bisque stage, porcelain has attained a greater level of strength, and the majority of the shrinkage has taken place to permit final contour adjustments and additional firing prior to glazing.

Visual indicators

Many porcelain manufacturers provide firing schedules complete with recommended temperature settings, but every porcelain furnace is different. Even with frequent calibration, temperatures will vary among units. The use of visual indicators gives technicians a tool to assess the performance of their porcelain furnace.

The technique is quite simple. The ceramic surface is visually assessed after each stage in the fabrication process: opaque applications, body and margin buildup, and a natural and an applied overglaze. The appearance of the work is visually compared with the porcelain manufacturer's recommended postfiring visual indicators.

> Restorations that appear different from the anticipated visual indicators should be analyzed carefully to determine if they have been under- or overfired.

If the general appearance of a restoration is in line with the desired appearance for each stage in the buildup process, technicians have some assurance that they are firing their work within an acceptable temperature range for each firing cycle. As a general rule, dental porcelain is transformed from a slight sheen or eggshell appearance (fired opaque) to a shiny appearance (body bisque bakes) to a smooth, satiny gloss or high gloss (glazed).

Restorations that appear different from the anticipated visual indicators should be analyzed carefully to determine if they have been under- or overfired. Temperature setting can then be modified accordingly and retested.

Number of firings

In the hands of an experienced ceramist, many single-unit crowns and even some fixed partial dentures can be fabricated with one to two buildups and firings. Yet you should not hesitate to make needed additions and correction firings. One study reported that repeated firings (up to nine times) may not compromise the shade of porcelain, but they can diminish porcelain's ability to autoglaze the veneer.[14]

Modern porcelains appear to be stable after multiple firings. Correction bakes may be a matter of routine until you gain more experience and improve your skills. As a rule, the same porcelain (eg, dentin, enamel, or translucent) that was initially placed in an area is used for additions to that same area. However, the firing temperature is usually lowered 10°C with each correction bake so the initial porcelain buildup is not affected. In addition, there is less bulk of porcelain with each subsequent correction, which allows for complete maturation at a slightly lower temperature. Again, follow the recommended firing schedule for each brand of dental porcelain.

Once these procedures are completed, inspect the inside of the crown for evidence of debris, and then reseat the restoration on the master cast, evaluating it for color and contours. Steam clean the restoration or place it in distilled water and an ultrasonic unit. At first glance, it is evident that this restoration will need a second bake to build up the mesio-incisal corner (see Fig 8-27). Rather than subject the crown to multiple firings, it is better to proceed to the adjusting and finishing procedures in the event that other areas also need modification. In this way, the second firing can correct all the deficiencies identified following the first bake. This restoration is now ready for occlusal adjustments and contouring (see chapter 9).

Alternative Buildup Techniques

Anterior single crown with lingual porcelain: Lateral segmental buildup technique

The standard dentin and enamel porcelain technique previously illustrated also can be used for anterior crowns when restoring the lingual surface in porcelain (Fig 8-28). For younger patients or individuals with increased incisal translucency, restorations can be fabricated with an alternative method, referred to as the *lateral segmental buildup technique* (Fig 8-29).[15]

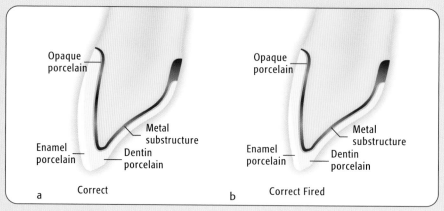

Fig 8-28 For restorations with porcelain lingual surfaces, layers of dentin and enamel porcelain are overbuilt slightly *(a)* to compensate for firing shrinkage, so the final restoration has the proper contours and esthetics *(b)*.

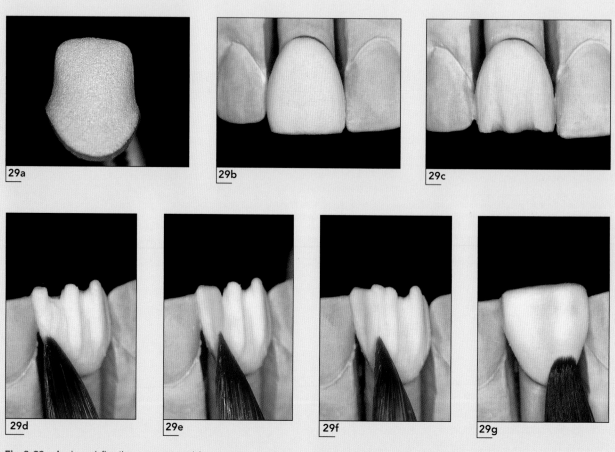

Fig 8-29a Apply and fire the opaque porcelain to create a uniform thickness that masks the underlying metal.

Fig 8-29b Complete and smooth the slightly overcontoured dentin buildup as described previously.

Fig 8-29c Create three developmental lobes using a pointed brush.

Fig 8-29d Invert the cast and place translucent porcelain in the two developmental grooves. Then add enamel porcelain to one interproximal area (mesial shown).

Fig 8-29e Working from left to right, apply a 50:50 mixture of enamel and translucent porcelain (color-coded pink) to the right of the enamel addition.

Fig 8-29f Place a second layer of enamel porcelain to the right of the 50:50 mixture of enamel and translucent porcelain and to the left of the translucent porcelain in the developmental groove area.

Fig 8-29g Continue this process until the entire crown is slightly over-built. Smooth the facial surface and then condense and blot the buildup. The tip of the brush was quickly flattened simply by moving the brush over a flat portion of the wet sponge.

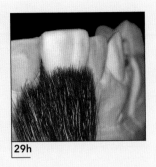
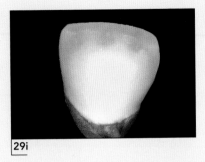
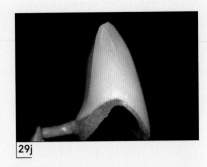

Fig 8-29h Use the whipping brush to gently smooth the porcelain buildup.

Fig 8-29i Once the porcelain has been fired, mamelons should be visible in the restoration (lingual view).

Fig 8-29j Well-condensed porcelain does not pull away from the porcelain-metal junction. Note the subtle blend from dentin to enamel porcelain. The cervical contour is refined in a second bake.

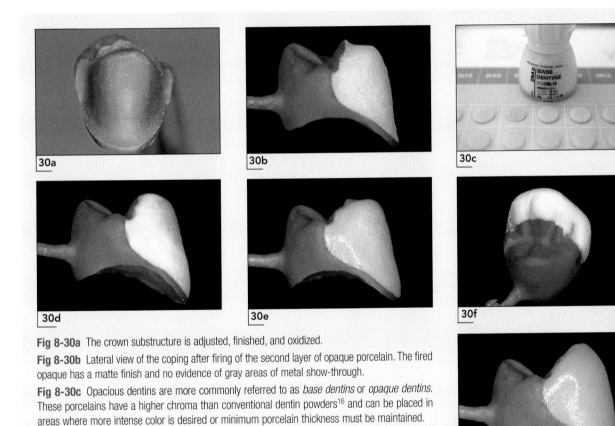

Fig 8-30a The crown substructure is adjusted, finished, and oxidized.

Fig 8-30b Lateral view of the coping after firing of the second layer of opaque porcelain. The fired opaque has a matte finish and no evidence of gray areas of metal show-through.

Fig 8-30c Opacious dentins are more commonly referred to as *base dentins* or *opaque dentins*. These porcelains have a higher chroma than conventional dentin powders[16] and can be placed in areas where more intense color is desired or minimum porcelain thickness must be maintained.

Fig 8-30d Lateral view of opacious dentin following application, condensing, and preparation for firing. Customarily, the opacious dentin is placed and fired together with the first body bake rather then separately, as shown here.

Fig 8-30e Lateral view of opacious dentin after firing. The desired visual indicator for fired opacious dentin is a shiny but unglazed appearance.

Fig 8-30f Occlusal view of the completed dentin and enamel porcelain buildup. The pointed porcelain brush was used to accent the anatomic form to minimize finishing in porcelain.

Fig 8-30g Lateral view after first porcelain firing. A natural internal color in the cervical third can be attributed to the opacious dentin.

Posterior single crown with metal occlusal surface

The technique for applying porcelain to a posterior crown with a metal occlusal surface is virtually the same as that used for anterior teeth. One major difference may be the need to incorporate a greater level of characterization to posterior teeth. Therefore, this example illustrates how to include opacious dentin porcelain (a body modifier) in the buildup (Fig 8-30).

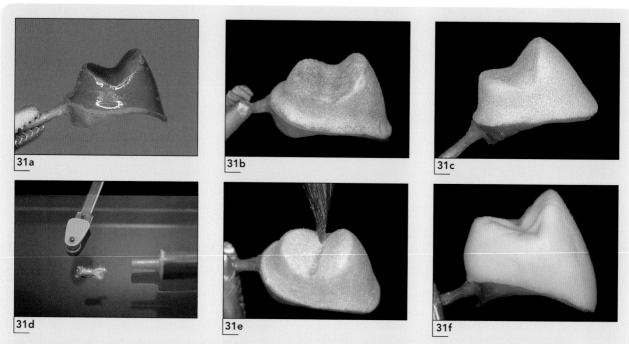

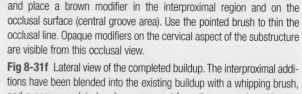

Fig 8-31a Wet the oxidized metal substructure with opaque liquid and remove the excess.

Fig 8-31b Lateral view of the coping after a thin layer of opaque porcelain was applied and fired.

Fig 8-31c Lateral view of coping after firing the second opaque layer. If areas of gray show through, avoid the tendency to apply so much opaque on the second application as to pool at the line angles and occlusal surface. The net result can be inadequate opaque coverage.

Fig 8-31d Premixed paste opaque modifiers are used to add more color internally to selected areas of a restoration. Because opaque modifiers are intense, mix only small quantities of the chosen colors. Tone down an effect simply by adding more opaque liquid to create a thinner mix.

Fig 8-31e Sparingly apply the opaque modifier to the cervical region, and place a brown modifier in the interproximal region and on the occlusal surface (central groove area). Use the pointed brush to thin the occlusal line. Opaque modifiers on the cervical aspect of the substructure are visible from this occlusal view.

Fig 8-31f Lateral view of the completed buildup. The interproximal additions have been blended into the existing buildup with a whipping brush, and excess porcelain has been removed from the exposed metal collar on the lingual, interproximal, and facial areas. Occlusal primary and secondary anatomy has been created at this stage to minimize grinding the fired porcelain. Any porcelain on the intaglio surface was removed.

Fig 8-31g Occlusal view of the restoration after the first body bake. The restoration closely approximates the proper crown outline and the natural occlusal anatomy. Both primary and secondary anatomy are evident in this first firing.

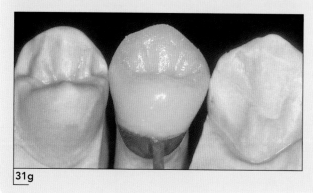

Posterior single crown with porcelain occlusal surface

As mentioned previously, the technique for applying porcelain to a posterior crown with either a metal or a porcelain occlusal surface is virtually the same as that used for ante-rior restorations. However, rather than modify the restoration with opacious dentins during the body buildup, the characterization process can begin earlier with the application of opaque modifiers (Fig 8-31).

Next, build the restoration to full contour with dentin porcelain. Perform this task on the master cast and use the

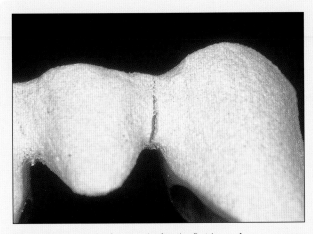

Fig 8-32a Inspect the framework after the first layer of opaque porcelain has been applied and fired. With multiple-unit cases, there is a greater likelihood that several porcelain applications will be necessary. Cracking on the facial surface in the connector area (as seen in this photograph) is not an uncommon occurrence, particularly if the fixed partial denture has been presoldered.

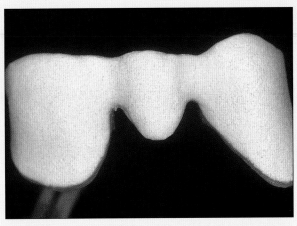

Fig 8-32b Apply and condense additional opaque porcelain over the crack in the connector area, cover any gray areas, and fire the prosthesis a second time.

adjacent teeth to provide perspective on axial contour and cusp placement. Cut back the dentin porcelain in preparation to apply a layer of enamel porcelain. Add the enamel and translucent porcelains, if desired, and condense the restoration well. Use a pointed porcelain brush tip or carving instrument to create the desired occlusal anatomy by sculpting the condensed porcelain. Take time to carve the desired anatomic form in the buildup with a sharp instrument (see Fig 8-31f). Remove the restoration, and apply either enamel or translucent porcelain to the interproximal areas to restore contact and complete the buildup process.

It is extremely important to make every effort to sculpt the outline form and occlusal anatomy in the condensed porcelain, rather than rely on firing a mass of porcelain on the substructure and "grinding in" the correct anatomy. When time and care are taken to skillfully develop a lifelike restoration in the first body bake, less time is required for gross adjusting and finishing, thereby minimizing the extent of corrections required in a second bake (see Fig 8-31g).

Fixed Partial Dentures: Porcelain Application

Anterior fixed partial denture

The steps involved in adding porcelain to a fixed partial denture differ only slightly, but are more complex, from those required for a single-unit restoration (Fig 8-32). It is recommended that you first master the basic skills required to successfully fabricate a single-unit crown before attempting to create multiple-unit restorations.

The opaque porcelain is applied as demonstrated with the single-unit crown. In inexperienced hands, the porcelain may dry out when fabricating fixed partial dentures because of the added time required to build multiple units simultaneously. To overcome this problem, try using a slightly wetter porcelain mixture for the first few fixed partial denture and other multi-unit cases. Also consider switching from distilled water to a modeling liquid for body porcelains to extend your working time.

Before firing the work, carefully remove the prosthesis from the master cast and examine it thoroughly from the facial and lingual aspects. Moistening the adjacent stone teeth and the tissue paper underneath the pontic may facilitate removal of the restoration. If the porcelain has dried and is sticking to the cast in any of these areas, wet the adjacent portions of the gypsum cast; this usually allows the porcelain to be released.

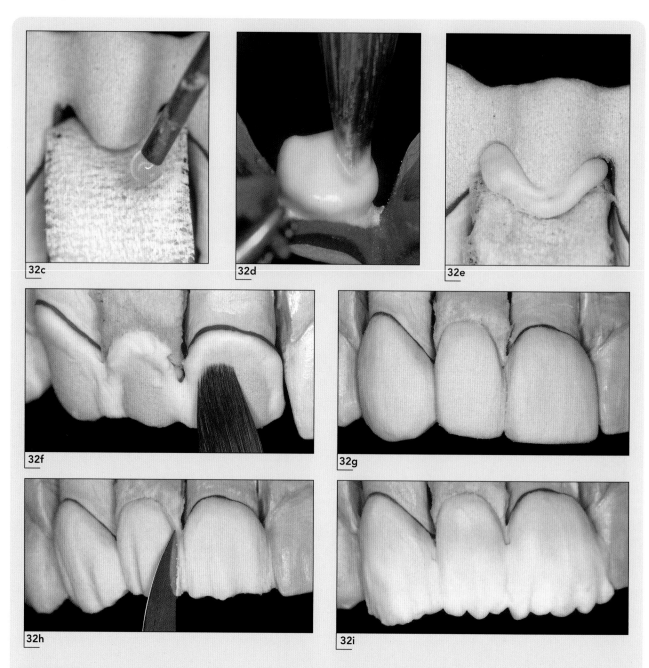

32c

32d

32e

32f

32g

32h

32i

Fig 8-32c Return the opaqued fixed partial denture to the master cast with a piece of moistened tissue paper cut to cover the entire pontic region and the labial surface of the gypsum cast. Tissue wetted with a drop or two of distilled water will cling to the edentulous ridge of the cast and prevent porcelain from sticking to it. In lieu of using wetted tissue paper, the edentulous area on the cast can be either sealed with cyano-acrylate or lubricated with a liquid porcelain-releasing agent.

Fig 8-32d Add a small portion of dentin porcelain to the underside of the pontic on the fixed partial denture framework. Use the pointed porcelain brush to move the porcelain over the opaqued surface and completely cover the tissue side of the pontic.

Fig 8-32e Return the framework to the master cast and gently rock it back and forth until it seats completely. Remove the framework and inspect the tissue side of the pontic. This area should be covered com-

pletely with well-condensed porcelain. You may wish to fill any voids in this fairly fragile part of the buildup because the gingival extension of the pontic is certain to require a subsequent correction bake. Some ceramists choose to slightly overbuild the pontic to compensate for shrinkage and then grind in the tissue contact on the working cast after firing (see chapter 9).

Fig 8-32f Place the framework back on the master cast, and apply dentin porcelain or add and condense opacious dentin to the cervical areas of the three components.

Fig 8-32g Complete the application of dentin porcelain.

Fig 8-32h Create the developmental lobes if desired. Use a thin razor knife to cut through the interproximal areas and individualize the teeth.

Fig 8-32i Add the enamel veneer using a standard buildup or a lateral segmental buildup.

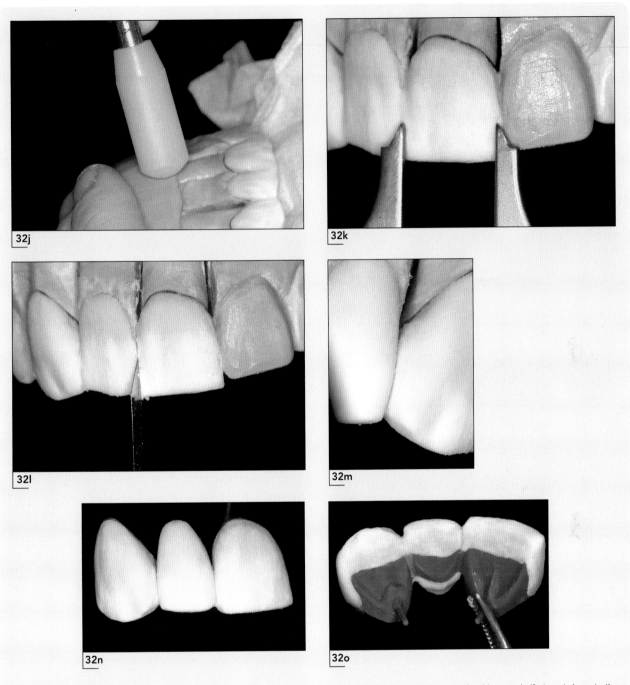

Fig 8-32j Condense the porcelain buildup using a small mallet (as shown) or another common technique.

Fig 8-32k Measure the mesial-distal width of each tooth with a Boley gauge, and compare it with the mesial-distal widths of porcelain buildups. Verify each tooth's width before firing to assure the buildups will allow for the estimated porcelain shrinkage.

Fig 8-32l Use a carving blade, knife, or other instrument to make necessary adjustments to the mesial-distal width of each buildup. Porcelain shrinks toward bulk, so the three units must be individualized to allow each to sinter separately, thus minimizing interproximal cracking. Some tears typically appear in the connector areas after the first bake due to fir-

ing shrinkage. To avoid this, use the thin razor knife to cut down to the opaque porcelain layer.

Fig 8-32m Interproximal cuts should be narrow to delicately form the interproximal line angles. In this way, the natural contours of these regions are preserved. As you acquire experience, you learn how to compensate for interproximal shrinkage through selective condensation of the initial porcelain layer in the embrasures themselves. Clean all exposed metal surfaces of any excess porcelain.

Fig 8-32n Facial view of the completed initial porcelain buildup.

Fig 8-32o Lingual view of the porcelain buildup. Do not forget to clean the lingual metal surface of excess porcelain and to remove any material from the intaglio surface.

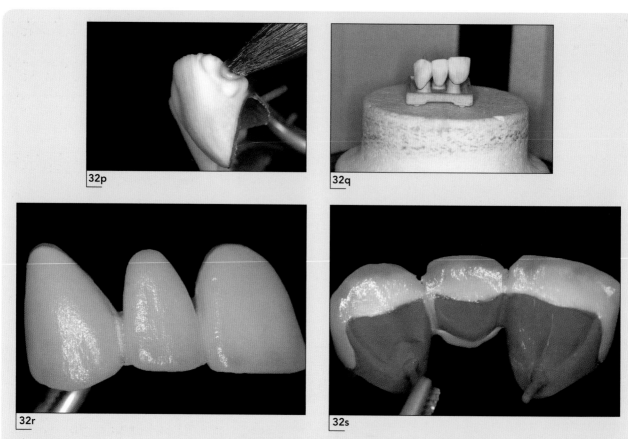

Fig 8-32p As a final step, add enamel or translucent porcelain to the interproximal contact areas, and blend the additions into the existing contour.

Fig 8-32q Place the restoration on an appropriate sagger tray. Be careful to properly balance the framework on the pegs, since many anterior fixed partial dentures have a tendency to tip labially because of their arch form. Obviously, a great deal of work can be lost very quickly if the unfired restoration falls off the pegs.

Fig 8-32r Labial view of the three-unit fixed partial denture after the first bake. In this case, the interproximal cuts were made, and the embrasure between the canine and lateral incisor opened slightly during firing. Yet, the same area between the central and lateral incisors retained a more

natural appearance. The successful visual indicator for fired porcelain is an orange peel surface, indicating that the firing schedule used was correct for this particular brand of porcelain.

Fig 8-32s Lingual view of the prosthesis. The porcelain was well condensed along the porcelain-metal junction and did not pull away from the metal substructure. The incisal edge reflects the layering of porcelain blends of enamel and translucent porcelain. The obvious separation in the canine interproximal region alone will necessitate the addition of a second application of porcelain. It is also possible that other portions of the prosthesis will require modifications. Rather than subject the prosthesis to unnecessary multiple firings, other adjusting and finishing techniques may be used, as discussed in chapter 9.

Summary

This chapter included the basic techniques for applying opaque and body porcelain to oxidized metal substructures. In addition to examples of several anterior and posterior substructure designs, the standard and lateral segmental buildup techniques were presented. As an added challenge, the fabrication of an anterior three-unit fixed partial denture

was illustrated to tax your talents once you have mastered the skills needed to construct satisfactory single-unit anterior and posterior restorations. The basics of internal color development were introduced through examples using opacious dentins and opaque modifiers.

Chapter 9 provides guidance on how to adjust and finish these fired porcelain restorations in preparation for second correction bakes, characterization (staining and glazing), and the final polish.

References

1. Müterthies K. Esthetic Approach to Metal Ceramic Restorations for Mandibular Anterior Region. Chicago: Quintessence, 1990.
   Custom metal-ceramic restorations are presented for patients of all ages.

2. Zhang Y, Griggs JA, Benham AW. Influence of powder/liquid ratio on porosity and translucency of dental porcelains. J Prosthet Dent 2004;91:128–135.

3. Naylor WP. Non-Gold Base Dental Casting Alloys. Vol II: Porcelain-fused-to-metal alloys [ADA173766]. Brooks AFB, TX: School of Aerospace Medicine, 1986:19–22.

4. Anusavice KJ. Phillips' Science of Dental Materials, ed 11. Philadelphia: Saunders, 2003.

5. Muia PJ. The Four Dimensional Tooth Color System. Chicago: Quintessence, 1982:160–162.

6. McLean JW. The Science and Art of Dental Ceramics. Vol I: The nature of dental ceramics and their clinical use. Chicago: Quintessence, 1979:42, 49.
   The addition of dry powder to a wet porcelain surface is not recommended for porcelain condensation (page 42). Bisque stages are discussed (page 49).

7. Barghi N, Lorenzana RE. Optimum thickness of opaque and body porcelains. J Prothet Dent 1982;48:429–431.
   Color comparison of test specimens with 0.3-mm opaque porcelain and from 0.5- to 1.0-mm body porcelain determines: (1) porcelain thicknesses vary among shades and brands; (2) a completely opaqued substructure does not produce the desired shade; (3) excess opaque porcelain does not affect shade, but excess body porcelain does; and (4) manufacturers should recommend porcelain thicknesses.

8. Tamura K. Essentials of Dental Technology. Fowler JA (trans). Chicago: Quintessence, 1987:366–368.
   Opaque powder is built to 0.4-mm thickness but reduced to 0.3 mm once fired.

9. Lacy AM. Ceramometal restorations. In: Eissmann HF, Rudd KD, Morrow RM (eds). Dental Laboratory Procedures. Fixed Partial Dentures, vol II. St Louis: Mosby, 1980:262–295.

10. Dykema RW, Goodacre CJ, Phillips RW. Johnston's Modern Practice in Fixed Prosthodontics, ed 4. Philadelphia: Saunders, 1986:296.

11. Avila R, Barghi N, Aranda R. PFM color changes caused by varied opaque firings [abstract 1249]. J Dent Res 1985;64(special issue):313.
    Refer to chapter 1 for summary.

12. Sinmazişik G, Ovecoğlu ML. Physical properties and microstructural characterization of dental porcelains mixed with distilled water and modeling liquid. Dent Mater 2006;22:735–745.

13. Berger RP. The art of dental ceramic sculpturing. Dent Clin North Am 1977;21:751–768.
    Use of metal spatulas and blades is depicted for porcelain application, rather than a pointed brush.

14. Barghi N. Color and glaze: Effects of repeated firings. J Prosthet Dent 1982;47:393–396.
    Firing up to nine times makes it difficult to glaze porcelain due to depletion of the glass matrix and reduced migration of that matrix to the surface.

15. McLaren E. The skeleton buildup technique: A systematic approach to the three-dimensional control of shade and shape. Pract Periodontics Aesthet Dent 1998;10:587–597.
    McLaren discusses shade selection, substructure design, porcelain techniques (including lateral segmental layering), porcelain contouring, and glazing.

16. Korson D. Natural Ceramics. Chicago: Quintessence, 1990:51–61.
    Author compares color-saturated dentin porcelains (eg, high chroma dentin) to opacious dentins.

Adjusting and Finishing the Metal-Ceramic Restoration

Applying and firing the porcelain veneer to a metal substructure only approximates the shape, contour, occlusion, and surface finish of the final restoration. The very nature of the application process, with the requirement to compensate for porcelain shrinkage, can result in a bulky (overcontoured) restoration. Even when you exercise great care, anatomically correct axial line angles and the final surface texture are difficult to achieve. Consequently, the fired porcelain requires adjustments to reduce any overcontoured areas and re-create a lifelike ceramic surface finish prior to the characterizing and glazing stages.

Adjusting, contouring, and finishing procedures for metal-ceramic restorations play a critical role in achieving both proper function and optimal esthetics. Occasionally, these tasks are viewed as mundane; however, anyone who has carefully observed an accomplished ceramist at work realizes that it is during these final phases of fabrication that a restoration comes to life. Subtle refinements in contouring, surface texture, and surface characterization often make the critical difference between a mediocre restoration and an exceptional restoration. Surprisingly, little equipment and few instruments are needed for the finishing procedures. When it comes to adjusting and contouring, knowing what to do and how to do it may be more important than which instruments are used.

Armamentarium

As with metal preparation, the simplest way to describe the armamentarium for adjusting and finishing the porcelain veneer and the metal substructure is to divide those items into three categories: *(1)* equipment, *(2)* instruments, and *(3)* materials.

Equipment

A wide variety of sophisticated equipment is available for individuals interested in establishing either a commercial dental laboratory or a small laboratory in a dental office. Some are essential to a basic operation; others are highly recommended. Several of the more important pieces of equipment can improve quality or facilitate production. When cost is a limiting factor, develop a budget and a long-term plan to purchase these pieces within a realistic timeframe.

As indicated in chapter 7, a laboratory microscope allows you to visualize areas needing adjustment, make necessary changes with more precision, and potentially save hours of work. Once you have used a microscope, you will likely find it to be an essential item in the laboratory for viewing restorations.

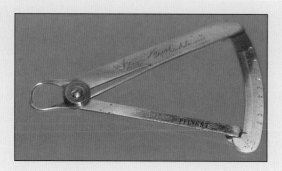

Fig 9-1 An Iwason metal caliper (Pfingst) can be used to determine the thickness of metal or metal and porcelain to a tolerance of approximately 0.1 mm.

Almost any type of dental handpiece can be helpful for contouring a porcelain restoration; however, some units have been designed specifically for this purpose, and their use will increase the probability of success. Select a variable-speed handpiece that operates at 50,000 rpm or below because it can be used for most adjusting and polishing procedures. High-speed, air-driven handpieces capable of operating at speeds greater than 50,000 rpm are useful when performing fine detail work such as sculpturing porcelain occlusal surfaces or refining primary and secondary anatomy. Yet they also have the ability to generate and transfer potentially damaging heat to the ceramic buildup, create internal stresses, and produce microcracks in the fired porcelain. Heat production can be minimized by making adjustments with light and intermittent pressure and not holding an abrasive in one location for a prolonged period of time.

Instruments

The principal instruments needed for any adjusting procedures are gauges that measure the length, width, or thickness of a given tooth or restoration. Measurement gauges permit accurate evaluation and adjustment of different dimensions of a restoration and decrease the amount of time required for contouring. For gross measurements (ie, those greater than 1.0 mm), use a metal caliper such as a Boley gauge. For a finer scale, an Iwanson metal caliper (Pfingst) is recommended to determine the thickness of metal or metal and porcelain to within approximately 0.1 mm (Fig 9-1).

> Measurement gauges permit accurate evaluation and adjustment of different dimensions of a restoration and decrease the amount of time required for contouring.

Materials

A wide selection of instruments and materials for adjusting, contouring, finishing, and polishing should become standard items in every ceramist's armamentarium

Abrasives

For the initial gross reduction, use either a diamond or a stone specifically designed for porcelain adjustment. These instruments are intended for use at slow to medium speeds and come in a variety of sizes and shapes. Care should be taken when using very coarse abrasives because they have the potential to chip and crack fired porcelain. Diamond abrasives also come in many different shapes and grits for use at all levels of finishing, from gross reduction to final contouring (Fig 9-2). Finer abrasives (eg, white stones) can be purchased separately if not found in porcelain adjustment kits (Fig 9-3). Diamond-impregnated wheels are highly recommended for performing a variety of tasks from gross contouring of ceramic and metal surfaces to final polishing (Fig 9-4). The choice of abrasives for creating surface texture depends on the type of characterization of each individual restoration. Some cases require a surface texture that is best re-created with a coarse diamond; others call for an extremely smooth and glossy finish best established with porcelain prepolishing wheels followed by mechanical polishing with a polishing agent. In the case of metal-ceramic crowns with porcelain margins, delicate ceramic margins can best be finished with diamond prepolishing wheels under light, intermittent pressure. Experience has shown that even the finest stone or sandpaper disks are capable of fracturing a delicate porcelain margin.

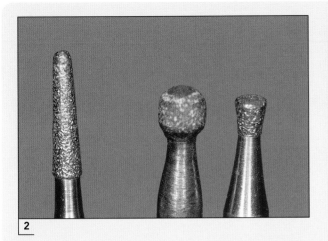

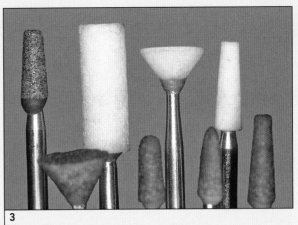

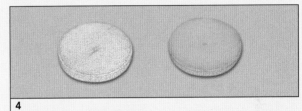

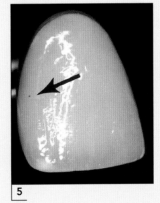

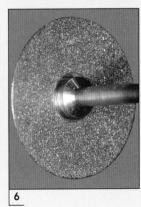

Fig 9-2 Diamond abrasive instruments are available in a variety of shapes, sizes, and grits, making them useful for all phases of adjusting and finishing.

Fig 9-3 Ceramic stones also come in different shapes, sizes, and grits for use on metal or porcelain.

Fig 9-4 Polishing wheels (Cerami-Pro Universal Polishers, Brasseler). The porcelain prepolisher wheel *(left)* is gray and may look similar to a coarse stone wheel. It is designed for adjusting ceramic surfaces without leaving a rough surface. The final polisher wheel *(right)* is diamond impregnated and has a distinctive pink color. It is excellent for creating a smooth porcelain surface. Both wheels are available in round and knife-edge designs.

Fig 9-5 Glazed porcelain surface contaminated with metal debris *(arrow)* appearing as a dark speck.

Fig 9-6 A diamond disk (Horico, Pfingst) is recommended for adjusting and contouring interproximal areas.

Regardless of the composition and shape of the stones used on ceramic materials, they should be clean and dedicated for use only with porcelain, never used interchangeably for finishing metal. Dedicating abrasive instruments to either metal or porcelain avoids the possibility of contamination. Otherwise, small particles of metal produced during metal grinding find their way into the ceramic veneer and discolor the porcelain surface or appear as black specks (Fig 9-5). Even when the stones have been used previously on acrylic resin, or any other material for that matter, residual particles may be transferred to the surface of the porcelain and become a physical contaminant in the fired restoration. Separating the porcelain finishing materials from the metal finishing and polishing materials minimizes potential sources of contamination.

Flexible diamond disks

For fixed partial dentures, diamond disks are required for shaping and contouring the interproximal areas between a pontic and its adjacent retainers (Fig 9-6). Diamond disks are available with a variety of characteristics: notched or unnotched, single-sided or double-sided diamond coating, various grit sizes, rigid or flexible, and large to small. Generally, the thinner the abrasive disk, the better: Ultra-thin disks (0.1 mm) flex and thus facilitate contouring the interproximal areas of fixed partial dentures.

Disclosing media

Many of the disclosing media mentioned in chapter 7 may be used in contouring and finishing procedures and add to the accuracy of the final restoration. To ensure that the interproximal and occlusal or incisal contacts on a restoration or cast are as close as possible to the patient's, use only the thinnest of materials. Because the restoration must be placed on its die and returned to the master cast, do not hesitate to use a disclosing medium, such as Occlude (Pascal), AccuFilm IV (Parkell), or Crown Fit Indicator (KerrLab), to verify complete seating.

Articulating film

Marking media of some sort should be included in a laboratory and clinical armamentarium. Products such as Accu-Film (Parkell) are ideal because they are thin (1/1,500 of an inch, or 3.8 μm) and available in either a single-sided or double-sided articulating film (AccuFilm I or AccuFilm II, respectively). The double-sided AccuFilm II is color-coded in three combinations: red/black, black/black, or red/red. This product is ideal for marking the occlusion and identifying the location of interproximal contacts. Avoid using actual articulating paper because paper products generally are too thick (up to 50 μm) and are prone to making false markings. Bear in mind that color-coded articulating films mark the location and size of a contact be it on the occlusal surface or in the interproximal area. They do not provide guidance on the intensity of those contacts.

Shimstock

One of the best products to use in the final check of interproximal and occlusal contacts is Artus Occlusal Registration Strips (Artus), often referred to as *shimstock* or *shim stock*. It is important to recognize that shimstock is available in a variety of dimensions, but the thicknesses reported for dental use range from 8 to 15 μm. For example, Anderson and Schulte[1] and Guichet et al[2] used 8-μm shimstock, while Boice et al[3] and Ogawa and Ogimoto[4] reported using shimstock that is 10 to 15 μm thick. Boice et al[3] adjusted proximal contact with 12.7-μm shimstock, and McDevitt and Warreth[5] reported using 13-μm shimstock when adjusting occlusion.

Shimstock can be used by both the laboratory technician and the dentist to check the fit of a restoration.[6,7] It is an excellent companion to articulating films that mark contact location because shimstock provides an indication of the relative intensity of that contact (ie, heavy, correct, light, or no contact). Furthermore, occlusal or proximal contacts located using articulating film can be verified using shimstock. However, it has been shown that even 8-μm thick shimstock cannot differentiate gaps that are between 0 and 4 μm in size.[6] In other words, articulating film indicates where to adjust, but it is shimstock's ability to hold or not hold such contacts that provides a rough approximation of how much adjustment to make, if any. Therefore, articulating film and shimstock should be used together for best results.

Laboratory vs clinical use of shimstock

Because shimstock is available in a variety of thicknesses, it is important that laboratory technicians recognize that differences in occlusion may exist if 15-μm shimstock is used in the dental laboratory and 8-μm shimstock is used by the clinician to evaluate the proximal contacts and occlusion on the patient. In other words, using the same indicating materials in the dental laboratory that are used in the mouth will ensure a more accurate restoration and reduce the insertion time for the dentist.

Anterior Single Crown with Metal Lingual Surface

Seating the casting

The first step to take before contouring a metal-ceramic restoration is to ensure that the metal substructure seats completely on the die. Even when care is taken during the porcelain application procedure, it is possible for small particles of porcelain powder to find their way inside a restoration and prevent complete seating. Therefore, inspect the intaglio surface of the work for porcelain residue. Do not rely exclusively on a gross visual examination: Use a microscope or some other form of magnification when checking the inside of the casting. Remember, particles of translucent porcelain will appear clear when fired and may not always be detectable to the naked eye. To remove any identified porcelain debris, use a small round carbide bur, diamond instrument, or ceramic stone, or airborne-particle abrade the area with 50-μm aluminum oxide. If you have a second die, coat it with a disclosing medium to expedite refitting the restoration.

After making the necessary adjustments, remove the die from the master cast and confirm the fit by gently seating the restoration on that die (Fig 9-7) before returning the die to the master cast. Do not proceed with the adjusting and

> To ensure that the interproximal and occlusal or incisal contacts on a restoration or cast are as close as possible to the patient's, use only the thinnest of materials.

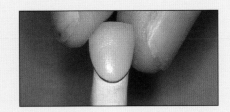

Fig 9-7 The restoration is returned to the master die to confirm complete seating and a proper fit.

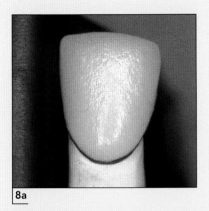

8a

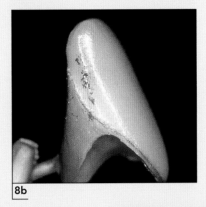

8b

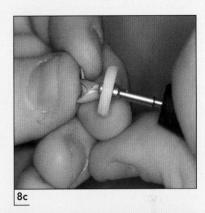

8c

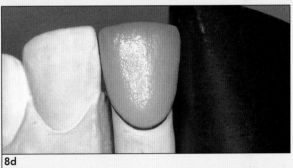

8d

Fig 9-8a Remove the die distal to the restoration, and mark the mesial interproximal contact using thin, double-sided articulating film (eg, Accu-Film II [Parkell]) or some other disclosing medium.

Fig 9-8b Remove the restoration from the master cast, and note how the marking material identifies the location and size of the contact (area in red). Use shimstock to determine if the contact is light, medium, or heavy.

Fig 9-8c Hold the restoration securely, protect the metal margins with your fingers, and make the necessary adjustments to the contact area. If gross reduction is necessary, select a coarse abrasive or use a prepolisher wheel. If only minor adjustments are required, use a final polisher wheel.

Fig 9-8d Return the distal die to the master cast. Mark and adjust the distal interproximal contact area following the same steps used for the mesial surface.

contouring without taking the time to verify the restoration's complete seating. If the interproximal and occlusal contacts are overcontoured, it is unlikely the restoration will seat completely in the patient's mouth.

Initial adjustment of the interproximal contacts

With the die in the master cast, position the restoration in its anatomically correct relationship to the adjacent teeth, if present. If complete seating cannot be achieved for any reason, do not force the restoration into place. Incomplete seating may be due to bulky interproximal contacts.

With the tooth distal to the crown removed, place a thin double-sided articulating film or one of the disclosing liquids

or sprays on the remaining interproximal areas and reseat the crown (Fig 9-8a). Remove the restoration from the cast. The double-sided articulating film should have transferred a marking to the proximal surface, indicating the location and area of any contact (Fig 9-8b). Repeat this step with shimstock to determine the intensity of that contact.

If the contact is too heavy, it may be necessary to recontour this interproximal area with a coarse abrasive. Minor adjustments are best made with a diamond-impregnated wheel because they smooth or polish the ceramic surface. Adjustments such as this are best made by holding the restoration securely in one hand (protecting the margins) and lightly removing contacts in unwanted areas marked by the articulating film (Fig 9-8c). As the contact area approaches the appropriate position and intensity, complete the initial adjustments with a diamond-impregnated final polishing wheel.

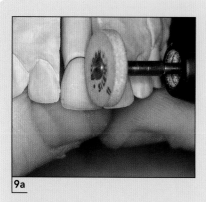
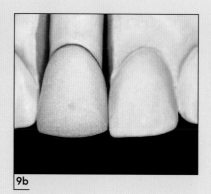
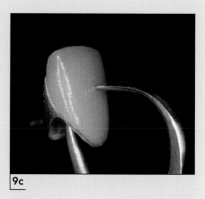

Fig 9-9a Adjust the axial contours of the facial surface using a coarse stone wheel (Busch Silent Stone, Busch) or a straight shank diamond instrument (see Fig 9-2). Use the contralateral tooth, the maxillary left central incisor, as a guide for outline form, contour, and surface texture (if it can be determined from the gypsum cast).

Fig 9-9b Once the initial (gross) reduction of the first body bake is completed, examine the restoration for areas in need of correction. In this case, the mesio-incisal corner and remainder of the incisal edge need to be lengthened. These and any other changes will be made in a second, corrective body bake.

Fig 9-9c Periodically check the thickness of the restoration to ensure that it is not over- or undercontoured.

Diamond-impregnated wheels make the necessary correction and leave behind a smooth ceramic surface as opposed to the rough surface created by ceramic stones or diamond instruments. To avoid possible overreduction, adjust one interproximal contact area at a time. After perfecting the mesial contact area, repeat the procedure on the distal contact area, first without and then with the adjacent stone teeth in place (Fig 9-8d). Use shimstock of a known thickness to confirm the amount of contact. At this stage, the goal is to ensure the proximal contacts do not prevent the work's complete seating.

If for any reason you find that a correction firing is required for one of the contact areas, first complete all of the finishing procedures. There may be other areas needing additions or correction, which can be incorporated in a subsequent bake.

Initial contouring of the facial surface

After the restoration has been seated on the working cast, its overall shape and contour should be evaluated carefully from different angles (ie, facial, occlusal/incisal, palatal, mesial, and distal). Any over- or undercontoured areas can be identified, so they may be reduced or corrected by an additional application of porcelain in a second body bake.

Begin the contouring by adjusting the axial surfaces with a straight-shank diamond cutting instrument or a stone wheel mounted in the slow-speed handpiece (Fig 9-9a). Use the same tooth on the contralateral side of the arch as a guide for proper shape, contour, and surface texture, if it is unrestored (Fig 9-9b). For most patients, the two teeth will be mirror images of one another. In the event the mesial and distal widths are not the same, the height of contour can be adjusted to give the illusion that both teeth are equivalent in size.

Adjust the lingual concavity and incisal edge. Be sure to periodically check the measurements of the restoration using a metal caliper (Fig 9-9c). Remember, the minimum facial thickness of the restoration is between 1.3 and 1.5 mm for both metal and porcelain. Dimensions below these values may result in a less desirable esthetic outcome.

Second porcelain application and body bake

The fitting of the interproximal areas and the initial (or gross) reduction of the facial surface should be accomplished quickly. From these two adjustments alone, you should be aware of what areas of the restoration are undercontoured or deficient (see Fig 9-9b). Use this second porcelain application to correct as many deficiencies as possible with one bake (Fig 9-10). This approach will allow you to proceed to final finishing and complete the restoration with a minimal number of firings.

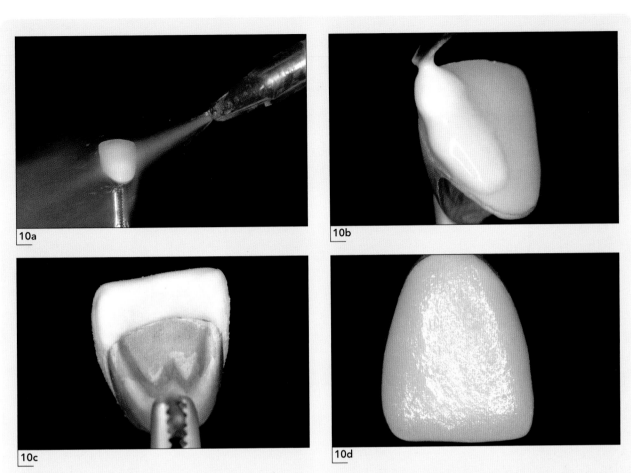

Fig 9-10a The restoration should be cleaned in preparation for the second application of porcelain. Airborne-particle abrade the porcelain-bearing surface with 50-μm aluminum oxide, and then steam clean or ultrasonically clean the crown to remove aluminum oxide or debris.[8]

Fig 9-10b Apply dentin and enamel porcelain to those areas to be corrected. Condense the porcelain well.

Fig 9-10c Examine the facial surface to ensure that the desired contour has been established. Inspect the lingual surface, the metal collar (if present), and the internal aspect of the crown. Remove excess porcelain from these areas before firing.

Fig 9-10d Adjust the porcelain firing schedule according to the porcelain manufacturer's recommendations for a second body bake. The fired porcelain should have a glossy or an "orange peel" appearance.

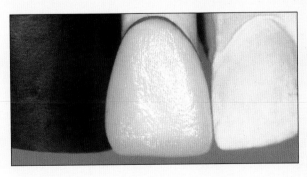

Fig 9-11 Check one interproximal area with the opposite stone teeth removed. After the mesial contact has been recontoured, finalize the distal interproximal contacts.

Perfecting interproximal contacts

Although the interproximal contact areas were already modified in the initial adjustment, the restoration has since received an additional application of porcelain. In the process of making corrections, the interproximal contact areas may have been modified. Therefore, recheck these areas to ensure complete seating and proper embrasure form on the master cast (Fig 9-11). As stated previously, another way to check the axial and occlusal contours is to

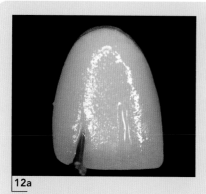
12a

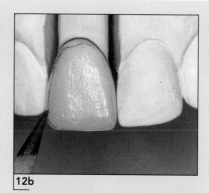
12b

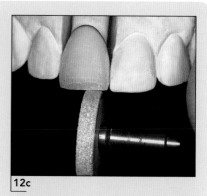
12c

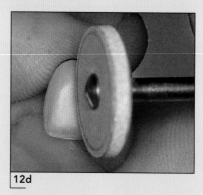
12d

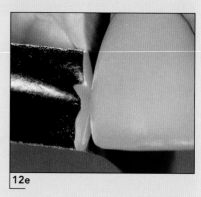
12e

Fig 9-12a As you approach the final stages of adjusting and contouring, periodically moisten the dental porcelain with distilled water. This simple step will aid your evaluation of the restoration's shape, color (shade), and level of translucency. During contouring, dry porcelain takes on a chalky appearance, and the true shade and translucency cannot be visualized and fully appreciated unless the surface is wet.

Fig 9-12b You may find it helpful to outline the final form you wish to create for the restoration. Use a pencil to mark the extent of the axial line angles on the facial surface and to identify the marginal ridges on the lingual surface.

Fig 9-12c Assess the amount of reduction needed and use either a coarse stone wheel or a porcelain prepolisher wheel to bring the facial surface to the desired final contour. Adjust the incisal edge to the proper length, shape, and angle (facial-lingual).

Fig 9-12d Smooth the facial surface of the porcelain with a diamond-impregnated prepolisher wheel (Vident Pre-Polisher Wheel shown).

Fig 9-12e After airborne-particle abrading and steam cleaning the restoration, return it to the master cast to check the contact areas with shimstock. Make any required refinements using the same procedures described previously. If a solid (uncut) cast is available, seat the restoration to evaluate the adjustments.

place the restoration on a cast that does not have removable dies. Generally, this gives you a better indication of how well the restoration will fit in the mouth. Many times the interproximal contacts are found to be too tight and need additional adjustment. This rechecking also will greatly decrease the dentist's time chairside for crown insertion. The procedure is the same as described previously (see Fig 9-9).

Final contouring of the facial surface

Adjusting procedures involve a serial polishing process that begins with a coarse instrument for contouring and shaping and ends with a fine polishing material to create a smooth surface finish (Fig 9-12). Once the axial and interproximal contouring have been completed, adjust the occlusion according to the requested occlusal scheme. There are dif-

ferent philosophies of occlusion, each with its unique requirements, so check the laboratory work authorization or call the requesting clinician for guidance on this subject.

Establishing surface texture

After the occlusion and contours have been perfected, attention can be devoted to re-creating facial anatomy and surface texture to mimic that of the adjacent natural teeth (Fig 9-13). The choice of instruments and technique to create the desired surface texture often depend on the shape and surface character desired. The cutting instruments used in this final phase may vary from coarse abrasives for very textured teeth to diamond prepolishers for teeth with a highly polished and glassy finish. More information on surface texture is presented at the end of this chapter.

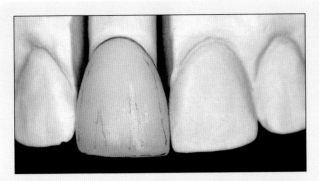

Fig 9-13a Mark the location and type of desired characterization directly on the facial surface with a pencil or other marking device. Select an abrasive with the appropriate shape and grit to create the sought-after changes.

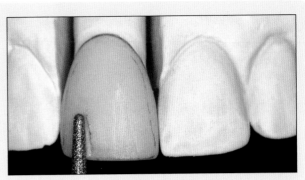

Fig 9-13b Avoid creating effects that appear abrupt and unnatural, because the crown will look more like a denture tooth than a natural tooth.

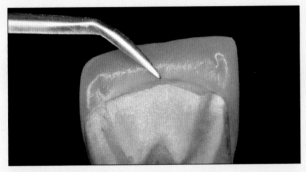

Fig 9-14a Examine the restoration for overextension of porcelain at the porcelain-metal junction. Use a fine stone, fine diamond abrasive, or prepolishing wheel to remove the porcelain without damaging the metal substructure.

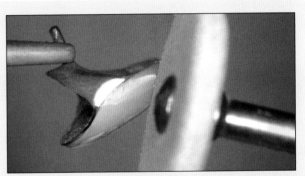

Fig 9-14b After removing a porcelain overextension, smooth the adjusted area with a prepolishing wheel because it will polish both the porcelain veneer and the metal substructure.

Once the desired texture has been created, run a diamond-impregnated wheel, fine-grit flexible diamond disk, or sandpaper disk over the facial porcelain to smooth and blend areas that appear too rough.

Finishing the porcelain-metal junction

The porcelain-metal junction of a restoration has the potential to have increased surface roughness. If this interface is not carefully finished and smoothed, it can irritate the patient's gingival tissues. Furthermore, overadjustment of the porcelain-metal junction may expose the rough layer of opaque porcelain. Once exposed, the opaque layer cannot be glazed or polished to the same level of smoothness as body porcelain. What results is a region on the occluding surface than can cause excessive wear of the opposing dentition, whether it be natural tooth structure (enamel or dentin) or restorative materials (eg, porcelain, gold, dental amalgam, or composite resin).

With the aid of some form of magnification, examine the restoration for any obvious porcelain overextensions at the porcelain-metal junction (Fig 9-14a). If overextensions exist, remove them through serial polishing, starting with a fine aluminum oxide stone, diamond instrument, or prepolishing wheel. Do not use a coarse stone wheel to remove a slight overextension; instead, select a fine ceramic stone or use a prepolisher if the overextension is accessible to this size wheel. Otherwise, you will have to repeat the finishing procedure with a series of sequential finishing points or stones of finer grit. Assuming any overextensions have been removed, use a diamond-impregnated prepolishing wheel to polish the porcelain and the metal of the porcelain-metal junction simultaneously (Fig 9-14b).

If this junction is not finished prior to glazing, porcelain overextensions will have to be removed during the final pol-

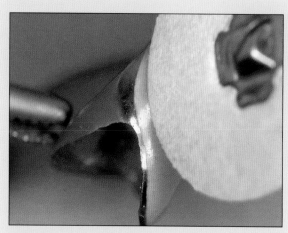

Fig 9-15 A fine-grit emery disk removes porcelain from the metal collar while smoothing both the metal and the adjacent porcelain.

ishing. The objective is to complete all adjusting and finishing before glazing. Grinding after glazing potentially can remove portions of the surface glaze and expose unglazed porcelain at the porcelain-metal junction. Unless careful porcelain polishing procedures are performed, this region will not be as smooth as the glazed porcelain itself. In addition, metal polishing compounds can contaminate these unglazed areas because particles of residual polishing agents are extremely difficult to remove (see Fig 9-5).

Finishing the labial margin

Finishing the labial margin is a delicate and tedious procedure for restorations with a fine metal margin. Any marginal finishing performed on the master die can abrade the gypsum and may result in a crown that fits the abraded die, but the margins may be short on the prepared tooth. It is safer to finish margins with the restoration on a second die, if available. In the case of a crown with a porcelain labial margin, it is recommended that marginal contouring be done with a diamond prepolishing wheel, preferably under magnification.

When great care is taken, it is possible to perform some of the marginal finishing procedures with the restoration held

> What we refer to simply as *color* actually is a complex science that was described by Munsell as having three dimensions: hue, value, and chroma.

securely in your fingers. Generally, a ⅝-in fine-grit emery disk works well in removing porcelain from the labial metal collar (Fig 9-15). Use caution in maintaining a proper emergence profile angle, and at the same time be careful not to damage the delicate metal margins.

Completion of the adjusting and finishing

At this point, carefully check the contouring, occlusal adjustment, and finishing at the porcelain-metal junction. The surface texture should harmonize with the adjacent teeth. If everything is in order, the restoration is ready for characterizing and glazing followed by polishing of the metal substrate.

Fundamentals of Color Science

Until you have mastered the techniques of internal color development, you will probably find that a metal-ceramic crown or fixed partial denture can be improved by surface characterization. In fact, there are instances where certain surface shade and stain modifications are responsible for a dramatic difference in the esthetics of the final restoration. Likewise, there are situations where attempts at color correction prove futile in remedying certain shade discrepancies. Knowing the difference between the two situations comes with experience as well as an understanding of color science and color correction techniques.

Very often, minor color adjustments can be achieved simply with small additions of surface stains. Too much surface staining, on the other hand, can reduce translucency by literally blocking light that would otherwise pass through areas of the porcelain. Inappropriate attempts at color correction can make a bad situation worse. Table 9-1 contains guidance on different types of modifications and how to approach making those changes.

To maximize the desired characterization or color correction for porcelain, you should understand fundamental color science, including dimensions of color and color systems, to appreciate the capabilities and limitations of color mixing. For additional information on color and esthetics, consult some of the more advanced texts.[9–19]

Table 19-1	Suggested guidelines for color modifications		
Desired change	Solution	How to do it	Secondary effects/Notes
Change a dominant yellow hue	Shift to a red/yellow (orange) hue	Add red	None
Change a dominant red/yellow (orange) hue	Shift to a yellow hue	Add yellow	None
Make a color more intense	Increase the chroma	Add the dominant hue	None
Make a color less intense	Decrease the chroma	Add the complementary color of the dominant hue	Decreases the value
Make a shade lighter	Increase the value	Add a stain of a higher value	Not recommended (remove the porcelain and start over)
Make a shade darker (grayer)	Decrease the value	Add the complementary color of the dominant hue	Decreases the chroma

Three dimensions of color

What we refer to simply as *color* actually is a complex science that was described by Munsell as having three dimensions: hue, value, and chroma.[9,16,20,21] Together, these three dimensions form a color solid that, if examined in cross section, give the appearance of an irregular sphere. Thus, it is common to find discussions of color science in which the three dimensions of color (hue, value, and chroma) are depicted as a wheel (Fig 9-16).

Hue

Hue is the dimension of color that enables you to distinguish one family of color from another. For example, green and red represent two different color families, so they are different hues. In the Munsell color ordering system,[20] hue makes up the rim of the color wheel. Think of *hue* as synonymous with the word *color*.[9]

Value

The second dimension of color, value, is independent of hue[16] and describes relative differences in whiteness or blackness. Value has a scale ranging from 0 (pure black) to 10 (pure white) in which the higher the number the greater the amount of reflected light and, thus, the higher the value.[9] A restoration with low value would be dark, while a crown with high value would appear bright by comparison. In other words, value can be used to describe a restoration in terms of its brightness, lightness, or brilliance. On the color wheel, value comprises the hub of the wheel.[9] By some accounts, value is the most important of the three dimensions of color.[23] The human eye is far more capable of detecting value differences than distinguishing subtle differences in hue or chroma. A simple clinical technique to discern value

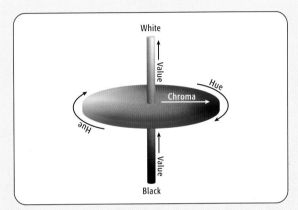

Fig 9-16 On the color wheel, hue makes up the wheel's rim, value serves as the hub, and chroma forms the spokes.

differences is to squint and take repeated, brief glimpses of the work being evaluated.

Chroma

The third dimension of color is chroma, which refers to what has been described as the relative concentration or strength,[16] saturation,[23] or intensity of a hue.[9,22] The more intense a color, the higher is its chroma level. In practical terms, *intensity* refers to the amount of light reflected back to the viewer.[9] Therefore, what is perceived as greater intensity actually means more wavelengths of that particular color emanate from the object and are perceptible. For example, when comparing two items, one navy blue and the other powder blue, the darker navy blue object has a higher blue chroma level. In color science, this means more reflected wavelengths in the blue range are seen by the viewer thus the object appears "blue." In the Munsell color ordering system,[20] chroma makes up the spokes of the color wheel.

181

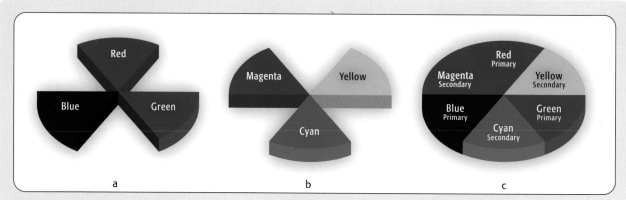

Fig 9-17 Color wheel of the additive color system with its primary colors *(a)*, its secondary colors *(b)*, and its combined color wheel *(c)*.

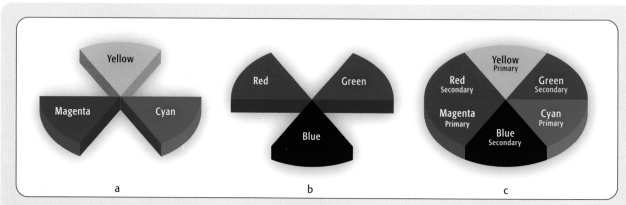

Fig 9-18 Color wheel of the subtractive color system with its primary colors *(a)*, its secondary colors *(b)*, and its combined color wheel *(c)*.

Color systems

Additive color-mixing system

When white light passes through a glass prism, the prism separates the light into individual colors of the visible light spectrum (ie, violet, blue, green, yellow, orange, and red). Looking very closely, the viewer would note three large color bands: blue, green, and red. These are the three primary colors, and because they are part of the visible light spectrum, they may more correctly be defined as the three additive primary colors (Fig 9-17a). Combining any two of the illuminant primary colors in the additive system produces a secondary color. For example, mixing red and green light produces the secondary color yellow. Combining green and blue yields cyan, and adding blue to red produces a magenta-colored light. These are all additive secondary colors (Fig 9-17b). When the primary and secondary colors are combined, they form a color wheel (Fig 9-17c).

It is important to note that the additive color system, also known as the *light-mixture color system*, only describes the color mixing of lights or illuminants and does not apply to the mixing of pigments.[16,22]

Subtractive color-mixing system

Combining paints or pigments describes the subtractive color system and is also known as the *pigment-mixture color system*. The subtractive color system is most helpful in explaining the effects obtained with extrinsic staining. Understanding the subtractive color system is easy because it is the direct opposite of the additive color system. In other words, the three primary colors of the subtractive color system (yellow, cyan, and magenta) are the secondary colors for the additive system (Fig 9-18a). The secondary colors of the subtractive color system (red, green, and blue) are the primary colors of the additive system (Fig 9-18b). The primary and secondary colors of the subtractive color system also combine to form a color wheel (Fig 9-18c). The pure subtractive color system is applicable if the pigments that are added permit light to pass through them.[16]

Partitive color-mixing system

Because dental porcelain colorants are opaque to some degree and can block light transmission, some color experts adhere to a third concept of color mixing—the partitive color system.[16,24] In the partitive color system, colors are separated into very small particles, and those color particles are remixed.[24] When color phenomena do not follow either the additive or the subtractive color mixing systems, the partitive system may be involved.[24] Owing to the complexity of the theory behind this third color system, it will not be discussed, but readers should be aware of its existence.

Complementary colors

Colors directly opposite one another on a color wheel are referred to as *complementary colors*. To locate a complementary color, draw an imaginary line from one color through the center of the color wheel, and it will pass through its complementary color. In the additive color system, the primary color red is the complement of the secondary color cyan. Green is the complement of magenta, and blue is the complement of yellow (see Fig 9-17c). Mixing any two complementary colors in the additive color system produces white light.

With the subtractive color system, colors opposite one another on the color wheel are also complementary colors, but when mixed together they produce black. The three possible combinations of complementary colors in the subtractive color system include yellow and blue, cyan and red, and magenta and green (see Fig 9-18c).

Color Correction of Dental Porcelain: Characterization

One of the first steps in color correction is to determine if the hue, chroma, or value of the restoration needs to be modified in any way (see Table 9-1). If only minor shade alterations or characterization of the porcelain are necessary, such adjustments generally can be accomplished by firing stains on the external surface of the restoration. Surface characterizing can be performed before or simultaneously with glazing. Therefore, the procedures commonly referred to as *staining* and *glazing* are discussed jointly because they are so intimately linked.

Definitions

Characterizing porcelain is a common adjunctive step to achieve minor color corrections, create unique features such as white opacifications, highlight pits and grooves, and add subtle color to the gingival and interproximal areas in otherwise high-value restorations. These color modifications can be achieved rather easily with surface stains. Although the process is often referred to as *staining*, some clinicians prefer to describe the procedure as a *characterization* of the final restoration when describing it to patients. Because patients have the perception that their metal-ceramic restoration will re-create an unrestored tooth, use of the word *staining* may take on a negative connotation.

The natural luster or sheen that must be developed for a lifelike restoration is achieved through glazing procedures and can be augmented with a mechanical polish. The two glazing methods involve a natural glaze and an overglaze.[25] Dental literature may contain references to the former terms *self-glaze*[12,13,19] (instead of natural glaze) or *applied glaze*[26] (instead of overglaze). Every ceramist should become familiar with these terms and their synonyms to appreciate which of the techniques is being discussed.

Natural glaze is a process in which the restoration is fired to a temperature that is usually equal to or slightly higher than the original firing temperature. This allows the surface to vitrify and take on a glassy appearance. Therefore, the formation of a glazed outer porcelain surface is created by heating porcelain in atmosphere without the application of any fluxes or glasses. Very often the high temperature setting for a natural glaze is above that used for an overglaze (see appendix A). Careful attention should be paid to using both the correct high temperature setting and hold time to avoid unwanted pyroplastic flow and deformation.

An overglaze involves the application of an artificial, low-fusing porcelain (fluxed glass) to the ceramic surface followed by sintering in atmosphere at a temperature that generally is 20°C to 60°C below that of the previous firing (see appendix A). This overglaze is basically a thin layer of clear porcelain that can artificially create a high sheen on the restoration. Surface stains may be applied and fired separately from an overglaze or, what is perhaps more common, fired in conjunction with sintering of an overglaze.

Although the methods of achieving a surface glaze may differ, the stains used for both glazing techniques are the same.

> If only minor shade alterations or characterization of the porcelain are necessary, such adjustments generally can be accomplished by firing stains on the external surface of the restoration.

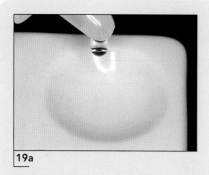 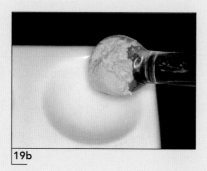 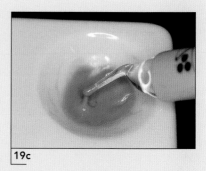

19a
19b
19c

Fig 9-19a To mix the stain powder with the liquid medium properly, place one or two drops of the liquid in a reservoir in a stain tray.

Fig 9-19b Using a metal spatula or glass mixing rod, slowly add the stain powder to the liquid and not vice versa. Thoroughly mix the two together with a small glass or plastic (nonmetallic) mixing instrument. Do

not use a brush when mixing stains (or porcelains for that matter) because the bristles contain air that can introduce bubbles into the mix.

Fig 9-19c Use the tip of a glass rod to test if the stain has been mixed to a thick, creamy consistency.

Materials

Porcelain surface stains consist of metallic oxides of varying hues in a vehicle of clear, low-fusing dental porcelain. The oxide pigments incorporated in the various stains are color stable at high temperatures. Consequently, what you see in the unfired state generally is comparable to, but not always exactly like, the appearance of the restoration after it has been fired.

Manufacturers and distributors of dental porcelain systems typically market the porcelain stain kit as a separate item. Fortunately, it is not always necessary to limit your use of specific stains to those accompanying a particular brand of dental porcelain. Stains are applied in such small amounts that usually they can be interchanged among brands of metal-ceramic porcelain. However, it is wise to use an entire ceramic system (ie, body porcelains, modifiers, and stains) from the same manufacturer.

The porcelain stains in a typical kit often are provided as a powder and accompanied by a bottle containing a slightly viscous fluid or stain medium.

> Using a metal spatula or glass mixing rod, slowly add the stain powder to the liquid and not vice versa.

Mixing stains

Invariably, the stain medium is nothing more than a mixture of glycerin and water (Fig 9-19a). This special liquid has the advantage of being slow to evaporate, which means the mixed stains do not dry out readily and can be stored long-term. However, mixed stains are best kept in a special tray

with an air-tight lid or, at least, a cover to protect them from contamination by laboratory dust and other debris.

If the mixed stains are too dilute, they tend to run when applied and lack intensity when fired. As a general rule, stains should be mixed thick but applied thin (Figs 9-19b and 9-19c). The liquid medium allows for even distribution of the stains once they have been applied to the prepared porcelain surface. When a large ceramic tray is used, you can prepare a palette of many different stains that allows mixing, blending, and diluting a variety of colors. A few manufacturers offer premixed stains that do not require mixing or wetting before use.

Characterizing technique

Regardless of whether you use conventional stain powder or premixed stains, the procedure for applying and firing those stains is the same. At this point, it is presumed that the restoration has been properly cleaned (ie, airborne-particle abraded and steam cleaned). So the first step in the characterizing procedure is to wet the porcelain surface with the clear stain medium. Apply only a thin, uniform layer. Moistening the ceramic surface also helps you to visualize what the crown will look like once it is glazed. In addition, this step makes it easier to apply the stains. Be careful to avoid using too much stain medium because it can cause the stains to run and pool (Fig 9-20).

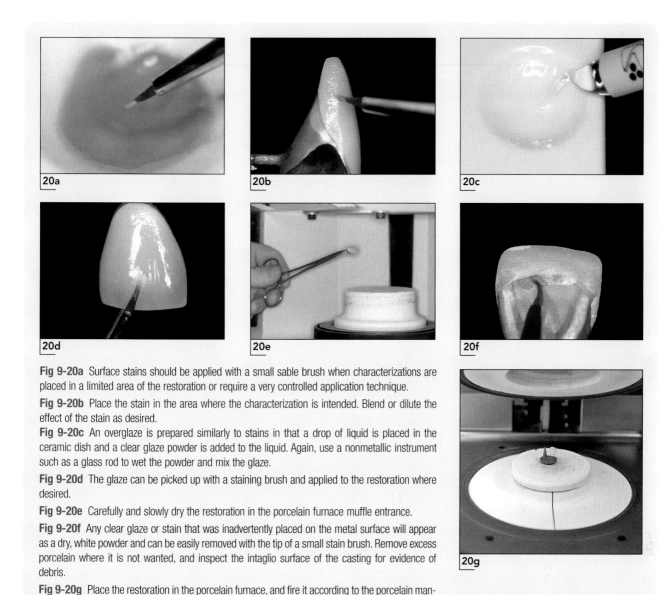

Fig 9-20a Surface stains should be applied with a small sable brush when characterizations are placed in a limited area of the restoration or require a very controlled application technique.

Fig 9-20b Place the stain in the area where the characterization is intended. Blend or dilute the effect of the stain as desired.

Fig 9-20c An overglaze is prepared similarly to stains in that a drop of liquid is placed in the ceramic dish and a clear glaze powder is added to the liquid. Again, use a nonmetallic instrument such as a glass rod to wet the powder and mix the glaze.

Fig 9-20d The glaze can be picked up with a staining brush and applied to the restoration where desired.

Fig 9-20e Carefully and slowly dry the restoration in the porcelain furnace muffle entrance.

Fig 9-20f Any clear glaze or stain that was inadvertently placed on the metal surface will appear as a dry, white powder and can be easily removed with the tip of a small stain brush. Remove excess porcelain where it is not wanted, and inspect the intaglio surface of the casting for evidence of debris.

Fig 9-20g Place the restoration in the porcelain furnace, and fire it according to the porcelain manufacturer's directions for time and temperature.

Natural glaze technique

For a natural glaze, the work is fired again after the stains are applied according to the porcelain manufacturer's instructions for the natural glaze technique (see appendix A). Use a porcelain firing program that slowly inserts the restoration into the furnace to the manufacturer's recommended natural glazing temperature. Once at temperature, the crown is either removed immediately from the porcelain furnace or

held at the recommended glazing temperature for a short period of time, usually 1 to 2 minutes, or until the outer surface of the porcelain develops the desired level of gloss.

Heating to achieve a natural glaze requires a firing cycle conducted at atmospheric pressure (ie, with no vacuum). During this firing cycle, the restoration is exposed to temperatures so high that the surface porcelain vitrifies and fuses just enough to fill in slight surface irregularities or porosities. The result is a smooth, glazed surface. Because a natural-glazed porcelain is based on a time-temperature relationship, the higher the temperature or the longer the work is held at that temperature, the smoother the surface will become. The glazing temperature and the length of the hold time varies from one brand of porcelain to another, depending on the maturation temperature and fluidity of the given dental porcelain.

If the porcelain is inadvertently raised to too high a temperature or held at the natural glazing temperature for too long a period, the porcelain can undergo pyroplastic flow, causing the restoration to lose natural contours, recrystallize, and even become opaque. These changes are particularly noticeable when sharp areas of porcelain, such as the mesial and distal corners of incisors, lose their original shape and become rounded. You may even notice regions of the porcelain that develop a white chalky appearance. These observations are more a reflection of problems with porcelains that are highly fluxed (ie, formulated to be more fluid at high temperatures).

To retain surface texture and avoid any loss of contour, the ceramist must be familiar with the manner in which each porcelain glazes at a given temperature in a specific porcelain furnace. For most dental porcelains, the ideal firing temperature produces the desired natural glaze within 2 minutes; larger work, such as long-span fixed partial dentures, may need to be held at temperature for longer periods of time.

When determining the ideal hold time, remember that it is preferable to underglaze rather than overglaze the porcelain initially. If after the first attempt the natural glaze is less than adequate, you may refire the restoration to a slightly higher maximum temperature or extend the hold time. Alternatively, you could mechanically polish the work to try to increase the level of glaze without subjecting the porcelain to another firing. However, if the glaze is excessive after the first attempt, it may require that the entire surface be recontoured and reglazed.

> The appearance of a glazed ceramic surface depends not only on the time and temperature to which the crown was fired but also on the extent of surface roughness or smoothness of that ceramic surface.

Overglaze techniques

When a restoration has been heavily characterized with external stains or a porcelain margin finish line has been selected for a case, you may not want to subject the porcelain to the high temperatures required to achieve a natural glaze. Fearing damage either to the stains or to a porcelain margin, you may wish to apply an overglaze to the ceramic veneer that is generally fired 20°C to 60°C below the firing temperature of the body porcelains. This can be achieved using two different techniques.

Technique No. 1

In the first technique, stains are applied to the ceramic surface and fired to the recommended fusion temperature after which the results are evaluated. Once the restoration has cooled, an applied glaze is placed over the stains and the work is fired again. This technique is time-consuming because it requires a second glaze firing, but it does have advantages. In fact, an applied glaze has been recommended by some authors because it slows the loss of surface characterization that results in a change in the appearance of the final restoration.

Technique No. 2

The second technique requires that the porcelain first be moistened with a clear overglaze, rather than the glaze medium used in the first technique. Stains are then applied directly to this wetted porcelain surface. The initial layer of clear glaze fills the surface pores and creates a uniformly moistened surface to accept any stain. The restoration is dried slowly in the porcelain furnace muffle entrance, as before, and heated to the recommended glazing temperature for an applied glaze.

Overglaze firing

As with natural glazing, overglazes are also air fired. Care must be taken when using such materials to prevent filling in of the surface texture that has been purposely adjusted to mimic the texture of the adjacent natural teeth. In addition, some overglazes discolor in areas where they are allowed to pool. When an acceptable glaze is finally achieved, the restoration should require only metal polishing before delivery to the patient. If the finishing procedures for the porcelain-metal junction have been accomplished properly, the final metal polishing procedure is very simple.

In all likelihood, an apprentice ceramist can achieve excellent esthetics and probably make satisfactory shade changes or color modifications when using surface stains in conjunction with an overglaze.

Evaluating the glaze and surface texture

After the restoration has been through the glazing cycle, carefully evaluate the finish to determine if the proper level of glaze and the desired amount of surface texture have been achieved. The appearance of a glazed ceramic surface

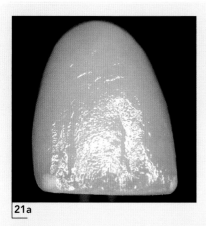 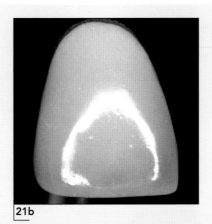 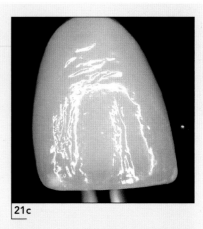

Fig 9-21a An underfired restoration typically retains much of its pebbly (orange peel) appearance with little evidence of surface changes.

Fig 9-21b An overfired crown possesses an extremely reflective, glossy surface devoid of surface characterization and shows signs of rounding of previously sharp corners.

Fig 9-21c There is no "correct" level of glaze because the amount of characterization depends on the features that must be reproduced to harmonize for each patient. However, this restoration has surface texture and the appearance of a more typical glaze, which lies somewhere between underglazing and overglazing.

depends not only on the time and temperature to which the crown was fired but also on the extent of surface roughness or smoothness of that surface (Fig 9-21). A medium glaze often is all that is required for a restoration to blend with surrounding unrestored teeth and look natural.[14] High glazing may look artificial, but mechanical polishing can help reduce a high sheen and smooth an otherwise rough surface.

> Polishing the metal substructure can be completed in three relatively easy steps: initial finishing, preliminary polishing, and final polishing.

The sequence of glazing and polishing procedures does make a difference. According to one laboratory study, the surface of incisal porcelain that was polished and then glazed naturally had more fine surface cracks than specimens that were only polished or only natural glazed.[27] Surface cracks can adversely affect the wear characteristics of a restoration. Therefore, it may be advisable to perform porcelain polishing as a final step after a natural glaze or an overglaze has been completed.

Mechanical polishing

Despite the outward appearance of an acceptable level of glaze, a more natural, lifelike restoration is obtained by mechanically polishing the ceramic surface following the glazing procedure. It makes no difference whether the crown has a natural glaze or an overglaze; polishing can be beneficial. At the very least, minor surface irregularities that are produced by an overglaze are removed, and surface smoothness is improved.

The true value of mechanical polishing probably lies in the ability to transform a glazed ceramic surface to approximate the look of human enamel. A highly glazed metal-ceramic restoration does not always capture the luster of a natural tooth because fired surfaces can take on a glassy appearance that needs to be toned down. Although glazing is helpful in creating a smooth surface with minimal microscopic voids and irregularities, mechanical polishing enhances a restoration by creating a more natural-looking luster.

With the flour of pumice and Brasso (Reckitt Benckiser) technique of mechanical polishing, it is important to apply the polishing paste liberally over the ceramic surface and use light, intermittent pressure to minimize heat production (Fig 9-22). Care should be taken when using Brasso with pumice or commercial polishing pastes because mechanical polishing can remove surface stains not well protected by a clear glaze.

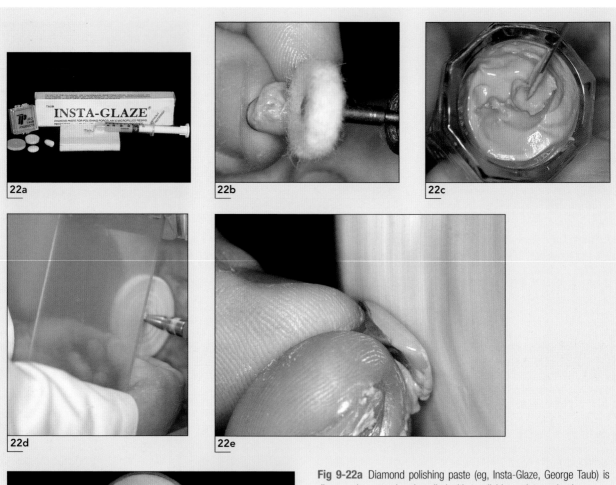

22a 22b 22c

22d 22e

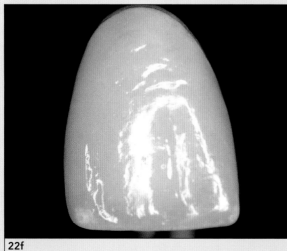

22f

Fig 9-22a Diamond polishing paste (eg, Insta-Glaze, George Taub) is dispensed on a pad and applied with a polishing point or wheel.

Fig 9-22b Hold the crown securely in one hand and apply intermittent pressure with the polishing wheel. Use a liberal application of diamond polishing paste to minimize heat production.

Fig 9-22c An inexpensive alternative to commercial diamond pastes is a mixture of Brasso (Reckitt Benckiser) and flour of pumice (Moyco). When combined, the two ingredients make a thick, creamy, and inexpensive polishing paste that can be stored in a resealable jar. A unit dose of the prepared paste can be placed in a dappen dish with a metal spatula for each case to avoid cross-contamination of the large container.

Fig 9-22d A large tight wet rag wheel run at high speed on a bench lathe is ideal for mechanical polishing, especially if the wheel is firm and offers resistance during polishing. Make certain the safety shield is in the correct position before operating to avoid liquid or paste spatter in the face. Apply a liberal amount of pumice and Brasso mixture to the ceramic surface.

Fig 9-22e Press the crown against the rotating wheel while protecting the crown margins at all times. Use light, intermittent pressure, and rotate the crown periodically to polish in all directions. Be sure to reapply more paste and water to prevent overheating of the porcelain.

Fig 9-22f Facial view of the crown in Fig 9-21c after mechanical polishing with flour of pumice and Brasso. Note the reduction in the glassy sheen and the natural rounding of the facial grooves. A lifelike luster is created in the ceramic, yet the surface characterization (white opacification) remains unaltered. Compare these results with Fig 9-21c (before polishing) to see the improvements from mechanical polishing.

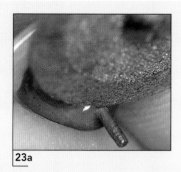
23a

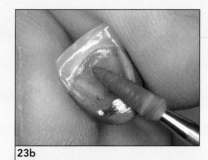
23b

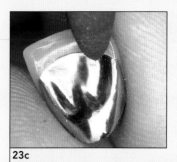
23c

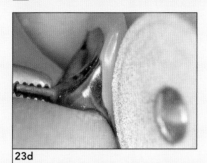
23d

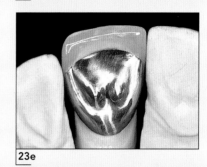
23e

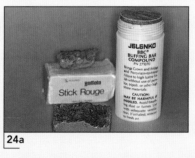
24a

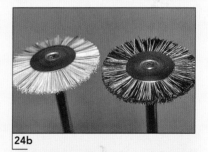
24b

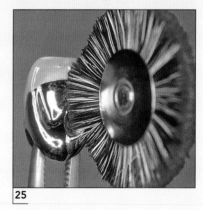
25

Fig 9-23a Cut off the metal handle using a thin carborundum disk.

Fig 9-23b Recontour the handle area with a ceramic stone. Finish the cingulum area with an appropriate abrasive until the surface is smooth and the proper contour is restored. Check the occlusion periodically to make certain the desired occlusal scheme is retained.

Fig 9-23c Use a green rubber polishing point to finish the remainder of the lingual surface, bringing the metal to a luster.

Fig 9-23d Use a porcelain prepolishing wheel to remove obvious scratches, irregularities, and oxidation from the metal's surface that appeared subsequent to the initial metal finishing. This wheel polishes both metal and porcelain at the porcelain-metal junction without marring the glazed ceramic veneer. If a more abrasive wheel is used, the surface glaze could be broken.

Fig 9-23e All metal surfaces should have a uniform, high sheen, and the glazed porcelain should remain unmarred. It is critical to finish the porcelain-metal junction prior to glazing (see chapter 7).

Fig 9-24a Polishing agents, such as tripoli compounds, rouge compounds, and Jelenko Buffing Bar Compound (Heraeus Kulzer) are needed for the polishing procedures.

Fig 9-24b Slowly rotate an appropriate brush in the polishing compound. Using light pressure and great care, polish the metal surfaces with the compound-loaded brush. Avoid bringing polishing compounds in contact with the glazed porcelain. Once the metal surface has been polished, remove residual polishing compound with a steam cleaner or ultrasonic cleaner.

Fig 9-25 With a second, soft-bristle brush, pick up a small quantity of rouge compound. Lightly polish the metal with rouge compound until the surface takes on a high luster (compare to Fig 9-23e). The labial metal collar can be mechanically polished quite adequately with fine green polishing wheels or other fine abrasives.

Polishing the Metal Substructure

Polishing the metal substructure can be completed in three relatively easy steps.

1. *Initial finishing.* The goal of this step is to remove handles, to reduce obvious surface irregularities and roughness with a ceramic stone, and to bring the metal to a high sheen with a diamond-impregnated wheel or point (Fig 9-23).

2. *Preliminary polishing.* The second step relies on polishing products (Fig 9-24) to transform the smooth metal surface left behind by the rubber wheels and points to a more highly polished state.

3. *Final polishing.* This final step creates a high shine and brings out the brilliant luster of the metal (Fig 9-25).

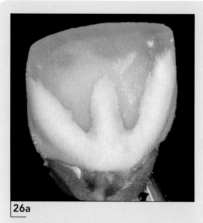

26a

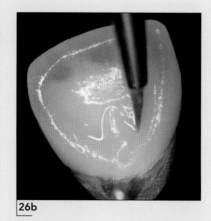

26b

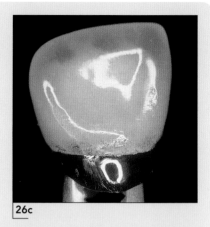

26c

Fig 9-26a Add the appropriate dentin, incisal, or translucent porcelain to those areas needing correction. The second body bake should restore adequate lingual contour and anatomy.

Fig 9-26b Recontour the restoration as necessary. Check and adjust the occlusion, then wet the porcelain with stain liquid. Characterize the facial and lingual surfaces as desired.

Fig 9-26c Overpolishing restorations with minimal metal collars can expose opaque porcelain, leave a roughened surface, and permit polishing agents to collect in surface irregularities. Unless the labial metal collar is fairly wide, be particularly careful if you use polishing compounds in that area. There is always the risk of embedding polishing compound in the porcelain surface, which can be very difficult to remove subsequently. Such contamination can result in an unacceptable appearance for the porcelain.

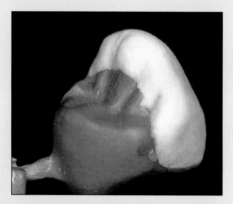

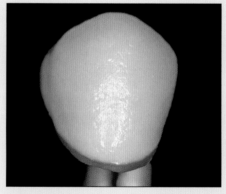

Fig 9-27a Occlusal view of crown with second porcelain application applied, condensed, and shaped to retain the desired anatomic form.

Fig 9-27b Facial view of the crown after the second body bake. The opacious dentin added across the cervical region provides a subtle blend of color through the middle and incisal thirds of the crown. The metal collar is uniform in dimension and free of excess porcelain, and there is a smooth transition from porcelain to metal. The restoration is ready to be polished using the materials and techniques described previously.

Anterior Single Crown with Porcelain Lingual Surface

This restoration is adjusted and contoured using the same materials and techniques described previously. For a cingulum that lacks sufficient form and contour, a corrective firing is needed (Fig 9-26a). In preparation for the second body buildup, airborne-particle abrade the porcelain and clean the restoration (Figs 9-26b and 9-26c).

Posterior Single Crown with Metal Occlusal Surface

After the first porcelain application, the restoration is adjusted and contoured as described previously (Fig 9-27a). Apply a second body buildup, and fire the restoration at a lower temperature (Fig 9-27b).

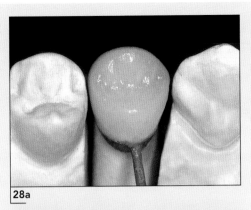
28a

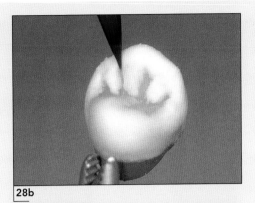
28b

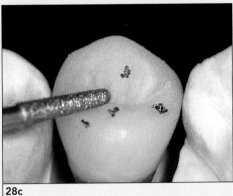
28c

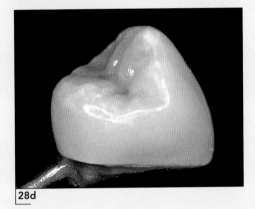
28d

Fig 9-28a Occlusal view of the restoration after the first body bake. The basic anatomic form was retained by the fired porcelain. However, the crown overbuilding (by 10% to 15%) to compensate for porcelain shrinkage may have been underestimated or the buildup was not well condensed.

Fig 9-28b Perform preliminary finishing of the porcelain contours and occlusal surface, then apply the second application of porcelain. Follow the anatomic outline established from the initial buildup.

Fig 9-28c Occlusal view of crown on the master cast after firing the second application of porcelain. Use articulating film to mark the occlusal

contacts and adjust the occlusion and contours according to the desired occlusal scheme. For redefining the anatomic detail, a set of fine diamond abrasives and a high-speed, air-driven handpiece are indispensable. Remember that the best-looking occlusal surface is of little value if all of the required occlusal contacts are removed.

Fig 9-28d Occlusal view of the characterized occlusal surface after glazing. Use of stains to highlight the occlusal pits and areas of hypocalcification (white) give a lifelike appearance to the porcelain.

Posterior Single Crown with Porcelain Occlusal Surface

Restorations with complete porcelain coverage undergo a greater amount of porcelain shrinkage than comparable restorations with a metal occlusal surface and a facial ceramic veneer (Fig 9-28a). Therefore, anticipate a second and perhaps even a third porcelain application to achieve the desired final contours, anatomic form, and occlusion.

Adjustment of the porcelain occlusal surface

Depending on porcelain building talents, the correction of a crown with a complete porcelain occlusal surface may require only slight adjustment (Figs 9-28b and 9-28c), or it may be a case of "the occlusal surface must be in there somewhere." Restorations that are overbuilt require a great deal of grinding to reveal the desired anatomy and occlusion.

Characterization

Use the same materials and techniques described previously to stain and glaze the facial, occlusal, and interproximal surfaces of this restoration (Fig 9-28d).

191

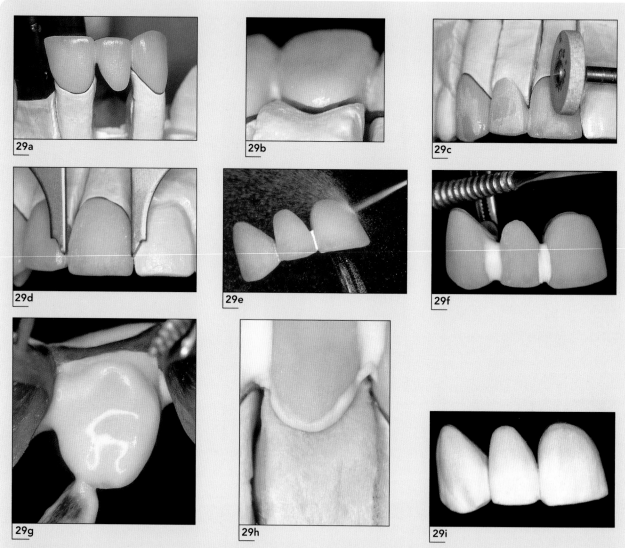

Fig 9-29a Remove the adjacent stone teeth and the pontic area, and mark and adjust one interproximal contact at a time. Adjust the opposite contact area in the same manner.

Fig 9-29b Replace the pontic area and seat the prosthesis on the master cast. Check the amount of shrinkage on the tissue side of the pontic from the facial and the lingual aspects. Porcelain shrinkage occurs in this area and requires a correction firing.

Fig 9-29c Adjust the facial contours using the natural teeth as guides. Carefully examine the prosthesis from all views (facial, palatal, incisal, mesial, and distal).

Fig 9-29d Measure the length and width of the adjacent natural tooth with a Boley gauge and compare those measurements with the adjacent porcelain restoration. Differences of as little as 0.5 mm can be visually detected as asymmetry and should be corrected.

Fig 9-29e Adjust and contour the interproximal areas using a flexible diamond disk before airborne-particle abrading the porcelain with non-recycled 50-μm aluminum oxide. Steam clean the prosthesis.

Fig 9-29f Add porcelain to the two connector areas and condense it well.

Fig 9-29g Lightly wet the tissue side of the pontic with distilled water. Apply additional porcelain as needed until the tissue side is covered completely.

Fig 9-29h Reseat the prosthesis on the master die with moist tissue paper over the pontic area, and condense the porcelain well. While the prosthesis is on the master cast, continue with the remainder of the second porcelain application.

Fig 9-29i Facial view of the completed second porcelain application. Ideally, the porcelain should be layered in such a way as to create proper embrasure spaces rather than being overbuilt and ground in.

Fixed Partial Dentures

Procedures for the adjustment of a fixed partial denture are similar to those for a single-unit restoration (Fig 9-29). However, there are areas that require additional attention. As stated previously, each retainer must first be seated on its individual die before seating of the fixed partial denture as one unit. Use a working cast with removable dies and a solid (uncut) cast to confirm final proximal contacts.

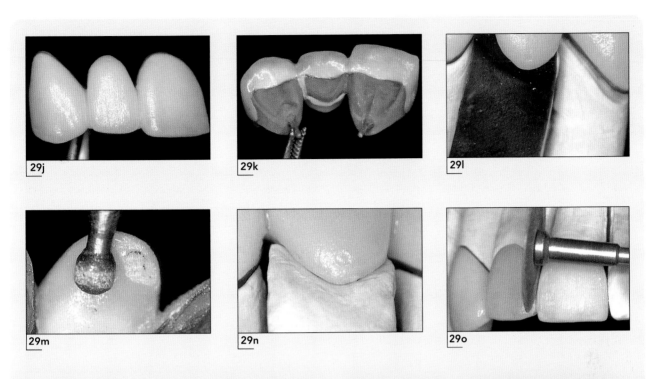

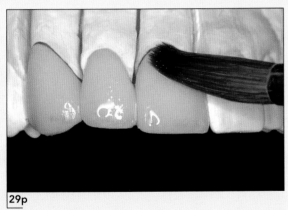

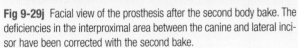

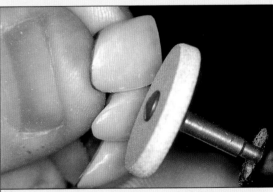

Fig 9-29j Facial view of the prosthesis after the second body bake. The deficiencies in the interproximal area between the canine and lateral incisor have been corrected with the second bake.

Fig 9-29k Lingual view of the prosthesis after the second body bake. The color difference of the soldered connector between the canine and the lateral incisor is normal.

Fig 9-29l Place articulating film underneath the pontic and mark the area of contact on the tissue side of the porcelain.

Fig 9-29m Adjust the porcelain on the tissue side to conform to the predetermined pontic design.

Fig 9-29n A modified ridge lap pontic (shown) should be well adapted to the edentulous ridge if it has been properly adjusted.

Fig 9-29o Refine the facial contours as needed. Adjust the interproximal line angles with a thin, flexible diamond disk, if necessary. Be sure to provide adequate space in the gingival embrasures for the papillae, but bear in mind that removing too much porcelain in these areas may result in large, dark triangular regions that can become apparent with a seated fixed partial denture in the dark oral cavity.

Fig 9-29p After the contouring has been completed, wet the porcelain to assess the esthetics.

Fig 9-29q Add surface texture, as needed, and go over the facial surfaces with a diamond-impregnated wheel.

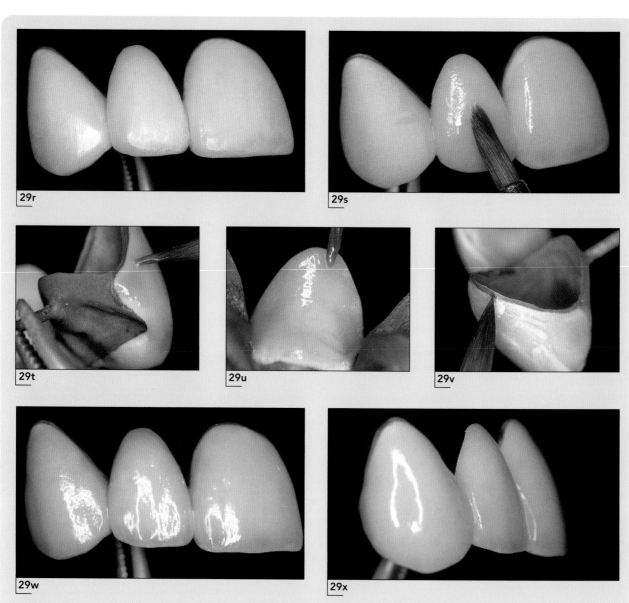

Fig 9-29r Facial view of the fixed partial denture after smoothing with a polishing wheel. Airborne-particle abrade with 50-µm aluminum oxide, and steam clean the prosthesis in preparation for characterizing and glazing. Create the desired surface roughness using preferred instruments (eg, carbide burs, diamond instruments, ceramic stones). Repeat the steam cleaning to remove surface debris.

Fig 9-29s Add a small amount of dark brown or gray stain to the connector areas to individualize the teeth. Lightly characterize the lateral and central incisors (shown).

Fig 9-29t Darken the canine more than the incisors. Add more chroma to the cervical and interproximal areas as the case requires to highlight the facial aspect of the restoration.

Fig 9-29u Continue the characterization onto the lingual surface and tissue side of the pontic. Dry the stains and overglaze at a porcelain furnace muffle entrance using the radiant heat.

Fig 9-29v Glaze and stain that have flowed onto the metal substructure are easy to identify because of their white appearance. Use a pointed brush to remove dried stain or glaze from metal surfaces.

Fig 9-29w Labial view of fixed partial denture after glazing with characterization in the cervical regions and interproximal areas.

Fig 9-29x Remember, the level of sheen and surface smoothness can be adjusted by additional mechanical polishing with a mixture of flour of pumice and Brasso. If the characterization is too pronounced, try mechanical polishing the affected areas to reduce or eliminate the amount of surface stains. If unsuccessful, remove both the stains and glaze and repeat the entire characterization process.

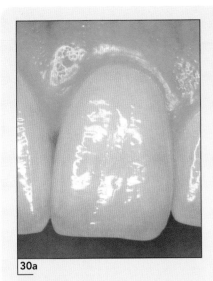
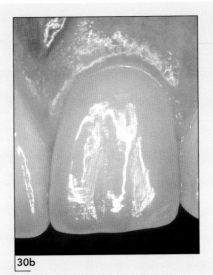
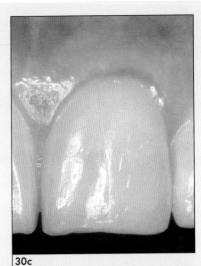
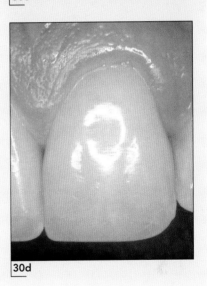

Fig 9-30a Maxillary left central incisor with a textured surface (horizontally), depressions (vertically), and an apparent groove running from the cervical to the incisal third (vertically).

Fig 9-30b Despite two vertical concavities, the more elevated areas on this maxillary central incisor are relatively smooth with a moderate gloss.

Fig 9-30c Maxillary left central incisor with surface irregularities, a prominent depression, and a low gloss.

Fig 9-30d Maxillary left central incisor with a relatively smooth surface and low gloss. Note the differences between the mesial- and distal-incisal line angles.

Reproducing Variations of Natural Teeth

The natural variability of teeth must be captured whether fabricating one or two teeth or an entire quadrant, arch, or dentition. Digital photographs greatly aid in the transmission of information other than shade alone and can be provided to support cases that pose esthetic challenges. Adolfi[28] has written one of the most outstanding textbooks devoted to a photographic depiction of teeth, particularly maxillary anterior teeth. The large, vivid photographs capture the characteristics found in teeth for patients of various ages. Differences in outline form, surface texture, and gloss are showcased throughout the book.

However, there are limitations to relying on a single view; it is highly recommended that ceramists request images from several angles.

The maxillary central incisors presented in Fig 9-30 vary substantially in appearance. Carefully examine each photograph to determine their similarities and differences. Note that natural teeth are not monochromatic but contain gradations of color. Study interproximal and cervical shading, and look for subtle gradations in color. Even a small amount of surface characterization in the interproximal embrasures and the area of the restoration at and just above the free gingival margin individualizes teeth and avoids the appearance of blocks of porcelain. This is true even for light, high-value restorations.

A metal-ceramic restoration should blend in with its given environment. Ceramists assess their ability to reproduce the natural esthetics by analyzing cases using a standardized, systematic approach. For optimum esthetics, a ceramist should evaluate any restoration in terms of outline form, surface texture, and level of glaze. Apprentice ceramists should challenge themselves and their ability to see differences using these three characteristics (Figs 9-30 to 9-32).

Outline form

The lateral incisors in Fig 9-31 vary substantially in overall appearance. Compare their outline form using the following criteria:

- Length
- Width
- Taper
- Incisal edge contour
- Incisal line angle sharpness/roundness

Note similarities and differences in outline form between maxillary incisors and canines (see Figs 9-30 to 9-32). As an exercise, transfer your interpretation of their outline form to a piece of paper, and then compare it to the actual photographs.

Surface texture

Differences in age and wear often mean that tooth surfaces vary widely in terms of surface texture. For example, when studying the appearance of lateral incisors, the enamel surface in Fig 9-31c looks rough and irregular whereas the surface texture in Fig 9-31d is smooth along the entire facial plane. Similar differences are apparent in the canines shown in Fig 9-32a and 9-32b. Look for similarities and differences in surface texture (see Figs 9-30 to 9-32). Continue this exercise by drawing the outline form of the two canines and adding your interpretation of the level and type of surface texture.

Level of glaze

To complete the evaluation, assess the level of glaze (sheen or gloss) of each of the lateral incisors in Fig 9-31 as well as the canines in Fig 9-32. If a final glaze comparable to the image in Fig 9-32b is produced for a tooth next to Fig 9-31d, the restoration will be too noticeable. The converse is also true. A low, dull glaze (see Fig 9-32d) would be unacceptable next to the canines in Fig 9-32a and 9-32b but would likely fit in well adjacent to the canine in Fig 9-32c. Again, look for similarities and differences in the level of glaze (see Figs 9-31 and 9-32). Complete the exercise by deciding what level of gloss you would wish as an outcome from glazing.

Porcelain Corrections

After completing the final adjusting and contouring of a crown (or fixed partial denture), it is not uncommon to find areas of the restoration that could benefit from minor corrections. In general, porcelain refinements can be addressed in three ways: *(1)* correct the problem before glazing the porcelain, *(2)* make the correction as part of the glazing procedure, or *(3)* glaze the restoration and correct the problem after the glazing has been completed. Correcting discrepancies as part of the characterizing and glazing process can be done, but it requires experience to be predictable. The apprentice ceramist may find it more practical to make corrections before the glazing procedure, but minor refinements are possible after glazing has been performed.

Corrections before glazing

During the contouring, adjusting, and finishing procedures, you may see areas of the restoration that could benefit from an additional porcelain firing. For example, there may be inadequate interproximal contact, the occlusion may no longer hold shimstock properly, or there may be an area of porosity. This is why it is best to wait until the final adjustments have been made, so you can remedy all the deficiencies with a correction bake before glazing. Then when the characterizing and glazing are performed, you can focus on those activities alone. Most porcelain kits contain a low-fusing, add-on porcelain. Prepare a 50:50 mix of add-on porcelain and enamel or dentin powder in the correct shade. Apply this add-on porcelain mixture in the normal manner, but take time to condense the porcelain properly. Poor condensing will result in excessive shrinkage and porosity. Then fire the porcelain according to the manufacturer's directions for a third firing. Usually this add-on firing is approximately 10°C below the temperature of the last body porcelain bisque bake. Allow the restoration to cool to room temperature; then adjust and finish the corrected areas before proceeding with the characterizing and glazing.

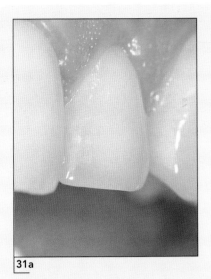

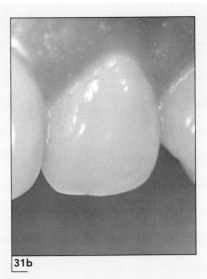

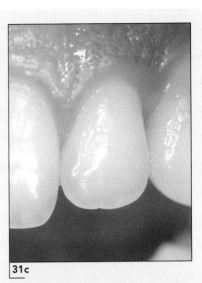

31a

31b

31c

Fig 9-31a Maxillary lateral incisor with a flat incisal edge, tapered cervical region, rounded distal-incisal line angle, and sharper mesial-incisal line angle. However, surface texture and level of glaze cannot be determined from this angle; photographs from different perspectives are needed.

Fig 9-31b This lateral incisor also has a tapered cervical region, but the tooth is short with rounded incisal line angles at both the mesial and distal. The tooth appears relatively smooth with a medium gloss.

Fig 9-31c Unlike Figs 9-31a and 9-31b, this lateral incisor with a tapered cervical region has different line angles, and the facial surface is slightly mottled with a medium gloss.

Fig 9-31d Lateral incisor with a cervical taper, rounded incisal line angles, and a smooth surface with a dull finish.

Fig 9-32a Maxillary left canine with an incisal edge that ends in a sharp point and a gentle cervical curve rather than an abrupt taper. The enamel is generally mottled (to match the adjacent teeth) with a high luster on the elevated surfaces.

Fig 9-32b Maxillary canine with uniformly smooth enamel with a subtle, natural luster. The cervical area is more tapered and the incisal edge is more worn than the canine in Fig 9-32a.

Fig 9-32c Maxillary left canine with distinct smooth facial surface, a slight depression on the mesial line angle in the cervical third, and a dull surface finish. The outline form depicts more incisal edge wear than Fig 9-32a and less chroma in the cervical region than Fig 9-32b.

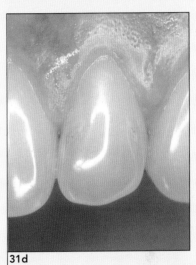

31d

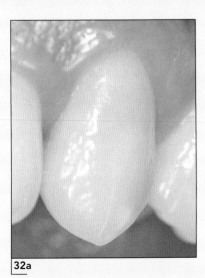

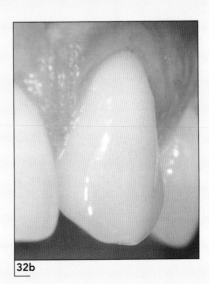

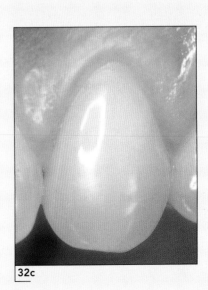

32a

32b

32c

Corrections after glazing

Minor contour corrections may be needed after the restoration has been stained or glazed. Airborne-particle abrading with 50-μm aluminum oxide can break the glaze, but it also may remove surface characterization and glaze. Because of this, it is best to avoid air-particle abrasion of any glazed porcelain surfaces. Instead, place a small amount of add-on porcelain on the area to be corrected, and fire it according to the recommended porcelain firing schedule for add-on bakes (see appendix A). The actual amount that the high temperature setting is reduced varies with the brand of porcelain, but expect to use a lower temperature setting than that used to stain and glaze.

Add-on porcelains are designed for situations requiring a quick fix, such as the correction of light interproximal contacts; they are not intended for large repairs. If a situation requires a major correction, it is always advisable to use the appropriate body porcelain (dentin or enamel) to restore the correct contours, even if that means removing the glaze and repeating a few steps. The quality of the restoration should not be compromised for expediency.

Capturing vitality

Over time, you can train your eye to discern the many features that constitute a natural-looking appearance and give teeth their vitality. The challenge comes in translating what your eye perceives and your brain interprets into what your hands can accomplish.

Delivery of the Completed Case

Every attempt should be made to deliver the restoration as well as the casts with the removable dies in the best possible condition. With some alloys, oxidation may build up inside the casting; this oxide layer should be removed before the restoration is delivered or cemented. Carefully airborne-particle abrade the casting with 50-μm aluminum oxide again, taking precautions to protect the marginal areas and glazed porcelain. It is also important to eliminate all polishing compounds from the restoration via steam or ultrasonic cleaning.

Hopefully, the master cast with removable dies has come through this ordeal without too much damage. If necessary, the master cast may also be steam cleaned to remove residual polishing debris. Steam cleaning has the potential to damage gypsum casts, so be careful.

Once the cleaning is complete, perform customary infection control procedures before returning the case. To prevent damage to the dies and restorations during shipping, remove them from the cast and store them in separate, cushioned containers.

Summary

This chapter completes your introduction to the basic metal-ceramic restoration. You have been given an overview of the procedures and techniques involved in the adjusting, finishing, and characterizing of both single-unit restorations and fixed partial dentures. Armed with this basic understanding, you can now combine this knowledge with your skills to fabricate single-unit metal-ceramic crowns and fixed-partial dentures.

References

1. Anderson GC, Schulte JK, Aeppli DM. Reliability of the evaluation of occlusal contacts in the intercuspal position. J Prosthet Dent 1993;70:320–323.
   Reliable clinical evaluation of occlusal contacts is accomplished with 8-μm shimstock.

2. Guichet DL, Yoshinobu D, Caputo AA. Effect of splinting and interproximal contact tightness on load transfer by implant restorations. J Prosthet Dent 2002;87:528–535.
   Ideal interproximal contacts are established with nonsplinted implant-supported restorations using 8-μm tin foil shimstock.

3. Boice PA, Niles SM, Dubois LM. Evaluation of proximal contacts with shim stock. J Oral Rehabil 1987;14:91–94.
   Shimstock at 0.0005-in (12.7-μm) thickness is passed through proximal contacts without tearing.

4. Ogawa T, Ogimoto T, Koyano K. Pattern of occlusal contacts in lateral positions: Canine protection and group function validity in classifying guidance patterns. J Prosthet Dent 1998;80:67–74.
   Authors record occlusal contacts with shimstock that is 10 to 15 μm in thickness.

5. McDevitt WE, Warreth AA. Occlusal contacts in maximum intercuspation in normal dentitions. J Oral Rehabil 1997;24:725–734.
   Occlusal contacts are checked with 13-μm-thick shimstock.

6. Harper KA, Setchell DJ. The use of shimstock to assess occlusal contacts: A laboratory study. Int J Prosthodont 2002;15:347–352.
   Shimstock that is 8- to 13-μm thick is thinner than articulating paper and can help to detect occlusal discrepancies in the 8- to 10-μm range.

7. Wassell RW, Barker D, Steele JG. Crowns and other extra-coronal restorations: Try-in and cementation of crowns. Brit Dent J 2002; 193(1):17–20, 23–28.
   The occlusion of restorations is evaluated clinically using 10-μm shimstock.

8. Winings JR. Using aluminous oxide abrasives in porcelain-bonded-to-metal fabrication. J Prosthet Dent 1981;46(3):345–347.
   Refer to chapter 5 for summary.

9. Chu SJ, Devigus A, Mieleszko A. Fundamentals of Color: Shade matching and Communication in Esthetic Dentistry. Chicago: Quintessence, 2004.

10. Hegenbarth EA. Creative Ceramic Color: A Practical System. Chicago: Quintessence, 1989.
    Hegenbarth emphasizes the re-creation of natural color and esthetics using restorations ranging from simple to complex.

11. Korson D. Natural Ceramics. Chicago: Quintessence, 1990.
    Proper tooth shaping, shade selection, communication, lighting, and tooth characterization are presented.

12. McLean JW. The Science and Art of Dental Ceramics. Vol I: The nature of dental ceramics and their clinical use. Chicago: Quintessence, 1979.
    Refer to chapter 2 for summary.

13. McLean JW. The Science and Art of Dental Ceramics. Vol II: Bridge design and laboratory procedures in dental ceramics. Chicago: Quintessence, 1980.
    Refer to chapter 2 for summary.

14. Muia PJ. The Four Dimensional Tooth Color System. Chicago: Quintessence, 1982.
    Muia discusses hue, value, and chroma. A fourth dimension of color—maverick—is added that can overpower hue and chroma. A medium glaze is recommended; a high glaze is to be avoided.

15. Müterthies K. Esthetic Approach to Metal Ceramic Restorations for Mandibular Anterior Region. Chicago: Quintessence, 1990.
    Refer to chapter 8 for summary.

16. Preston JD, Bergen SF. Color Science and Dental Art. St Louis: Mosby, 1980.

17. Rinn LA. The Polychromatic Layering Technique: A Practical Manual for Ceramics and Acrylic Resins. Chicago: Quintessence, 1990.

18. Ubassy G. Shape and Color: The Key to Successful Ceramic Restorations. Chicago: Quintessence, 1993.

19. Yamamoto M. Metal-Ceramics: Principles and Methods of Makoto Yamamoto. Chicago: Quintessence, 1985:401.
    Author contends that a "self-glazed" surface has irregularities and is not a smooth surface microscopically.

20. Munsell AH. A Color Notation. Baltimore: Munsell Color, 1936.

21. Sproull RC. Color matching in dentistry. I. The three-dimensional nature of color. J Prosthet Dent 1973;29:416–424.
    Sproull reviews "the color language and the necessary tools to approach color matching problems" logically.

22. Preston J. The elements of esthetics-application of color science. In: McLean JW (ed). Dental Ceramics. Proceeding of the First International Symposium on Ceramics. Chicago: Quintessence, 1983:491–520.

23. Dykema RW, Goodacre CJ, Phillips RW. Johnston's Modern Practice in Fixed Prosthodontics, ed 4. Philadelphia: Saunders, 1986: 330–340.
    Authors note that value is the most critical component when comparing a restoration to a tooth.

24. McPhee ER. Extrinsic coloration of ceramometal restorations. Dent Clin North Am 1985;29:645–666.
    McPhee discusses three color systems: additive, subtractive, and partitive.

25. The glossary of prosthodontic terms. J Prosthet Dent 2005;94: 10–92.

26. Kuwata M. Theory and Practice for Ceramo Metal Restorations. Chicago: Quintessence, 1980.

27. Edge MJ, Wagner WC. Surface cracking identified in polished and self-glazed dental porcelain. J Prosthodont 1994;3(3):130–133.
    Fine surface cracks were found in porcelain that was first polished and then natural glazed; no surface cracks were found in specimens that were only polished or natural glazed.

28. Adolfi D. Natural Esthetics. Chicago: Quintessence, 2002.
    Color photographs depict differences in outline form, surface texture, gloss, and characterization in anterior teeth.

Glossary of Technical Terms

A

airborne-particle abrading Finishing of a metal or porcelain surface with an abrasive material (eg, aluminum oxide, glass beads, sand) under pressure. The grit size of powder abrasives used in dentistry typically range from 25 to 100 µm in diameter. *Syn: airborne-particle abrasion*.

air firing Process of sintering in a porcelain furnace without a vacuum.

alloy Substance possessing metallic properties and composed of two or more chemical elements, of which at least one is an elemental metal comprising the majority of the mixture.

aluminum oxide (Al_2O_3) Important addition to dental porcelain to increase overall strength and viscosity of the melt, yet it is only slightly soluble in low-fusing porcelain. Because aluminum oxide has a low, linear coefficient of thermal expansion ($9 \times 10^{-6}/°C$) compared to metal-ceramic alloys (13.5 to $15.5 \times 10^{-6}/°C$), glass modifiers such as potassium, sodium, and calcium oxide are added to the mix to raise the coefficient of thermal expansion of a low-fusing porcelain. *Syn: alumina*.

applied glaze —*See overglaze*.

autoglaze —*See natural glaze*.

B

base metal Element that is non-noble and has little intrinsic value (eg, chromium, copper, nickel, tin, zinc). Base metals are added to high-noble metal alloys to produce the oxide layer for porcelain bonding.

bond Attachment or union between dental porcelain and the metal substructure.

brilliance Luster or sheen of a ceramic/porcelain surface.

Brinell hardness Measure of the hardness of a material obtained via laboratory test in which a hardened steel ball is pressed into the polished surface of a material under a measured load. The amount of indentation is computed according to the load and assigned a Brinell hardness number (BHN). The smaller the indentation, the harder the material, and the higher the BHN. *Compare with Vickers hardness*.

C

cameo surface Exterior surface of a restoration.

carat (K) Unit of measure of gold. The carat of an alloy is determined by the parts of pure gold in the alloy of 24 parts. Thus, *18K gold* means that 18/24 or 75% of the alloy is gold. The term is never used to describe nongold alloys.

casting temperature Temperature, usually 100°F to 150°F above the melting or fusing range of an alloy, that compensates for heat loss during the casting procedure.

ceramometal restoration —*See metal-ceramic restoration*.

characterization Addition of surface texture, porcelain stains, and a glaze to the ceramic veneer of a metal-ceramic restoration in an effort to blend the work into the surrounding dentition. This term is preferred over *staining and glazing*.

chroma Component of color that identifies the relative intensity/saturation of a particular hue. The greater the reflection of wavelengths for a particular color, the greater the perceived chroma of that color.

color Quality with respect to reflected light, composed of three components: hue, value, and chroma.

conductivity Property of transferring thermal and electric energy, which is important to pulpal tissues. Noble alloys containing elements such as gold, silver, and copper are good thermal conductors. Base metal alloys containing nickel, chromium, and cobalt are poor thermal conductors.

coping Metal substructure of a single-unit metal-ceramic restoration.

corrosion Process in which the surface of a metal restoration deteriorates through a reaction with its environment.

crucible The container in which alloys are melted for casting. High-heat zircon-alumina or quartz crucibles are recommended for metal-ceramic alloys. Clay crucibles should be limited to Type III or IV gold alloys.

D

degassing —*See oxidation*.

delamination Porcelain bond failure where the veneering porcelain becomes separated from the metal substructure.

density Weight of a substance as compared with the weight of the same volume of water. The standard is 1 cc of water (at 4°C) is equal to a density of 1. The density of pure gold is 19 g/cm^3, whereas many of the base metal alloys have a density between 7.75 and 8.5 g/cm^3. *Syn: specific gravity.*

devitrification Return of some of the dental porcelain components to a crystalline form. This transformation is caused by repeated firing and overfiring, which can produce increased cloudiness (opacification). *Syn: recrystallization.*

discoloration Alterations in the shade on the porcelain surface formed by unwanted chemical reactions between the veneering porcelain and oxides produced by the metal substructure during a porcelain firing cycle. Usually associated with silver-containing alloys, the color changes are more typically yellow or brown rather than "green," as described in some publications.

ductility Quality of withstanding permanent deformation without rupture under a tensile (pulling) load. It is the property of a metal that permits it to be drawn into a wire without breaking. Gold and silver are very ductile; nickel and chromium are not. *Compare with malleability.*

E

elastic limit —*See modulus of elasticity.*

elongation Measure of the ductility of a metal or an alloy. *Percentage of elongation* refers to the amount an alloy will increase in length when drawn from a zero load to its breaking point. The higher the percentage, the greater the ductility; the lower the percentage, the less likely the metal margins in a cast restoration can be burnished.

etching Process by which surface metal is electrolytically or chemically removed (usually with acids) to create microscopic three-dimensional relief for micromechanical retention. A resin cementing medium is permitted to flow into the etched metal surface to provide mechanical retention of the prosthesis.

extraneous oxidation Oxidation that forms on nonporcelain areas of the metal substructure (ie, occlusal/lingual surface, metal collar).

F

feldspar Key ingredient in dental porcelains that adds translucent qualities to fired restorations. It exists in two forms: *(1)* potassium alumino-silicate (K_2O-Al_2O_3-6SiO_2), also known as *potash feldspar*, or *(2)* sodium alumino-silicate (Na_2O-Al_2O_3-6SiO_2), also known as *sodium feldspar.* Refer to chapter 2 for an expanded discussion.

feldspathic porcelain Low-fusing porcelains typically designed to veneer compatible metal-ceramic substructures.

fineness Measure of precious metal. Alloy fineness is the parts per 1,000 that are gold. Although this term may be used to describe gold-based alloys, it is generally limited to describing dental solder.

flexibility Amount of bending movement, or distortion, an alloy can withstand and still be able to return to its original shape *without* evidence of distortion. An alloy that possesses a low modulus of elasticity but a high yield strength offers great flexibility.

framework One-piece substructure composed of either several copings attached to one or more pontics or multiple single units connected as a single structure. Often used in reference to fixed partial dentures.

frit Fragments of porcelain produced by the fritting process. *See fritting.*

fritting Manufacturing process that produces dental porcelain. The minerals used to make low-fusing and medium-fusing porcelain are mixed together in a specified proportion, heated to a molten state, and held at a specified temperature for a given amount of time to allow chemical reactions to occur. The molten glass is then quenched, which results in the production of fractured pieces of feldspathic porcelain that are ground to the desired particle size for the product to be made.

G

galvanism Production of small electric currents in the mouth as a result of contact by restorations of dissimilar metals (eg, gold onlay opposing an amalgam restoration). Galvanism may cause tooth sensitivity.

gassing Release of entrapped gases from a metal substrate during a firing procedure, resulting in voids or bubbles in the opaque or body porcelains.

glaze —*See natural glaze, overglaze.*

grain 1. Microscopic component that makes up a metal. Thousands of individual grains create a polycrystalline structure and make up the metal. An alloy composed of many small similar grains is often referred to as a *microfine homogeneous metal* and exhibits better physical and mechanical properties than a macro-grain heterogeneous alloy. Manufacturing and handling of the alloy by the technician affects the grain structure. *Syn: crystal.* 2. Unit of mass. Noble alloys are frequently weighed to calculate the volume of metal used to produce a given restoration. Since 24 grains are in each pennyweight (dwt), and 20 dwt are in each troy ounce (ozt), 480 grains are in 1 ozt. In metric measurements, 1 grain equals 200 mg; 24 grains equal 1.5552 g; and 480 grains (1 ozt) equal 31.1035 g.

grain growth Formation of larger grains. Overheating an alloy, or subjecting it to prolonged heating, may permit the grains or crystals of the metal to merge, thus forming larger grains. Large-grain alloys are weaker than small or microfine grain metals. Slow cooling after casting can permit such grain growth.

gram (g) Basic unit of weight in the metric system, with 28.3495 g in each avoirdupois ounce and 31.1035 g in each troy ounce.

H

hardness Resistance of an alloy to surface penetration. As hardness increases, resistance to surface wear also increases. Values for hardness are most often reported as either a Vickers or a Brinell hardness number. *See Brinell hardness, Vickers hardness.*

high-fusing porcelain Ceramic material used to produce porcelain denture teeth.

hue Component of color that is equivalent to the word *color.*

I

intaglio surface Internal surface of a restoration.

investment (gypsum-bonded) Material consisting of a gypsum binder (alpha calcium sulfate hemihydrate) and a refractory material (silica). In general, gypsum investments should not be heated to temperatures higher than 1,292°F (700°C) for fear of investment breakdown and the increased potential for alloy contamination.

investment (phosphate-bonded) Material consisting of a phosphate binder (an ammonium phosphate compound), magnesium oxide, and a refractory material (silica). These investments are not only considerably stronger than gypsum-bonded investments but are also capable of withstanding temperatures well above 1,292°F (700°C).

K

kaolin Clay formed from igneous rock (hydrated aluminum silicate [$Al_2O_3 \cdot 2SiO_2 \cdot 2H_2O$]) that served as a binder to allow porcelain to be built and shaped (molded) in the unfired state. Mention of kaolin is made solely for historical benefit because it has long since disappeared from dental porcelain yet continues to be mentioned in dental materials textbooks. Refer to chapter 2 for expanded discussion.

L

liquidus Temperature above which an alloy is entirely molten.

liquidus range Temperature range from the time a casting alloy becomes semiliquid until it is completely molten, without overheating the metal and burning off trace elements.

low-fusing porcelain Feldspathic porcelain used in metal-ceramic technology that is fired below 850°C (contemporary classification). Refer to chapter 2 for expanded explanation.

M

malleability Quality of withstanding permanent deformation without rupture under compressive forces (compression). *Compare with ductility*.

mechanical properties Properties of an alloy or metal that reveal elastic or inelastic behavior when a loading force is applied (eg, percentage elongation, hardness, ultimate tensile strength, and yield strength).

medium-fusing porcelain Dental porcelains often used to produce prefabricated pontics.

melting range Range (of 50°F to 200°F) over which alloys melt. The lower limit indicates the initial melt temperature while the upper limit represents the temperature at which the alloy should be totally fluid (molten).

metal-ceramic restoration Restoration in which dental porcelain is fired onto a metal substructure. *Syn: ceramometal restoration, porcelain-fused-to-metal (PFM) restoration.*

modulus of elasticity Measure of the rigidity of an alloy. The higher the modulus, the more difficult it is to alter the shape (deform) of a restoration under function. This term is preferred over *elastic limit*.

N

natural glaze Naturally occurring surface glaze obtained by air-firing dental porcelain in a porcelain oven to a recommended temperature and maintaining it at that temperature for a specific period of time. *Syn: self-glaze, autoglaze.*

noble metal Element that is corrosion and oxidation resistant due to an inherent chemical inertness. The seven noble elements include gold, platinum, palladium, iridium, osmium, rhodium, and ruthenium.

O

ounce (avoirdupois) (oz) One ounce is equal to 28.3495 g.

ounce (troy) (ozt) One ounce is equal to 20 dwt or 31.1035 g. *See troy weights.*

overglaze Translucent low-fusing porcelain (fluxed glass) applied to the dental porcelain surface and air-fired for a specified period of time. *Syn: applied glaze.*

oxidation Process of heat treating a metal-ceramic alloy to produce an oxide layer on the metal surface for porcelain bonding. Whether the oxidation firing is accomplished in air or in a vacuum depends of the requirements of the particular alloy system. There is no standard oxidation procedure, and manufacturers specify the technique for each of their alloys. Formerly called *degassing*.

oxide layer Colored microscopic film that forms on the cameo and intaglio surfaces of a metal ceramic alloy after the metal has been heat treated. The oxide layer on porcelain-bearing areas is used to bond the dental porcelain to the metal substructure.

P

pennyweight (dwt) Composed of 24 grains and representing 1/20th of a troy ounce. In metric terms, 20 dwt represent one troy ounce or 31.1035 g.

PFM —*See porcelain-fused-to-metal.*

physical properties Properties inherent to a metal or an alloy (eg, casting temperature, density, melting range).

porcelain-fused-to-metal (PFM) Term in general use to describe the metal-ceramic restoration. *Syn: metal-ceramic restoration, ceramometal restoration.*

porosity Presence of holes, voids, and pits, either within a material or on its surface.

postsoldering Soldering of two or more metal components after the application of the porcelain. *Syn: postceramic soldering.*

presoldering Soldering of two or more metal components before the application of the porcelain. *Syn: preceramic soldering.*

processing Procedures involved in the production of a metal ceramic restoration—from waxup to the final finish.

proportional limit Amount of stress a metal or alloy will withstand before permanent deformation. This property is indicative of the relative strength and toughness of a material.

pyroplastic flow Loss of form of a ceramic material due to flow of molten glass. *Syn: slumping.*

Q

quartz (SiO_2) Key ingredient in dental porcelains with a high fusion temperature that helps prevent the buildup from undergoing pyroplastic flow during firing and also strengthens the porcelain. Refer to chapter 2 for the expanded discussion. *Syn: silica.*

quench To immerse a heated alloy or invested casting in water to stop atomic diffusion. In other words, quenching prevents a certain constituent in the alloy, which is soluble at a high temperature but less so at a lower temperature, from precipitating out of solid solution.

R

recrystallization *—See devitrification.*

resiliency Ability of an alloy to spring back to its original shape or form after receiving a sudden blow. Resilient alloys have a high yield strength and low modulus of elasticity.

S

sag resistance Ability of the cast form of a fixed partial denture to resist distortion during soldering and repeated firings at elevated temperatures. This quality is of particular concern with long-span metal-ceramic fired partial dentures in which multiple pontic areas are unsupported. In general, the lower-density alloys with higher Brinell and Vickers hardness numbers offer greater sag resistance due to their increased strength.

self-glaze *—See natural glaze.*

sintering Firing of dental porcelain. *Syn: firing.*

slumping *—See pyroplastic flow.*

solidus Temperature at which a metal or an alloy begins to melt. *Syn: incipient melting point.*

solubility Ability of a material to be dissolved in another material. For example, palladium is known to dissolve gasses readily, especially hydrogen, while silver has an affinity for oxygen. Consequently, it is important to properly mix and evacuate all phosphate-bonded investments and not overoxygenate the flame when casting metal-ceramic alloys.

specific gravity *—See density.*

T

tarnish Formation of a discoloration or other alteration to the surface finish of a metal restoration in the mouth. Food items (eg, eggs and fish that are rich in sulfur) can form copper or silver sulfides. Pigment-producing bacteria, iron, mercury-containing drugs, and absorbed food debris can also form stains or discolor dental restorations.

toughness Ability of an alloy to withstand sudden blows or shocks that may stress the alloy beyond its yield strength yet not beyond its breaking strength. Generally, it is found in those alloys with a high percentage of elongation and a high ultimate tensile strength.

troy weights One troy ounce (ozt) is made up of 20 pennyweight (dwt), and each dwt contains 24 grains of metal. All precious metal weights should be recorded in both pennyweights and grains.

U

ultimate tensile strength Greatest amount of tensile stress an alloy can withstand before it fractures.

V

vacuum-firing Firing of dental porcelain in a furnace in which the air or atmosphere has been removed to create a denser porcelain restoration (ie, less air between porcelain grains).

value Component of color that defines the relative brightness or darkness of a hue using a scale from 0 (pure black) to 10 (pure white). Correspondingly, the greater the value, the more visible light is reflected toward the viewer.

Vickers hardness Measure of the hardness of a material obtained via laboratory test in which a pyramid-shaped diamond is used instead of a steel ball. The higher the Vickers hardness number (VHN), the greater the hardness, although the VHN for an alloy is usually greater than its Brinell hardness number, solely because of the testing method. Therefore, compare similar test results when evaluating different alloys. *Compare with Brinell hardness.*

vitrification Development of a liquid phase that, on reaction or cooling, provides a glassy phase. In other words, the formation of a glass, or glasslike, structure by fusion due to heat.

volatility Vaporizing of a substance into a gas that can occur when an alloy is melted, particularly if it is inadvertently overheated. Vaporization can re-alloy the metal and change the properties of the alloy before it is even cast.

Y

yield strength Greatest amount of stress a metal or alloy can withstand and retain its original shape or form when the stress is removed.

Appendices

Appendix A Dental Porcelain Firing Schedules*

Ceramco 3 (Dentsply)

Porcelain	Drying time (min)	Preheat time (min)	Rate of rise °C (°F)	Type of environment (mm Hg)	Low temperature °C (°F)	Vacuum release temperature °C (°F)	High temperature °C (°F)	Hold time (min)	Rate of cooling	Visual indicators	Thickness (mm)
Opaque											
Paste	5	3	100 (180)	Vacuum (720)	500 (932)	975 (1,787)	975 (1,787)	0	Fast	Rough, reflective surface	0.1
Powder											
First firing	3	3	70 (126)	Vacuum (720)	650 (1,202)	970 (1,778)	970 (1,778)	0	Fast	Slight sheen, but not glazed	0.1
Second firing	3	3	70 (126)	Vacuum (720)	650 (1,202)	970 (1,778)	970 (1,778)	0	Fast	Dull sheen or slight matte finish	0.1
Dentin, enamel, opacious dentin, body modifiers											
First firing	5	5	55 (99)	Vacuum (720)	650 (1,202)	960 (1,760)	960 (1,760)	0	Fast	Shiny but *not* glazed or milky	As needed
Second firing	5	5	55 (99)	Vacuum (720)	650 (1,202)	960 (1,760)	960 (1,760)	0	Fast	Shiny but *not* glazed or milky	As needed
Margin porcelain											
First and second firing	5	5	70 (126)	Vacuum (720)	650 (1,202)	965 (1,769)	965 (1,769)	1	Fast	Shiny but *not* glazed or milky	As needed
Final firing (with overglaze)	3	3	70 (126)	Air	650 (1,202)	—	935 (1,715)	0	Fast	Shiny but *not*	As needed glazed or milky
Final firing (with natural glaze)	3	3	70 (126)	Air	650 (1,202)	—	945 (1,733)	0	Fast	Shiny but *not* glazed or milky	As needed
Overglaze											
First firing	3	3	70 (126)	Air	650 (1,202)	935 (1,715)	935 (1,715)	0.5	Fast	High gloss[†]	Thin layer
Natural glaze											
First firing	3	3	70 (126)	Air	650 (1,202)	945 (1,733)	945 (1,733)	0.5	Fast	Satiny gloss	Thin layer
Add-on porcelain											
First firing	5	5	70 (126)	Air	650 (1,202)	940 (1,724)	940 (1,724)	0	Fast	Shiny but *not* glazed or milky	As needed

*Times and temperatures are approximate. Call Dentsply for specific instructions for your porcelain furnace. Visually inspect your work after each firing to evaluate each firing program.

†The actual level of gloss for the glaze cycle should be based on the individual patient.

Appendix A Dental Porcelain Firing Schedules*

Finesse (Dentsply)

Porcelain	Drying time (min)	Preheat time (min)	Rate of rise °C (°F)	Type of environment	Low temperature °C (°F)	Vacuum release temperature °C (°F)	High temperature °C (°F)	Hold time (min)	Rate of cooling	Visual indicators	Thickness (mm)
Opaque											
Paste	5	3	90 (162)	Vacuum	450 (842)	790 (1,454)	790 (1,454)	0	Fast	Sandpaper or emery board appearance	0.1
Powder											
First firing	3	3	90 (162)	Vacuum	450 (842)	800 (1,472)	800 (1,472)	1	Fast	Slight sheen but *not* glazed	0.1
Second firing	3	3	90 (162)	Vacuum	450 (842)	800 (1,472)	800 (1,472)	1	Fast	Slight sheen but *not* glazed	0.1
Dentin, enamel, opacious dentin, body modifiers											
First firing	5	5	35 (63)	Vacuum	450 (842)	760 (1,400)	760 (1,400)	0.5	Fast	Shiny with slight texture	As needed
Second firing	5	5	35 (63)	Vacuum	450 (842)	750 (1,382)	750 (1,382)	0	Fast	Shiny with slight texture	As needed
Correction of opaque dentin, opacious dentin, body modifiers											
First firing	5	5	35 (63)	Vacuum	450 (842)	760 (1,400)	760 (1,400)	0.5	Fast	Shiny with slight texture	As needed
Margin porcelain											
First firing	5	7	35 (63)	Vacuum	675 (1,247)	770 (1,418)	770 (1,418)	0	Fast	Shiny but *not* glazed or milky	As needed
Second firing	5	7	35 (63)	Vacuum	675 (1,247)	770 (1,418)	770 (1,418)	0	Fast	Shiny but *not* glazed or milky	As needed
Overglaze											
First firing	3	3	70 (126)	Vacuum	450 (842)	750 (1,382)	750 (1,382)	0	Fast	High gloss†	Thin layer
Natural glaze											
First firing	3	3	70 (126)	Air	450 (842)	750 (1,382)	750 (1,382)	0	Fast	Satiny gloss	Thin layer
Dentin correction porcelain											
First firing	5	5	70 (126)	Air	450 (842)	710 (1,310)	730 (1,346)	0	Fast	Smooth satiny gloss	As needed

*Times and temperatures are approximate. Call Dentsply for specific instructions for your porcelain furnace. Visually inspect your work after each firing to evaluate each firing program.

†The actual level of gloss for the glaze cycle should be based on the individual patient.

Appendix A Dental Porcelain Firing Schedules*

IPS d.SIGN (Ivoclar Vivadent)

Porcelain	Drying time (min)	Preheat time (min)	Rate of rise °C (°F)	Type of environment	Low temperature °C (°F)	Vacuum start temperature °C (°F)	Vacuum release temperature °C (°F)	High temperature °C (°F)	Hold time (min)	Rate of cooling	Visual indicators	Thickness (mm)
Opaque paste												
First firing (wash)	6	—	80 (144)	Vacuum	403 (757)	450 (842)	899 (1,650)	900 (1,652)	1	Normal[†]	Eggshell gloss	0.1
Second firing (slightly higher than first firing)	6	—	80 (144)	Vacuum	403 (757)	450 (842)	889 (1,632)	890 (1,634)	1	Normal[†]	Eggshell gloss	0.1
Dentin, enamel, opacious dentin, body modifiers												
First firing	—	4–9	60 (108)	Vacuum	403 (757)	450 (842)	869 (1,596)	870 (1,598)	1	Normal[†]	Shiny but *not* glazed or milky	As needed
Second firing	—	4–9	60 (108)	Vacuum	403 (757)	450 (842)	869 (1,596)	870 (1,598)	1	Normal[†]	Shiny but *not* glazed or milky	As needed
Margin porcelain												
First firing	—	6	60 (108)	Vacuum	403 (757)	450 (842)	889 (1,632)	890 (1,634)	1	Normal[†]	Shiny but *not* glazed or milky	As needed
Second firing	—	6	60 (108)	Vacuum	403 (757)	450 (842)	889 (1,632)	890 (1,634)	1	Normal[†]	Shiny but *not* glazed or milky	As needed
Overglaze (glaze paste)												
First firing	—	4	60 (108)	Vacuum	403 (757)	450 (842)	829 (1,524)	830 (1,526)	1–2	Normal[†]	High gloss[‡]	Thin layer
Natural glaze												
First firing	—	4	60 (108)	Vacuum	403 (757)	450 (842)	869 (1,596)	870 (1,598)	0.5–1	Normal[†]	Satiny gloss	Thin layer
Add-on porcelain												
First firing	—	4	60 (108)	Vacuum	403 (757)	450 (842)	749 (1,380)	750 (1,382)	1	Normal[†]	Shiny but *not* glazed or milky	As needed

*Times and temperatures are approximate. Call Ivoclar Vivadent for specific instructions for your porcelain furnace. Visually inspect your work after each firing to evaluate each firing program.

[†]When the alloy coefficient of thermal expansion is very low, then fast cooling is recommended. When it is very high, slow cooling is recommended.

[‡]The actual level of gloss for the glaze cycle should be based on the individual patient.

Appendix A Dental Porcelain Firing Schedules*

Vita VM13 (Vident)

Porcelain	Drying time (min)	Preheat time (min)	Rate of rise °C (°F)	Type of environment (mm Hg)	Low temperature °C (°F)	Vacuum release temperature °C (°F)	High temperature °C (°F)	Hold time (min)	Rate of cooling	Visual indicators	Thickness (mm)
Opaque paste											
First firing (wash)	2	4	75 (135)	Vacuum (720)	500 (932)	890 (1,634)	890 (1,634)	2	Fast	Rough, reflective surface	Thin skim
Second firing	2	2	75 (135)	Vacuum (720)	500 (932)	890 (1,634)	890 (1,634)	1	Fast	Rough, reflective surface	Thin skim
Opaque powder											
First firing (wash)	2	2	75 (135)	Vacuum (720)	500 (932)	890 (1,634)	890 (1,634)	2	Fast	Slight sheen but *not* glazed	Covered layer
Second firing	2	2	75 (135)	Vacuum (720)	500 (932)	890 (1,634)	890 (1,634)	1	Fast	Light surface glaze	0.1
Dentin, enamel, opacious dentin, body modifiers											
First firing	6	6	55 (100)	Vacuum (720)	500 (932)	880 (1,616)	880 (1,616)	1	Fast	Slight luster (eggshell)	As needed
Second firing	6	6	55 (100)	Vacuum (720)	500 (932)	870 (1,598)	870 (1,598)	1	Fast	Slight luster (eggshell)	As needed
Margin porcelain											
First firing	6	6	55 (100)	Vacuum (720)	500 (932)	890 (1,634)	890 (1,634)	2	Fast	Slight luster (eggshell)	As needed
Second firing	4	6	55 (100)	Vacuum (720)	500 (932)	880 (1,616)	880 (1,616)	1	Fast	Slight luster (eggshell)	As needed
Overglaze											
First firing	4	4	80 (144)	Air	500 (932)	880 (1,616)	880 (1,616)	1	Fast	High gloss[†]	Thin layer
Vita Akzent	4	4	80 (144)	Air	500 (932)	880 (1,616)	880 (1,616)	1	Fast	High gloss[†]	Thin layer
Natural glaze											
First firing	0	0	80 (144)	Air	500 (932)	880 (1,616)	880 (1,616)	2	Fast	Satiny gloss	Thin layer
Add-on porcelain											
First firing	4	4	50 (90)	Air	500 (932)	800 (1,472)	800 (1,472)	1	Fast	Shiny but *not* glazed or milky	As needed

*Times and temperatures are approximate. Call Vident for specific instructions for your porcelain furnace. Visually inspect your work after each firing to evaluate each firing program.
[†]The actual level of gloss for the glaze cycle should be based on the individual patient.

209

Appendix A Dental Porcelain Firing Schedules*

Willi Geller Creation (Creation North America)

Porcelain	Drying time (min)	Preheat time (min)	Rate of rise °C (°F)	Type of environment (mm Hg)	Low temperature °C (°F)	Vacuum release temperature °C (°F)	High temperature °C (°F)	Hold time (min)	Rate of cooling	Visual indicators	Thickness (mm)
Opaque											
First firing	0.5	6	80 (144)	Vacuum (720)	550 (1,022)	980 (1,776)	980 (1,776)	1	Fast	Slight sheen but *not* glazed (granular texture)	70% coverage
Second firing	0.5	6	80 (144)	Vacuum (720)	550 (1,022)	950 (1,742)	950 (1,742)	1	Fast	Slight sheen but *not* glazed (granular texture)	100% coverage
Dentin, enamel, opacious dentin, body modifiers											
First firing	6	6	55 (100)	Vacuum (720)	580 (1,076)	920 (1,688)	920 (1,688)	1	Fast	Shiny look but *not* glazed or milky	1.0–1.5 mm
Second firing	4	4	55 (100)	Vacuum (720)	580 (1,076)	910 (1,670)	910 (1,670)	1	Fast	Shiny look but *not* glazed or milky	As needed
Margin porcelain											
First firing	2	2	80 (144)	Vacuum (720)	600 (1,112)	950 (1,742)	950 (1,742)	1	Fast	Shiny look but *not* glazed or milky	As needed
Second firing	2	2	80 (144)	Vacuum (720)	600 (1,112)	950 (1,742)	950 (1,742)	1	Fast	Shiny look but *not* glazed or milky	As needed
Third firing (if needed)	1	2	80 (144)	Vacuum (720)	600 (1,112)	945 (1,733)	945 (1,733)	1	Fast	Shiny look but *not* glazed or milky	As needed
Add-on porcelain											
First firing	4	2	55 (100)	Air	580 (1,076)	900 (1,652)	900 (1,652)	0	Fast	Smooth satiny gloss	As needed
Overglaze											
First firing	0.5	2	45 (81)	Air	480 (896)	880 (1,616)	880 (1,616)	1	Fast	High gloss†	Thin layer
Natural glaze											
First firing	0.5	2	55 (100)	Air	600 (1,112)	930 (1,706)	930 (1,706)	0	Fast	Satiny gloss	Thin layer

*Times and temperatures are approximate. Call Creation North America for specific instructions for your porcelain furnace. Visually inspect your work after each firing to evaluate each firing program.
†The actual level of gloss for the glaze cycle should be based on the individual patient.

Appendix B Celsius-Fahrenheit Conversion Chart

°C	°F	°C	°F	°C	°F
				1,010	1,850
0	32			1,020	1,868
50	122			1,030	1,886
100	212			1,040	1,904
300	572			1,050	1,922
310	590	660	1,220	1,060	1,940
320	608	670	1,238	1,070	1,958
330	626	680	1,256	1,080	1,976
340	644	690	1,274	1,090	1,994
350	662	700	1,292	1,100	2,012
360	680	710	1,310	1,110	2,030
370	698	720	1,328	1,120	2,048
380	716	730	1,346	1,130	2,066
390	734	740	1,364	1,140	2,084
400	752	750	1,382	1,150	2,102
410	770	760	1,400	1,160	2,120
420	788	770	1,418	1,170	2,138
430	806	780	1,436	1,180	2,156
440	824	790	1,454	1,190	2,174
450	842	800	1,472	1,200	2,192
460	860	810	1,490	1,210	2,210
470	878	820	1,508	1,220	2,228
480	896	830	1,526	1,230	2,246
490	914	840	1,544	1,240	2,264
500	932	850	1,562	1,250	2,282
510	950	860	1,580	1,260	2,300
520	968	870	1,598	1,270	2,318
530	986	880	1,616	1,280	2,336
540	1,004	890	1,634	1,290	2,354
550	1,022	900	1,652	1,300	2,372
560	1,040	910	1,670	1,310	2,390
570	1,058	920	1,688	1,320	2,428
580	1,076	930	1,706	1,330	2,446
590	1,094	940	1,724	1,340	2,464
600	1,112	950	1,742	1,350	2,482
610	1,130	960	1,760		
620	1,148	970	1,778		
630	1,166	980	1,796		
640	1,184	990	1,814		
650	1,202	1,000	1,832		

Conversion formulas

$°C = 5/9(°F - 32)$

$°F = 9/5(°C) + 32$ *or* $°F = 1.8(°C) + 32$

Appendix C Percentage Composition of Historical Metal-Ceramic Alloys*

High-Noble Alloys

Gold-platinum-palladium	Au	Pd	Pt	Ag	Sn	In		Other elements	Color
SMG-2 (JM Ney)	87	5	7	–	< 1	< 1		–	Yellow
Ultra-Gold (JF Jelenko)	87.5	1	10	–	+	+		–	Yellow
Rx Y-Ceramic (Jeneric/Pentron)	84	6	7	1	0.7	0.5		–	Yellow

Gold-palladium-platinum	Au	Pd	Pt	Ag	Sn	In		Other elements	Color
Image (JM Ney)	85	5	5	4	< 1	–		–	Yellow

Gold-platinum	Au	Pd	Pt	Ag	Sn	In	Rh	Other elements	Color
Rx G (Jeneric/Pentron)	87	–	10	–	+	+	1.5	–	Yellow

Gold-palladium-silver	Au	Pd	Pt	Ag	Sn	In		Other elements	Color
Rx WCG (Jeneric/Pentron)	52	28	–	14	1	3		–	White

Gold-palladium	Au	Pd	Pt	Ag	Sn	In	Co	Cu	Ga	Other elements	Color
500SL (Leach & Dillon)	51.5	38.5	–	–	–	8.5	–	–	1.5	–	White
Deva M (Degussa)	46.5	44.5	–	–	–	–	–	–	–	–	White
SF 45 (Jeneric/Pentron)	45	45	–	–	3.5	5	–	–	–	–	White

Noble Metal Alloys

Palladium-silver	Au	Pd	Pt	Ag	Sn	In	Co	Cu	Ga	Zn	Other elements	Color
Paladent B (Jeneric/Pentron)	–	60	–	28	2.5	6.5	–	–	1.5	–	–	White
100SL (Leach & Dillon)	–	54	–	37	8.5	0.5	–	–	–	–	–	White
Rx 91 (Jeneric/Pentron)	–	53.3	–	37.5	8.5	0.5	–	–	–	–	–	White

High-palladium

High-palladium–cobalt	Au	Pd	Pt	Ag	Sn	In	Co	Cu	Ga	Other elements	Color
PTM-88 (JF Jelenko)	–	88	–	–	–	–	4	–	8	–	White
APF (Jeneric/Pentron)	–	79	–	–	6	4	8	–	1.5	–	White

High-palladium–copper	Au	Pd	Pt	Ag	Sn	In	Co	Cu	Ga	Other elements	Color
PG-82 (Unitek/3M)	2	80.5	–	–	–	5.5	–	5	6.9	–	White
Albabond E (Degussa)	2	78	–	–	< 1	< 2	–	11	7.5	–	White
Liberty (JF Jelenko)	2	76.5	–	–	6	–	–	10	5.5	–	White

High-palladium–silver-gold	Au	Pd	Pt	Ag	Sn	In	Cu	Co	Ga	Other elements	Color
Legacy (JF Jelenko)	2	86	–	< 1	–	+	–	–	10	–	White
Degupal G (Degussa)	4.5	77.5	–	7	4	–	–	–	6	–	White
Aspen (Jeneric/Pentron)	5.5	75	1	6.5	–	+	–	–	+	–	White

Predominantly Base Metal Alloys

Nickel-chromium

Nickel-chromium-beryllium	Ni	Co	Cr	Be	Al	Mo	Ti	Ru	V	Other elements	Color
Biobond II (Dentsply)	80.7	–	13.5	1.8	–	–	–	–	4	–	White
Litecast B[†] (Williams Dental)	77.5	–	12.5	1.7	–	4	–	–	–	–	White

Nickel-chromium beryllium-free	Ni	Co	Cr	Be	Al	Mo	Nb	W	Fe	Cb	Other elements	Color
Forte[†] (Unitek/3M)	64	–	22	–	–	9	–	–	–	–	–	White
Neptune (Jeneric/Pentron)	62	–	22	–	–	8.5	–	–	–	3.5	–	White

Cobalt-chromium	Ni	Co	Cr	Be	Al	Mo	Si	Ru	W	Other elements	Color
Genesis II (Jelenko)	–	53	27	–	–	–	–	3	–	–	White
Novarex (Jeneric/Pentron)	–	55	25	–	+	–	–	5	10	–	White
Ultra 100 (Unitek/3M)	–	52	28	–	–	–	–	–	–	–	White
Rexillium-NBF (Jeneric/Pentron)	–	52	25	–	+	–	–	–	14	–	White

*Exact alloy formulations are considered proprietary information and are not always available for publication. Many of these alloys also contain trace amounts of other base metals that serve as grain refiners (eg, ruthenium), oxide scavengers (eg, boron, silicon), and strengtheners (eg, iron), to mention just a few.
†Rated acceptable by the ADA Acceptance Program.
+ Elements present in unspecified amounts.
– Elements not identified as being present.

Appendix D Wax Pattern–Alloy Conversion Tables

Weigh your wax pattern(s) with the entire sprue system before investing. Record the weight in grams (g) or pennyweights (dwt), and multiply that number by the specific gravity (density) of the alloy that you plan to use. Refer to the conversion tables below for approximations of examples of high-noble, noble, and predominantly base metal alloys.

(Pennyweight and grain measures are listed as follows: 5^{12} represents 5 dwt and 12 grains, or 5.5 dwt [1 dwt = 24 grains]).

If you elect to use plastic sprue formers, multiply the estimated weight of the alloy by 0.33, and add that value to obtain the final alloy weight.

High-Noble Alloy Conversion Table*

Weight of wax pattern																								
(g)	0.2	0.4	0.6	0.8	1.0	1.2	1.4	**1.6**	1.8	2.0	2.2	2.4	2.6	2.8	3.0	**3.2**	3.4	3.6	3.8	4.0	4.2	4.4	4.6	**4.8**
(dwt^{grains})	0^3	0^6	0^9	0^{12}	0^{15}	0^{18}	0^{21}	**1**	1^3	1^6	1^9	1^{12}	1^{15}	1^{18}	1^{21}	**2**	2^3	2^6	2^9	2^{12}	2^{15}	2^{18}	2^{21}	**3**
Weight of alloy (dwt^{grains})	2^6	4^{12}	6^{18}	9	11^6	13^{12}	15^{18}	**18**	20^6	22^{12}	24^{18}	27	29^6	31^{12}	33^{18}	**36**	38^6	40^{12}	42^{18}	45	47^6	49^{12}	51^{18}	**54**

*Assumes a density of 18 g/cm^3.

Noble Alloy Conversion Table†

Weight of wax pattern																								
(g)	0.2	0.4	0.6	0.8	1.0	1.2	1.4	**1.6**	1.8	2.0	2.2	2.4	2.6	2.8	3.0	**3.2**	3.4	3.6	3.8	4.0	4.2	4.4	4.6	**4.8**
(dwt^{grains})	0^3	0^6	0^9	0^{12}	0^{15}	0^{18}	0^{21}	**1**	1^3	1^6	1^9	1^{12}	1^{15}	1^{18}	1^{21}	**2**	2^3	2^6	2^9	2^{12}	2^{15}	2^{18}	2^{21}	**3**
Weight of alloy (dwt^{grains})	1^9	2^{18}	4^3	5^{12}	6^{21}	8^6	9^{15}	**11**	12^9	13^{18}	15^3	16^{12}	17^{21}	19^6	20^{15}	**22**	23^9	24^{18}	26^3	27^{12}	28^{21}	30^6	31^{15}	**33**

†Assumes a density of 11 g/cm^3.

Predominantly Base Metal Alloy Conversion Table‡

Weight of wax pattern																								
(g)	0.2	0.4	0.6	0.8	1.0	1.2	1.4	**1.6**	1.8	2.0	2.2	2.4	2.6	2.8	3.0	**3.2**	3.4	3.6	3.8	4.0	4.2	4.4	4.6	**4.8**
(dwt^{grains})	0^3	0^6	0^9	0^{12}	0^{15}	0^{18}	0^{21}	**1**	1^3	1^6	1^9	1^{12}	1^{15}	1^{18}	1^{21}	**2**	2^3	2^6	2^9	2^{12}	2^{15}	2^{18}	2^{21}	**3**
Weight of alloy (dwt^{grains})	1	2	3	4	5	6	7	**8**	9	10	11	12	13	14	15	**16**	17	18	19	20	21	22	23	**24**

‡Assumes a density of 8 g/cm^3.

Appendix E List of Equipment, Instruments, and Materials

Type	Manufacturer/ Distributor*	Characteristics/ Function
Equipment		
Laboratory microscope		
KRX	Denerica	Step magnification of 10× and 20×
EMZ-2	Meiji	Zoom magnification of 7× to 45×
SMZ-1	Nikon	Zoom magnification of 7× to 30×
Low-speed electric handpiece (≤ 50,000 rpm)		
Dynamo Plus	Henry Schein	Designed for adjusting and finishing metal or porcelain
X50 Brushless Electric	Buffalo	1,000 to 50,000 rpm
X35 Premium Electric Lab	Buffalo	0 to 35,000 rpm
XL-230	Osada	900 to 30,000 rpm
EXL-M40	Osada	1,000 to 40,000 rpm
Z500	NSK America	1,000 to 50,000 rpm
High-speed air-driven handpiece (≥ 50,000 rpm)		
Presto and Presto II Standard	NSK America	Designed for adjusting and finishing metal or porcelain
Steam cleaners		
Steam Clean	Williams Dental	Steam clean die, casts, casting, and porcelain
Portable Steamer	Belle de St Claire	Steam clean die, casts, casting, and porcelain
Airborne particle–abrasion units		
MicroBlaster MB 1000	Comco	Single-tank airborne-particle abrasion (metal or porcelain) with aluminum oxide, glass beads, and other abrasive powders
MicroBlaster MB 1002	Comco	Dual-tank airborne-particle abrasion (metal or porcelain) with aluminum oxide, glass beads, and other abrasive powders
Instruments		
Measurement devices		
Boley gauge caliper	Salvin Dental Specialties	Measurements in 1.0-mm increments
Iwanson Spring Caliper for Metal	Most distributors	Metal or porcelain thickness in 0.1-mm increments
Iwanson Spring Caliper for Wax	Most distributors	Wax measurements in 0.1-mm increments
Porcelain instrument kits		
Instrument set	KerrLab	Instruments for porcelain buildup
Instrument set	Renfert	Instruments for porcelain buildup
Porcelain sculpturing kit	Tanaka Dental	Instruments for porcelain buildup
Vita expert instrument set	Vident	Instruments for porcelain buildup
Materials		
Aluminum oxide	Most distributors	Metal and porcelain surface treatment
Carborundum disks	Most distributors	Despruing and gross metal reduction
Carbide burs	Brasseler USA	Metal reduction

(cont.)

Type	Manufacturer/ Distributor*	Characteristics/ Function
Ceramic abrasives		
Busch Silent Stone	Pfingst	Metal and porcelain adjustment and contouring
Stones	Shofu	Metal and porcelain adjustment and contouring
Diamonds	Brasseler USA	Metal and porcelain adjustment and contouring
Disclosing agents and marking materials		
AccuFilm IV	Parkell	Fit restorations and mark contacts
Crown Fit Seating Indicator	Belle de St Claire	Fit restorations and mark contacts
Pascal Occlude Spray	Most distributors	Fit restorations and mark contacts
AccuFilm I and II	Parkell	Mark interproximal and occlusal contact areas
Artus Occlusal Registration Strips	Most distributors	Shimstock to assess occlusal and interproximal contact
Finishing materials and polishing agents		
Burlew wheels	Most distributors	Rubber wheeling metal
Green points	Dedeco	
Pre-Polisher Wheels (gray)	Vident	Adjusting and smoothing porcelain
Final Polisher Wheels (pink)	Vident or Brasseler USA	Mechanically polish porcelain
Sandpaper disks	Most distributors	
BBC Buffing Bar Compound	Most distributors	Preliminary metal polishing
Tripoli	Most distributors	
Rouge	Most distributors	Final metal polishing
Stone		
Busch Silent Stone	Mizzy USA	Gross adjustment
Heatless Stone	Henry Schein	
Laboratory vacuum for precious metals		
Hippo Portable Hand-held Vac	RE Williams	Recovery of precious metal grindings/dust
Pattern resins		
DuraLay	Reliance Dental	Acrylic resin for patterns
GC Pattern Resin LS	GC Corporation	Acrylic resin for patterns
Prefabricated sprue formers (direct and indirect)		
Ready Sprues	KerrLab	Wax sprue formers for spruing and ringless casting
PowerCast System	Whip Mix Corp	Wax sprue formers for spruing and ringless casting
Tri-Wax	Ivoclar Vivadent	Wax sprue formers for spruing and ringless casting

*See appendix F for a list of manufacturers and distributors.

Appendix F List of Manufacturers and Distributors

The following is a partial listing of manufacturers and distributors of the products mentioned in the text. Some of these companies either sell their products directly or maintain a sales force in the field. However, many manufacturers are not involved in direct sales, and their products may be purchased through local dental distributors or mail order houses. Contact the companies directly for additional information.

Manufacturer/Distributor	Contact information	Products
3M ESPE 3M Center, Bldg 275-2SE-03 Saint Paul, MN 55114	(800) 634-2249 www.3mespe.com	Ceramics, Rocatec
Aalba Dent 400 Watt Dr Fairfield, CA 94534	(800) 227-1332 (707) 864-3334 www.aalbadent.com	Dental alloys
Argen Corporation 5855 Oberlin Dr San Diego, CA 92121	(800) 255-5524 (858) 455-7900 www.argen.com	Dental alloys
Artus Corporation PO Box 511 Englewood, NJ 97631	(201) 568-1000 (no direct sales) www.artuscorp.com	Shimstock
Belle de St Claire Products	*See KerrLab*	
Bolton Dental Manufacturing 50 Goebel Ave Cambridge, ON N3C 1Z1, Canada	(800) 667-3770 (519) 651-2444 www.bdmcan.com	Abrasives, burs, polishing compounds, waxes, and laboratory equipment
Brasseler USA One Brasseler Blvd Savannah, GA 31419	(800) 841-4522 (912) 925-8525 www.brasselerusa.com	Diamond instruments, polishing points, and wheels
Buffalo Dental Manufacturing PO Box 678 Syosset, New York 11791	(800) 828-0678 (516) 496-7200 www.buffalodental.com	Polishing rouge and lab equipment
Ceramco	*See Dentsply Ceramco*	
Comco 2151 N Lincoln St Burbank, CA 91504	(800) 796-6626 (818) 841-5500 www.comcoinc.com	Abrasive powders (aluminum oxide, crushed glass, glass beads, walnut shells)
Dedeco International Route 97 Long Eddy, NY 12760	(888) 433-3326 (845) 887-4840 www.dedeco.com	Abrasives, carbide burs, diamond instruments, polishers, separating disks, stones for finishing metal, and wheels for finishing porcelain
Dentsply Ceramco 570 W College Ave York, PA 17404 Technical Center Six Terri Ln Burlington, NJ 08016	(800) 487-0100 (800) 354-8251 (technical information) ceramcomkting@dentsply.com www.ceramco.com	Ceramics, dental alloys, porcelains, equipment, and laboratory supplies

Manufacturer/Distributor	Contact information	Products
Dentsply International 221 W Philadelphia St PO Box 872 York, PA 17405	(800) 877-0020 (717) 845-7511 (800) 354-8251 (technical information)	Dental alloys, equipment, and dental porcelains (wide range of products)
Dillon Company Leach & Dillon Products 161 Comstock Pkwy Cranston, RI 02921	(800) 535-2633 (401) 464-5850 www.leachdillon.com	Ceramics, dental porcelains, alloys, and laboratory supplies
Elephant USA	*See European Dental Imports*	
European Dental Imports 49 Emerson Rd Durham, NH 03824	(800) 648-0035 (603) 868-3306 www.elephantusa.com	Dental alloys, dental porcelains, and supplies
GC America 3737 W 127th St Alsip, IL 60803	(800) 323-7083 www.gcamerica.com	Ceramics, dental stone; GC Pattern Resin, investments, metal primer, and separator
George Taub Products & Fusion 277 New York Ave Jersey City, NJ 07307	(800) 828-2634 (201) 798-5353 www.taubdental.com	Die spacer, Insta-Glaze diamond polishing paste for porcelain, and equipment
Henry Schein 135 Duryea Rd Melville, NY 11747	(800) 496-9500 (631) 843-5500 www.henryschein.com	Wide range of laboratory supplies and equipment
Heraeus Kulzer 99 Business Park Dr Armonk, NY 10504	(800) 431-1785 (914) 273-8600 www.heraeus-kulzer-us.com	Gypsum products, investments, porcelain systems, and a variety of consumable laboratory products (abrasive powders, burs, finishing disks and wheels, mounted stones, polishing points, porcelain accessories)
Hu-Friedy Chicago 3232 N Rockwell Chicago, IL 60618	(800) 483-7433 (773) 975-1683	Dental instruments including Iwanson Spring Calipers (for metal and wax), spatulas, wax carvers and other laboratory instruments (eg, PK Thomas waxing instruments)
International Dental Supply 8205 W 20th Ave Hialeah, FL 33014	(800) 437-6455 (305) 817-2800 www.idsdental.stores.yahoo.net	Distributor of a variety of laboratory products and equipment
Ivoclar Vivadent 175 Pineview Dr Amherst, NY 14228	(800) 533-6825 (716) 691-2283 www.ivoclarvivadent.us.com	Dental alloys, ceramics, dental porcelains, equipment, and laboratory supplies
Jensen Premium Dental Products 50 Stillman Rd North Haven, CT 06473 10288 South Jordan Gateway South Jordan, UT 84095	(800) 243-2000 (203) 239-2090 (801) 619-0660 www.jensendental.com	Dental alloys, articulators, and dental porcelains
KerrLab 1717 W Collins Orange, CA 92867	(888) 766-7650 (714) 766-7650 www.kerrlab.com	Wide range of laboratory equipment and supplies (includes the former Belle de St Claire product line)

Manufacturer/Distributor	Contact information	Products
Kerr Manufacturing Sybron Corporation 28200 Wick Rd PO Box 455 Romulus, MI 48174	(800) 537-7123 (734) 946-7800 www.sybrondental.com (888) 766-7650 www.kerrlab.com	Casting supplies, equipment, porcelain accessories, supplies, and waxes
Leach & Dillon	*See Dillon Company*	
Meiji Techno America 3010 Olcott St Santa Clara, CA 95054	(800) 832-0060 (408) 970-4799 www.meijitechno.com	Microscopes, cameras, and accessories
Mizzy 616 Hollywood Ave Cherry Hill, NJ 0802	(800) 333-3131 (856) 663-4700 www.keystoneind.com *(no direct sales)*	Abrasives, ceramic brushes, die lubricant, dowel pins, hollow sprue formers, laboratory supplies, porcelain trays, and waxes (all types)
EC Moore 13325 Leonard Dearborn, MI 48126	(800) 331-3548 (313) 581-7878 www.ecmoore.com	Abrasives (finishing and polishing) and laboratory burs
Moyco Technologies 200 Commerce Dr Montgomeryville, PA 18936	(800) 331-8837 (215) 855-4300 www.moycotech.com	Abrasive and finishing materials (eg, aluminum oxide, disks)
NSK America 700B Cooper Ct Schaumburg, IL 60173	(800) 585-4675 (847) 843-7664 www.nskamericacorp.com	Low- and high-speed handpieces
Nikon Instruments 1300 Walt Whitman Rd Melville, NY 11747	(800) 526-4576 (631) 547-8500 www.nikoninstruments.com	Microscopes, cameras, and accessories
Osada 3000 S Robertson Blvd, Ste 130 Los Angeles, CA 90034	(800) 426-7232 (310) 841-2220 www.osadausa.com	Low-speed (high torque) electric handpieces and accessories
Parkell 300 Executive Dr Edgewood, NY 11717	(800) 243-7446 (631) 249-1134 www.parkell.com	AccuFilm I, AccuFilm II, AccuFilm, brush-on liquid, and separating film
Pascal Company 2929 NE Northup Way Bellevue, WA 98004	(800) 426-8051 (425) 827-4694 www.pascaldental.com	Occlude aerosol indicator marking spray (red and green)
Pentron Ceramics 500 Memorial Dr Somerset, NJ 08873	(732) 563-4755	Ceramics and dental porcelains
Pfingst & Company 105 Snyder Rd South Plainfield, NJ 07080	(908) 561-6400 www.pfingstco.com	Abrasives, burs, diamond instruments, and laboratory equipment
RE Williams Contractor 29021 Sherman Ave, Ste 103 Valencia, CA 91355	(888) 845-6597 (611) 775-5979 www.rewci.com	Hippo Portable Hand-Held Vac

Manufacturer/Distributor	Contact information	Products
Reckitt Benckiser PO Box 225 Parsippany, NJ 07054	(800) 333-3899 www.reckittbenckiser.com	Brasso polish
Reliance Dental Manufacturing PO Box 38 Worth, IL 60482	(708) 597-6694 www.reliancedental.net	DuraLay resin
Renfert USA 3718 Illinois Ave St Charles, IL 60174	(800) 336-7422 www.renfertusa.com	Dental products and equipment
Salvin Dental Specialties 3450 Latrobe Dr Charlotte, NC 28211	(800) 535-6566 (704) 442-5400 www.salvin.com	Boley gauge
Sybron Dental Specialties	*See KerrLab*	
Shofu Dental Corporation 1225 Stone Dr San Marcos, CA 92078	(800) 827-4638 (760) 736-3277 www.shofu.com	Porcelains, diamonds, equipment, finishing stones and carbide burs, and polishing instruments
Talladium 27360 W Muirfield Ln Valencia, CA 91355	(800) 221-6449 (661) 295-0900	Dental alloys, gypsums, investments, supplies, and waxes
Tanaka Dental 5135 Golf Rd Skokie, IL 60077	(800) 325-5266 (847) 679-1610	Brushes for porcelain, casting products, and diamonds
Vident 3150 E Birch St Brea, CA 92821	(800) 828-3839 (888) 249-1640 (technical support) www.vident.com	Ceramics, dental porcelains, equipment, and laboratory supplies
Whip Mix Corporation 361 Farmington Ave PO Box 17183 Louisville, KY 40217	(800) 626-5651 (502) 637-1451 www.whipmix.com	Articulators, casting supplies, dental stones, equipment, investments, and laboratory supplies
Williams Ivoclar Vivadent	*See Ivoclar Vivadent*	
Zahn Dental Laboratory Division	*See Henry Schein*	

Index